Oxford American Handbook of **Rheumatology**

Second Edition

Philip Seo

Director, The Johns Hopkins Vasculitis Center
Director, Johns Hopkins Rheumatology Fellowship
Associate Professor of Medicine
Division of Rheumatology
The Johns Hopkins University School of Medicine

with

Alan J. Hakim
Gavin P.R. Clunie
Inam Haq

OXFORD
UNIVERSITY PRESS

OXFORD
UNIVERSITY PRESS

Oxford University Press is a department of the University of Oxford.
It furthers the University's objective of excellence in research, scholarship,
and education by publishing worldwide.

Oxford   New York
Auckland   Cape Town   Dar es Salaam   Hong Kong   Karachi
Kuala Lumpur   Madrid   Melbourne   Mexico City   Nairobi
New Delhi   Shanghai   Taipei   Toronto

With offices in
Argentina   Austria   Brazil   Chile   Czech Republic   France   Greece
Guatemala   Hungary   Italy   Japan   Poland   Portugal   Singapore
South Korea   Switzerland   Thailand   Turkey   Ukraine   Vietnam

Oxford is a registered trademark of Oxford University Press
in the UK and certain other countries.

Published in the United States of America by
Oxford University Press
198 Madison Avenue, New York, NY 10016

Library of Congress Cataloging-in-Publication Data
Seo, Philip.
Oxford American handbook of rheumatology / Philip Seo.—2nd ed.
    p. ; cm.—(Oxford American handbooks)
Handbook of rheumatology
Adapted from: Oxford handbook of rheumatology / Alan J. Hakim,
Gavin P.R. Clunie, Inam Haq. 2nd ed. 2006.
Includes bibliographical references and index.
ISBN 978 0 19 990799 1 (alk. paper)
I. Hakim, Alan. Oxford handbook of rheumatology. II. Title. III. Title:
Handbook of rheumatology. IV. Series: Oxford American handbooks.
[DNLM: 1. Rheumatic Diseases—Handbooks. WE 39]
LCClassification not assigned
616.7′23—dc23   2012035653

9 8 7 6 5 4 3 2 1
Printed in the United States of America
on acid-free paper

Foreword

Patients with rheumatic disorders present so many different challenges that almost every practicing physician needs some familiarity with rheumatology. An abbreviated litany of common rheumatic symptoms and signs—arthralgias, myalgias, weakness, back pain, and neck pain—reinforces the observation that rheumatic disorders are among the most frequent reasons patients present to family physicians, general internists, geriatricians, and orthopedists. Although many rheumatic diseases are temporary nuisances, others can cause life-threatening, multisystem diseases that can be encountered by hospitalists, critical care specialists, nephrologists, cardiologists, neurologists, and a myriad of other consultants. Distinguishing among the more than 150 different forms of arthritis, although often challenging, is important, given the recent dramatic increase in specific and effective therapies that are now available.

Fortunately, this handbook will offer any physician substantial help in meeting the challenges posed by rheumatic diseases. The liberal use of bulleted summary points and tables makes this handbook both concise and thorough. Physicians eager to improve their clinical skills will enjoy the excellent photographs that illustrate important aspects of the musculoskeletal physical examination. The chapter on rheumatic emergencies will be especially useful to hospitalists.

I believe this handbook will allow many physicians to experience the joy and sense of accomplishment that can come from diagnosing and treating patients with rheumatic diseases.

David B. Hellmann, M.D., M.A.C.P.
Aliki Perroti Professor of Medicine
Vice Dean, Johns Hopkins Bayview Medical Center
Chairman, Department of Medicine Johns Hopkins Bayview
The Johns Hopkins University School of Medicine

Preface

Rheumatology is one of the last great frontiers in medicine. In this modern era, in which we hear less about neck veins and more about BNP levels, rheumatology remains the exception to the rule. Despite the growing number of diagnostic tests we have at our disposal, they remain a mere adjunct to the patient evaluation. This is one of the last subspecialties in which it is not only common, but appropriate, to ignore a positive ANA or joint space narrowing, and instead listen to what the patient has to say.

That said, rheumatology is a field in transition. Long behind us are the days in which clinical trials compared the efficacy of one NSAID to another. The advent of biologic agents in particular has led to a new era in therapeutics in which largely nonspecific immunosuppressive drugs are being replaced by progressively more nuanced agents. The day that molecular phenotyping of patients joins clinical phenotyping as a way of selecting treatment strategies cannot be far behind.

During the last few years, the rate of transitions has occurred at breakneck speed. Since the publication of the first edition, new classification criteria have been published for systemic lupus erythematosus, Sjögren's syndrome, polymyalgia rheumatica, and rheumatoid arthritis. For the first time, we have FDA-approved agents for the treatment of both systemic lupus erythematosus and ANCA-associated vasculitis. Finally, we are starting to see oral biologic agents hit the market, allowing patients to take advantage of our most advanced therapeutics without subjecting them to the needle.

For the present, rheumatology encompasses a dizzying amount of information; no book can be expected to replace years of clinical experience. I believe and hope, however, that this book will find a home in many white-coat pockets, from the attending who just needs to refresh his or her memory on a few details, to the trainee who is looking for some way of getting a toehold in this daunting field.

More than anything else, this book is meant to provide you with an approach to the patient, and a framework on which you can build. This book represents just the beginning of a continually evolving, continuously changing story that never fails to fascinate.

Philip Seo, MD, MHS
Director, the Johns Hopkins Vasculitis Center
Director, Johns Hopkins Rheumatology Fellowship
Associate Professor of Medicine
Johns Hopkins University School of Medicine

Acknowledgments

Last year, I became Director of the Rheumatology Fellowship at Johns Hopkins, and with that new position came a deep sense of obligation to improve my general understanding of rheumatology—no small feat after many years of seeing only patients with systemic vasculitis.

My new position has allowed me to work even more closely with my colleagues, and has left me awestruck by the depths of both their knowledge and their generosity.

As I have said before, the greatest gift that a fellow academic can give is his or her time. I am therefore pleased to thank publicly my friends and colleagues who graciously reviewed these chapters during airport layovers and other moments stolen from far more deserving obligations: Alan Baer, Clifton (Bing) Bingham, Lisa-Christopher-Stine, Fred Wigley, Grant Louie, Laura Hummers, Khalil Ghanem, Michelle Petri, Geeta Sood, and Sangeeta Sule.

This motley crew gently (or not so) informed me when I was woefully misinformed—which was more often than I would like to admit—and credit for many of the improvements to this second edition really belongs to them.

I also wish to thank Antony Rosen and David Hellmann, whose avuncular support has provided my career with a second act.

I continue to be grateful to Alan Hakim, Gavin Clunie, and Inam Haq, who wrote the original Oxford Handbook of Rheumatology, and provided the backbone (and much of the meat) for this current edition. Also, I would be remiss if I did not thank Andrea Seils, Senior Editor of Clinical Medicine at Oxford University Press, whose encouragement and support have been invaluable.

Finally, I dedicate this work to my family, who mean more to me with each passing year: Kyung Hwa Seo, Hae Ja Yoon Seo, Susan Seo, and Ellen Seo. I also dedicate this work to my niece and nephew, Avery Pusey and Jackson Pusey, who—as they pointed out to me—I had neglected to name in the first edition, but are never far from my heart.

Philip Seo
Baltimore
February 2013

Contents

Detailed contents

List of color plates

Plate 1 MR scan of the neck showing loss of height and signal affecting several discs with multisegmental spondylotic bars, compression of the cord from protrusion of the C5/6 disc and myelopathic changes (high signal) in the cord.

Plate 2 Patterns of radiographic abnormality in chronic SAI: sclerosis and cystic changes in greater tuberosity.

Plate 3 Dactylitis, nail changes, and DIP joint arthritis in psoriatic arthritis.

Plate 4 (a) Normal nailfold capillaries. (b) Nailfold capillaries in scleroderma showing avascular areas and dilated capillaries in an irregular orientation (original magnification 65x).

Plate 5 Diffuse arm and hand swelling in chronic regional pain syndrome (reflex sympathetic dystrophy).

Plate 6 Slight flexion of fourth and fifth fingers as a result of an ulnar nerve lesion at the elbow. The area of sensory loss is indicated by the dotted line.

Plate 7 Psoriatic spondylitis: Nonmarginal and "floating" (nonattached) syndesmophytes.

Plate 8 Spondylolysis. The defect in the pars interarticularis (black arrows) may only be noted on an oblique view. The patient has had a spinal fusion (open arrows).

Plate 9 Testing passive hip flexion and rotational movements (a) and hip abduction (b).The pelvis should be fixed when testing abduction and adduction.

Plate 10 Bone scintigraphy showing osteonecrosis of the left femoral head (on the right-hand side as this is an anterior view). Photopenia (an early sign) corresponds to ischemia.

Plate 11 The "patellar tap" test. Any fluid in the suprapatellar pouch is squeezed distally by the left hand. The patella is depressed by the right hand. It will normally tap the underlying femur immediately. Any delay in eliciting the tap or a feeling of damping as the patella is depressed suggests a joint effusion.

Plate 12 Injection of the glenohumeral joint via the anterior route.

Plate 13 Injection of the subacromial space.

Plate 14 Injection of tennis elbow (lateral humeral epicondylitis/enthesitis).

Symbols and abbreviations

⚠	alert/warning
1°	Primary
2°	Secondary
↑	increase/raise
↓	decrease/reduce
♂	male(s)
♀	female(s)
±	plus or minus
α	Alpha
β	Beta
ACA	Anticentromere antibody
AC(J)	Acromioclavicular (joint)
ACR	American College of Rheumatology
ADM	Abductor digiti minimi
ALP	Alkaline phosphatase
ALT	Alanine transaminases
ANA	Anti-nuclear antibody
ANCA	Antineutrophil cytoplasmic antibody
AP	Anteroposterior
APB	Abductor pollicis brevis
APL	Abductor pollicis longus
APS	Antiphospholipid (antibody) syndrome
ARA	American Rheumatism Association
AS	Ankylosing spondylitis
AST	Aspartate transaminase
ASOT	Antistreptolysin O titer
ASU	Avocado/soybean unsaponifiable
AZA	Azathioprine
BCP	Basic calcium phosphate (crystals)
bid	Twice daily
BJHS	Benign joint hypermobility syndrome

BMC	Bone mineral content
BMD	Bone mineral density
BSR	British Society of Rheumatology
C	Cervical (e.g., C6 is the sixth cervical vertebra)
CA	Coracoacromial
CBC	Complete blood count
CINCA	Chronic, infantile, neurological, cutaneous, and articular syndrome
CK	Creatine phosphokinase
CMC(J)	Carpometacarpal (joint)
CMP	Comprehensive metabolic panel
CMV	Cytomegalovirus
CPPD	Calcium pyrophosphate deposition (arthritis)
CREST	Calcinosis, Raynaud's, Esophageal dysmotility, Sclerodactyly, Telangiectasia (syndrome)
CRP	C-reactive protein
CS	Congenital scoliosis
CSS	Churg–Strauss syndrome
CT	Computed tomography
CTS	Carpal tunnel syndrome
CXR	Chest radiograph
dcSScl	Diffuse cutaneous systemic sclerosis
DEXA/ DXA	Dual-energy X-ray absorptiometry
DIP(J)	Distal interphalangeal (joint)
DISH	Diffuse idiopathic skeletal hyperostosis
DLCO	Diffusion capacity for carbon monoxide
DM	Dermatomyositis
DMARD	Disease-modifying antirheumatic drug
DVT	Deep vein thrombosis
EA	Enteropathic arthritis
EBV	Epstein–Barr virus
ECG (EKG)	Electrocardiogram
ECM	Erythema chronicum migrans

ECRB	Extensor carpi radialis brevis
ECRL	Extensor carpi radialis longus
ECU	Extensor carpi ulnaris
ED	Extensor digitorum
EDL	Extensor digitorum longus
EDM	Extensor digiti minimi
EDS	Ehlers–Danlos syndrome
EHL	Extensor hallucis longus
EI	Extensor indicis
ELMS	Eaton–Lambert myasthenic syndrome
EMG	Electromyography
EN	Erythema nodosum
ENA(S)	Extractable nuclear antigen(s)
EPB	Extensor pollicis brevis
EPL	Extensor pollicis longus
ERA	Enthesitis-related arthritis
ESR	Erythrocyte sedimentation rate
ESSG	European Spondyloarthropathy Study Group
EULAR	European League Against Rheumatism
FCR	Flexor carpi radialis
FCU	Flexor carpi ulnaris
FDP	Flexor digitorum profundus
FDS	Flexor digitorum superficialis
FHB	Flexor hallucis brevis
FM	Fibromyalgia
FMF	Familial Mediterranean fever
FPL	Flexor pollicis longus
FR	Flexor retinaculum
GARA	Gut-associated reactive arthritis
GBS	Guillain Barré syndrome
GCA	Giant cell arteritis
GFR	Glomerular filtration rate
GI	Gastrointestinal

GOA	Generalized osteoarthritis
HA	Hydroxyapatite
HIV	Human immunodeficiency virus
HLA	Human leukocyte antigen
HO	Hypertrophic osteoarthropathy
HSP	Henoch–Schönlein purpura
HTLV	Human T-cell leukemia virus
IL	Interleukin
ILAR	International League of Associations for Rheumatology
IM	Intramuscular(ly)
INR	International normalized ratio
ITB	Iliotibial band
ITP	Idiopathic thrombocytopenic purpura
JCA	Juvenile chronic arthritis
JIA	Juvenile idiopathic arthritis
JIO	Juvenile idiopathic osteoporosis
KD	Kawasaki disease
L	Lumbar (e.g., L5 is the fifth lumbar vertebra)
LCL	Lateral collateral ligament
LDH	Lactate dehydrogenase
LFTS	Liver function tests
lcSScl	Limited cutaneous systemic sclerosis
MCP(J)	Metacarpophalangeal (joint)
MCL	Medial collateral ligament
MCTD	Mixed connective tissue disease
MG	Myasthenia gravis
MND	Motor neuron disease
MPA	Microscopic polyangiitis
MR	Magnetic resonance
MTP(J)	Metatarsophalangeal (joint)
MTX	Methotrexate
NMS	Neuromuscular scoliosis
NSAID	Nonsteroidal anti-inflammatory drug
OA	Osteoarthritis

OI	Osteogenesis imperfecta
PAN	Polyarteritis nodosa
PBC	Primary biliary cirrhosis
PCR	Polymerase chain reaction
PIN	Posterior interosseous nerve
PIP(J)	Proximal interphalangeal (joint)
PL	Palmaris longus
PLM	Polarized light microscopy
PM	Polymyositis
PMN	Polymorphonuclear neutrophil
PMR	Polymyalgia rheumatica
PSA	Psoriatic arthritis
PSA	Prostatic specific antigen
PTH	Parathyroid hormone
PV	Plasma viscosity
PVNS	Pigmented villonodular synovitis
qhs	Every night, at bedtime
qid	Four times daily
RA	Rheumatoid arthritis
RF	Rheumatoid factor
RNP	Ribonucleoprotein
RP	Raynaud's phenomenon
REA	Reactive arthritis
RSD	Reflex sympathetic dystrophy (algo/osteodystrophy)
RSI	Repetitive strain injury
RS_3PE	Remitting seronegative symmetrical synovitis with pitting edema
RTA	Renal tubular acidosis
sACE	Serum angiotensin converting enzyme
SAI	Subacromial impingement
SAPHO	Synovitis, acne, palmoplantar pustulosis, hyperostosis, aseptic osteomyelitis (syndrome)
SARA	Sexually transmitted reactive arthritis
sq	Subcutaneous(ly)
SC(J)	Sternoclavicular (joint)

SI(J)	Sacroiliac (joint)
SLE	Systemic lupus erythematosus
SpA	Spondyloarthritis
SS	Sjögren's syndrome
SScl/Scl	Systemic sclerosis/Scleroderma
T	Thoracic (e.g. T5 is the fifth thoracic vertebra)
TB	Tuberculosis
Tid	Three times daily
TENS	Transcutaneous electrical nerve stimulation
TFTs	Thyroid function tests
TIA	Transient ischemic attack
TM(J)	Temporomandibular (joint)
TNF(α)	Tumor necrosis factor (alpha)
TPMT	Thiopurine S-methyltransferase
TRAPS	Tumor necrosis factor-associated periodic syndrome
TSH	Thyroid stimulating hormone
UC	Ulcerative colitis
US	Ultrasound
UV	Ultraviolet
WG	Wegener's granulomatosis
WHO	World Health Organization

Part I

The presentation of rheumatic disease

Chapter 1

Evaluating musculoskeletal pain

Introduction

Pain is the most common musculoskeletal symptom. It is defined by its subjective description, which may vary depending on its physical (or biological) cause, the patient's understanding of it, its impact on function, and the emotional and behavioral response it invokes. Pain is also often colored by cultural, linguistic, and religious differences. Therefore, pain is not merely an unpleasant sensation; it is in effect an emotional change. The experience is different for every individual. Patients who think of themselves as having a high pain threshold may have the hardest time coping.

In children and adolescents, the evaluation of pain is sometimes complicated further by the interacting influences of the experience of pain within the family, school, and peer group.

Localization of pain and pain patterns

- Adults usually localize pain accurately, although there are some situations worth noting in rheumatic disease where pain may be poorly localized (see Table 1.1).
- Adults may not clearly differentiate between periarticular and articular pain, referring to bursitis, tendonitis, and other forms of soft tissue injury as "joint pain." Therefore, it is important to confirm the precise location of the pain on physical examination.
- Pain may be well localized but caused by a distant lesion, e.g., interscapular pain caused by mechanical problems in the cervical spine, or right shoulder pain caused by acute cholecystitis.
- Pain caused by neurological abnormalities, ischemic pain, and pain referred from viscera are harder for the patient to visualize or express, and the history may be more difficult to interpret.
- Bone pain is generally constant despite movement or change in posture—unlike muscular, synovial, ligament, or tendon pain—and often disturbs sleep. Fracture, tumor, and metabolic bone disease are all possible causes. Such constant, localized, sleep-disturbing pain should always be investigated.
- Patterns of pain distribution are associated with certain musculoskeletal conditions. For example, polymyalgia rheumatica (PMR) typically affects the shoulder girdle and hips, whereas rheumatoid arthritis (RA) affects the joints symmetrically, with a predilection for the hands and feet.
- Patterns of pain distribution may overlap, especially in the elderly, who may have several conditions simultaneously. For example, hip and/or knee osteoarthritis (OA), peripheral vascular disease, and degenerative lumbar spine all may cause lower extremity discomfort.

The quality of pain

Some individuals find it hard to describe pain or use descriptors of severity. A description of the quality of pain can often help determine the cause. Certain pain descriptors are associated with nonorganic pain syndromes (see Table 1.2):

- Burning pain, hyperpathia (i.e., an exaggerated response to painful stimuli), and allodynia (i.e., pain from stimuli that are normally not painful) suggest a neurological cause.
- A change in the description of pain in a patient with a long-standing condition is worth noting, since it may denote the presence of a second condition, e.g., a fracture or septic arthritis in a patient with established RA.
- Repeated, embellished, or elaborate description (i.e., "catastrophizing") may suggest nonorganic pain, but be aware that such a presentation may be cultural.

Table 1.1 Clinical pointers in conditions where pain is poorly localized

Diagnosis	Clinical pointer
Periarticular shoulder pain	Referred to deltoid insertion
Carpal tunnel syndrome	Nocturnal paresthesias and/or pain, often diffuse
Trochanteric bursitis	Nocturnal pain lying on affected side
Hip Synovitis	Groin/outer thigh pain radiating to the knee

Table 1.2 Terms from the McGill pain scale that help distinguish between organic and nonorganic pain syndromes

Organic	Nonorganic
Pounding	Flickering
Jumping	Shooting
Pricking	Lancinating ("Shooting")
Sharp	Lacerating
Pinching	Crushing
Hot	Searing
Tender	Splitting
Nagging	Torturing
Spreading	Piercing
Annoying	Unbearable
Tiring	Exhausting
Fearful	Terrifying
Tight	Tearing

Changes in pain on examination

Eliciting changes in pain by the use of different examination techniques may be used to provide clues to the diagnosis:

- Palpation and comparison of active and passive range of motion can be used to reproduce pain and localize pathology. This requires practice and a good knowledge of anatomy.
- Many of the classic physical exam signs and maneuvers have a high degree of interobserver variability. Interpretation should take into account the context in which the examination is done and the effects of suggestibility.
- Palpation and passive range of motion exercises are performed while the patient is relaxed. The concept of passive movement is the assumption that when the patient is completely relaxed, the muscles and tendons around the joint are removed as potential sources of pain; in theory, passive range of motion is limited only by pain at the true joint. This assumption has its own limitations, however, especially since passive movements of the joint will still cause some movement of the soft tissues. In some cases, e.g., shoulder rotator cuff disease, the joint may be painful to move passively because of subluxation or impingement due to a musculotendinous lesion.
- The clinician should be aware of myofascial pain when palpating musculotendinous structures, especially around the neck and shoulder regions. Myofascial pain is said to occur when there is activation of a trigger point that elicits pain in a zone stereotypical for the individual muscle. It is often aching in nature.
- Trigger points are associated with palpable, tender bands of skeletal muscle that are hyperirritable. Trigger points are tender to palpation, and pressure may induce a stereotyped pattern of referred pain. This is different from the tender points characteristic of fibromyalgia, which tend to be present symmetrically throughout the body and do not induce referred pain.
- Local anesthetic infiltration at the site of a painful structure is sometimes used to help localize pathology, e.g., injection under the acromion may provide substantial relief from a "shoulder impingement syndrome." However, the technique is reliable only if localization of the injected anesthetic can be guaranteed. Few, if any, rigorously controlled trials have shown it to give specific results for any condition.

The assessment of pain in young children

The assessment of pain in young children is often difficult:
- Young children often localize pain poorly. Careful identification of the painful area is necessary through observation and palpation.
- A child may not admit to pain but will withdraw the limb or appear anxious when the painful area is examined.
- Observing a child's facial expression during an examination is very important, as is the parent's response.
- Quantification of pain often requires nonverbal clues, such as the child's behavior. Pain rating scales are often helpful (see Figure 1.1).
- Turning the examination into a form of play may put the child at ease and assist with the examination. For example, asking the child to imitate your own movements may help you gauge range of motion.
- The trappings of a clinic setting may make young children nervous, and removing a white coat or stethoscope from sight may also help place the patient at ease.

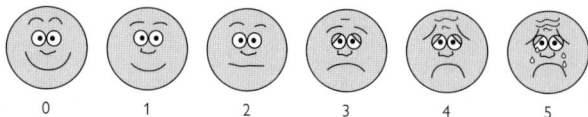

Fig. 1.1 Pain assessment in children—the faces rating scale.

Regional musculoskeletal conditions: making a working diagnosis

Introduction

This chapter provides a guide to constructing an appropriate differential diagnosis for the patient who presents with regional musculoskeletal symptoms. It does not make reference to all possible diagnoses, only to the most common. This section is divided into discussions of the neck, upper limb (shoulder, elbow, wrist), hand, thoracolumbar spine, lower limb (pelvis, groin, thigh, knee), and foot.

General considerations

- Findings from conventional clinical examination and imaging of the musculoskeletal system usually occur when the patient is at rest, and therefore only minimally symptomatic. Examination in the context of function (i.e., carrying, lifting, walking, bending, etc.) is not easy, although it is arguably more appropriate. Therefore, a thorough history utilizing deep knowledge of functional anatomy is the best alternative and an invaluable way of obtaining good information about abnormal function and its causes.
- Time spent obtaining a detailed account of the onset of symptoms is often helpful, regardless of whether the symptoms are of recent onset, or chronic, or obviously associated with trauma. Patients usually have a clearer concept of injury-induced disease and may try to rationalize the appearance of nontrauma-related symptoms by association with an event or injury.
- Weakness (as a symptom) may be due to a neuropathic or myopathic condition or it may be perceived according to the impact of other symptoms such as pain.
- With children, it is important to obtain a history from both the child and a care provider. Second-hand information, even if provided by the mother, may be less reliable than direct information from someone who has the opportunity to observe the child during the day.
- Regional musculoskeletal lesions may be a presenting feature of a systemic disorder such as an autoimmune rheumatic disease, malignancy or infection. Clinical suspicion should guide the evaluation.
- Screening for disseminated malignancy, lymphoma, myeloma, and infection should at least include a CBC, CMP, serum and urine protein electrophoresis with immunofixation, ESR and CRP. Thereafter, tests should be directed specifically toward the clinical scenario.

Corticosteroid injections and rehabilitation, as part of regional pain treatment, are discussed in general terms at appropriate points in the text. The practical approach to these therapies is presented at the end of this chapter.

Neck pain

Background epidemiology

- About 10% of the adult population has neck pain at any one time, although many people do not seek medical help.
- About 1% of adult patients with neck pain develop neurologic deficits, but overall levels of disability are lower than for patients with low back pain.
- Isolated neck pain in children and adolescents is unusual. More commonly, it accompanies thoracic spine pain or pathology.
- A continuum of radiological appearances exists in relation to age: intervertebral disc narrowing, marginal end-plate osteophytes, and facet joint changes. The appearances are often termed degenerative; however, their correlation with the presence and severity of pain is poor.

Functional anatomy

- The neck is the most mobile (37 separate articulations) but least stable part of the spine. There are seven vertebrae (C1–C7) and five intervertebral discs (C2/3–C6/7). The C5/6 disc is most often associated with radicular symptoms. If it occurs, cord compression is most likely in this region, although atlantoaxial (C1–C2) subluxation may produce the same picture, especially among patients with RA.
- Minor congenital abnormalities are not infrequent and increase the risk of degenerative changes.
- Nerve roots C2 and C3 cover sensation over the back of the head, the lower jaw line, and the neck.
- Nerve roots C4–T1 leave the spine in dural root sleeves, traverse the intervertebral foramina, and form the brachial plexus.
- Cervical nerves have a dermatomal representation (see Figure 2.1) and supply the upper limb musculature in a predictable way.

Taking a history

The site, radiation, and description of pain

- Nerve root (radicular) pain is usually sharp and reasonably well localized in the arms. It is often described as "burning" and associated with paresthesias and numbness. Nerve root irritation and compression by an intervertebral disc are common causes of radicular pain. However, in older adults and those who suffer recurrent bouts of pain, it is usually due to stenosis of the exit foramen caused by vertebral end-plate osteophytes, facet joint osteophytes, thickened soft tissue, or fibrosis.
- Pain from deep cervical structures is common. It often localizes poorly across the upper back. It can be referred to the upper arms, is typically described as "heavy" or "aching," and is more diffuse than nerve root pain.
- Muscle spasm often accompanies various lesions. It can be very painful.
- Pain from the upper cervical spine (C1–C3) can be referred to the temporomandibular joint (TMJ) or retro-orbital regions. Conversely,

Table 2.1 The major causes of neck pain in adults

Soft tissue lesions (posture, psychogenic issues, and overuse as modifiers)	Neck strain
	Torticollis
	Myofascial pain
	Trauma (e.g., acute flexion—extension injury [whiplash]))
	Cervicothoracic interspinous bursitis
Degenerative and mechanical lesions	Spondylosis
	Disc prolapsed
	Thoracic outlet syndrome
	Diffuse idiopathic skeletal hyperostosis (DISH)
Inflammatory conditions	Rheumatoid arthritis (RA)
	Spondyloarthropathy (associated with fracture and inflammatory discitis) (Chapter 8)
	Juvenile idiopathic arthritis (Chapter 7)
	Polymyalgia rheumatica (PMR) (Chapter 14)
	Myelitis
Bone lesions	Traumatic fracture
	Osteomyelitis (e.g., TB)
	Osteoporosis (fragility fracture) (Chapter 16)
	Osteomalacia (bone disease or muscle pain)
	Paget's disease
Nonosseous infections	General systemic infection (general/cervical myalgias)
	Meningitis
	Discitis
Malignancy	Primary (rare) or primary tumors (and pathological fracture)
	Myeloma, lymphoma, leukemias
Brachial plexus lesions	Trauma
	Thoracic outlet syndromes (e.g., cervical rib)
Referred pain from	Acromioclavicular or temporomandibular joint
	Heart and major arteries (e.g., angina, thoracic aorta dissection)
	Pharynx (e.g., infection, tumors)
	Lung and diaphragm (e.g., Pancoast tumor, subphrenic abscess)
	Abdomen (e.g., gallbladder, stomach, esophageal, or pancreatic disease)
	Shoulder (e.g., adhesive capsulitis) (Chapters 2 and 19)

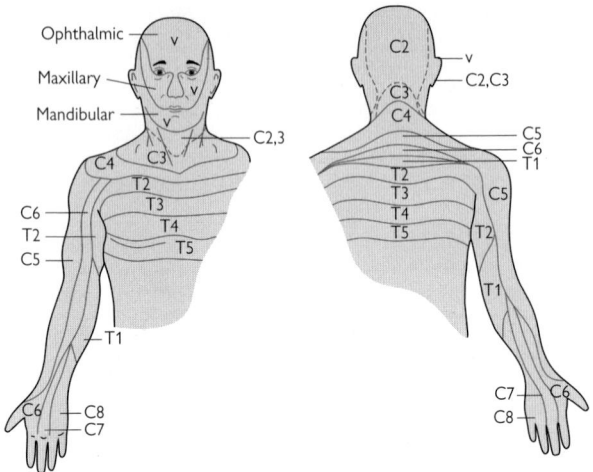

Fig. 2.1 Dermatomal distribution of the cervical and upper thoracic nerves reflecting the radicular pattern of nerve root lesions.

pain from TMJ disorders or as a result of dental malocclusion can be referred to the neck.
- Pain from the lower neck may be referred to the interscapular and anterior thoracic wall regions. The latter may mimic cardiac ischemic pain.
- Florid descriptions of the pain and of its extent and severity ("catastrophizing") are associated with prominent psychological modulators of pain.
- Evaluation of the shoulder joint is often necessary as pathology there often coexists and symptoms around the shoulder often complicate neck evaluation.
- Occipital headache is a common manifestation.

Acute neck pain with trauma
- Acute neck pain with trauma requires urgent assessment even if there are no obvious neurologic symptoms.
- Acute trauma requires urgent evaluation and consideration of fracture, spinal cord damage, and vertebral instability. About 80% of serious injuries occur from an accelerating head hitting a stationary object.
- An abrupt flexion injury may fracture the odontoid (this occurs less commonly with extension); however, fewer than one in five injuries at C1/C2 produce neurologic deficit because of the wide canal at this level.
- If not traumatic or osteoporotic (the latter being relatively rare in the cervical spine), fractures may occur in bone invaded by malignancy.

New and/or associated symptoms

Ask about associated leg weakness and new bladder or bowel symptoms. New onset acute neck pain with neurologic features needs urgent evaluation. Neurologic symptoms may also accompany chronic neck pain:

- Spinal osteomyelitis, meningitis, discitis (infection or inflammation), myelitis, and fracture may all present with acute or subacute neck pain. All may cause cord compression. Myelopathy due to spondylosis typically presents with a slowly progressive disability over weeks to months, although it can be acute, particularly if associated with central disc prolapse.
- Subacute pain, flaccid paralysis, and profound distal neurologic signs may suggest myelitis, a condition caused mainly by infections and autoimmune diseases.
- Tinnitus, gait disturbance, blurring of vision, and diplopia associated with neck pain are all ascribed to irritation of the cervical sympathetic nerves.
- The vertebral arteries pass close to the facet joints just anterior to emerging nerve roots. Disruption of vertebral blood flow may cause dizziness in severe cases of neck spondylosis.

Previous trauma

Ask about previous trauma—it often precedes and influences chronic pain:

- Acute and occupational (chronic overuse) trauma is a common antecedent of chronic neck pain.
- Cervical dystonia (torticollis) can occur 1 to 4 days after acute trauma. It responds poorly to treatment and can be longstanding. It may also complicate arthropathy such as in RA or Parkinson's disease.
- Whiplash injury is associated with chronic myofascial pain.
- In some patients with chronic pain following (sometimes trivial) trauma, there may be dissatisfaction with the quality of care received at the time of the injury.
- Unresolved litigation associated with trauma correlates with the persistence of neck pain and reported disability.

Occupational and leisure activities

Some occupations and sports/activities are associated with recurrent neck pain:

- Neck pain (and early spondylosis) is prevalent among people whose occupations require persistent awkward head and neck postures, e.g., professional dancers.
- Although biomechanical factors may be an important influence in initiating and aggravating neck pain, there may also be an underlying genetic predisposition to OA and/or hypermobility.

Other points

Establish whether the pain started or varies with any nonmusculoskeletal symptoms:

- Cardiac ischemia, dyspepsia, or abdominal pain can result in referred pain to the neck (see Table 2.2).

Examination

Functionally, the neck is part of the upper limb, and symptoms in the arms and legs may be relevant. Neurologic examination of the arms is important to the assessment of the neck.

- An adequate examination cannot be performed in a clothed patient. Despite the inconvenience, it is important to have the patient change into an examination gown to avoid missing potentially relevant clues.
- Inspection from front and back may reveal specific muscle wasting or spasm and poor posture.
- Observing active movements reveals little if the patient has severe pain or muscle spasm. Inability to move the neck even small distances is characteristic in advanced ankylosing spondylitis (AS) (Chapter 8).
- Tenderness often localizes poorly in degenerative disease. Exquisite tenderness raises the possibility of a disc lesion, osteomyelitis, or malignancy (the latter two are rare).
- There may be trigger points in neck stabilizer and extensor muscles. Activation of a trigger point elicits myofascial pain in a zone that is stereotypical for the individual muscle.
- Tender points (localized, nonradiating pain elicited by pushing with the thumb), notably at the occipital origin of the trapezius, the medial scapular border, and the mid-belly of the trapezius, are features of fibromyalgia (FM) (Chapter 18). It is not clear whether tender and trigger points are the same.
- Examination of passive mobility may be helpful primarily if it reveals gross asymmetry. The normal range of movement varies depending on age, sex, and ethnicity. Generally, at least 45° of lateral flexion and 70° of rotation should be achieved in a middle-aged adult. Global loss of passive mobility is nonspecific and occurs with increasing age. The range of movement that might indicate hypermobility has not been established.
- Care should be taken if neck instability is a possibility (e.g., after trauma, or in a patient with a history of RA). Vigorous passive examination of forward flexion may exacerbate disc lesions.
- Examination of the shoulder is important to evaluate any referred pain or associated articular lesion (e.g., adhesive capsulitis) (Chapter 19).
- Neurologic examination of upper and lower limbs is important in all cases in which pain is referred to the arms and/or the legs if cord compression is a possibility: look for increased tone, clonus, pyramidal weakness, and extensor plantar response. It is also important to check for a cervicothoracic sensory level.

Diagnostic procedures

Radiographs

Radiographs should be requested with specific objectives in mind:

- A lateral neck film may demonstrate soft tissue thickening (characteristic of infection or synovitis), spondylitis (i.e., syndesmophytes, discitis, and periosteal apposition), and the severity of spondylosis.
- Oblique views centered on the suspected level may show nerve root foramen stenosis from bony encroachment in patients with radiculopathy. There may be underlying OA (Chapter 6).

- High cervical flexion and extension views and a "through-the-mouth" (odontoid) view are useful to demonstrate odontoid pathology.
- In a patient with RA, if the distance between the anterior arch of the atlas and odontoid process is >3 mm on a lateral film taken in flexion, there is likely to be C1/C2 AP subluxation.
- On a lateral film, superior odontoid subluxation in RA can be judged from a reduced distance from the anteroinferior surface of C2 to a line drawn between the hard palate and base of the occiput (McGregor's line). The distance should be >34 mm in men and >29 mm in women. Lateral odontoid subluxation is best demonstrated with magnetic resonance (MR) imaging.
- Stepwise vertebral subluxation throughout the cervical spine demonstrated on a lateral film is characteristic of advanced RA.
- There may be only a few but important signs of spinal infection such as a soft tissue mass or isolated loss of joint space.

Magnetic resonance (MR) and computed tomography (CT)

- MR has largely superseded CT, arthrography, and CT–arthrography in assessing cervical spine/nerve, dural, vertebral, disc, and other soft tissue lesions in the neck.
- In many cases the relevance of some MR findings is still being established—patterns of signal abnormality do occur in asymptomatic people. The frequency of these effects increases with age.
- MR is the technique of choice for imaging disc prolapse, myelopathy (Plate 1), myelitis, and for excluding infection or tumors. MR is used to help evaluate the need for neurosurgical intervention in RA patients with high cervical instability.
- MR may show soft-tissue swelling around the odontoid in CPPD disease (Chapter 15) but the diagnosis is best made with CT, which shows calcification around the odontoid and of adjacent ligaments ("crowned dens syndrome").
- In patients with the combination of unexplained radiographic signs and generalized symptoms, MR is an important investigation. Cases of spinal infection (such as TB or brucellosis) and lymphoma and can be detected using MR (Chapter 17).

Bone scan

- Scintigraphy has little role in diagnosing neck lesions.
- Despite improved image quality and tomographic images, the neck is poorly imaged by bone scan.

Treatment

Figure 2.2 shows the principles of treating mechanical cervical syndromes and the timing of MR scanning.

- Remember to review the diagnosis if pain is persistent despite treatment and symptoms seem disproportionate to the results or reports of imaging. In our experience, inflammatory psoriatic-related neck pains are often mistaken for cervical spondylosis. This may be because the clinician too readily assumes the latter diagnosis and/or radiologists misinterpret radiographs.

Fig. 2.2 The principles of treating mechanical neck syndromes and the timing of MR scanning.

MECHANICAL CERVICAL SPINE LESION

NO NEUROLOGICAL SIGNS

CHRONIC OR RECURRENT

FIRST
Mobilization physiotherapy
Other physiotherapy—traction, hydrotherapy
postural advice and home exercise
cervical pillow
Pain control*
intermittent soft collar

THEN
Tricyclic agent at night
Inject 'trigger' points

IF NO BETTER

MR SCAN
Scan normal—epidural injection
Scan abnormal—neurosurgical
referral or review diagnosis

IF STILL NO BETTER
Pain clinic

ACUTE

Rest or bedrest
Soft collar
Pain control*
Muscle relaxant
Physiotherapy—heat. etc.
Tricyclic agent at night

Gentle mobilization
Other physiotherapy

MR SCAN
Scan normal—epidural injection
Scan abnormal—neurosurgical
referral or review diagnosis

Pain clinic

WITH NEUROLOGICAL SIGNS

MYELOPATHY

Collar—firm or soft
Pain control*
Muscle relaxant
? rest or bedrest

URGENT MR SCAN

Scan abnormal—neurosurgical
referral or review diagnosis
Scan normal—review diagnosis
walking aid

Pain clinic

RADICULOPATHY

Collar—firm or soft
Pain control*
Muscle relaxant
Tricyclic agent at night
?rest or bedrest

Gentle traction

MR SCAN
Scan normal—further traction
and/or epidural injection
Scan abnormal—neurosurgical
referral or review diagnosis

Pain clinic

*=simple analgesics and/or
anti-inflammatory

Shoulder pain

Anatomy of the shoulder (see Figure 2.3)

- The glenohumeral joint is a ball and socket joint. The shallow glenoid cavity permits a wide range of movement. The circular fibrocartilagenous labrum sits on the glenoid, increases the articular surface area, and acts as a static joint stabilizer.
- Normal glenohumeral movements include depression, then glide and rotation of the humeral head under the coracoacromial (CA) arch to enable elevation of the arm. As the arm elevates, there is smooth rotation and elevation of the scapula on the thoracic wall.

(a)

Acromion

Subacromial (subdeltoid) bursa

Greater tuberosity of humerus

Deltoid muscle

Humerus

Supraspinatus muscle

Labrum

Glenohumeral joint space

Glenoid fossa (scapula)

Axillary recess

Joint capsule

(b)

Acromioclavicular joint

Acromion

Coracoacromial ligament

Transversehumeral (intertubercular) ligament

Tendon and synovial sheath of the long head of the biceps

Humerus

Clavicle

Coracoclavicular ligament

Coracoid process

Subscapularis bursa

Scapula

Fig. 2.3 (a) Major shoulder structures. (b) The relationship of the joint capsule to its bony surround and the coracoacromial arch.

- Shoulder movements are a synthesis of four joints: glenohumeral, acromioclavicular (AC), sternoclavicular (SC), and scapulothoracic.
- Movements at AC and SC joints enable slight clavicular rotation, shoulder elevation/depression, and protraction/retraction.
- The rigid CA arch protects the glenohumeral joint from trauma; it and the overlying deltoid are separated from the capsule by the subacromial (subdeltoid) bursa.
- A cuff of muscles surrounds the glenohumeral joint capsule. These rotator cuff muscles are the supraspinatus, infraspinatus, teres minor, and subscapularis.
- The supraspinatus initiates abduction by depressing the humeral head, then elevating the arm alone for the first 10° of movement. The more powerful deltoid then takes over abduction. The infraspinatus/teres minor externally rotates the arm, and the subscapularis internally rotates the arm (see Figure 2.4).
- Production of powerful shoulder movements requires some degree of arm elevation, since the larger muscles such as the deltoid, latissimus dorsi (extensor), and teres major (adductor) work inefficiently with the arm in the anatomical position. The rotator cuff muscles act synchronously as joint stabilizers throughout the range of shoulder movement.
- The long head of biceps tendon originates above the glenoid (usually attached to the labrum) and runs within the glenohumeral joint capsule anteromedially in a bony groove.

Pain and shoulder lesions (see Chapter 19)

- Shoulder pain is common and may have its origin in articular or periarticular structures or may be referred from the cervical or thoracic spine, the thoracic outlet, or subdiaphragmatic structures (see Table 2.2).
- Shoulder lesions often produce pain referred to the humeral-deltoid insertion, which the patient will interpret as pain in the upper arm.
- Periarticular disorders, mainly subacromial/shoulder impingement (SAI) disorders, are the most common cause of shoulder pain in adults (>90% of cases).
- Traumatic or inflammatory lesions of many different shoulder structures and conditions that result in neuromuscular weakness of the rotator cuff or scapular stabilizers may result in impingement pain.
- Pain from subacromial impingement syndrome is thought to be generated by the "squashing" of subacromial structures between the greater tuberosity of the humeral head and the ca arch during rotation/elevation of the humeral head.

Taking a history

When did the pain start?

Shoulder injuries are common and may be acute or chronic (overuse).

- Rotator cuff lesions (inflammation, degenerative weakness, or tear) are often associated with activities and occupations that involve straining the arm in abduction or forward flexion. A history of an acute

Fig. 2.4 The muscles of the shoulder: (a) anterior view; (b) posterior view.

Table 2.2 The most common causes of shoulder pain

Periarticular lesions (often manifest as subacromial impingement pain)	Rotator cuff tendonitis/tears (very common age 40y+)
	Calcific tendonitis
	Bicipital tendonitis
	Subacromial bursitis
	Milwaukee shoulder (basic calcium phosphate crystal periarthritis)
	Periarticular muscle weakness
Articular lesions	Synovitis (glenohumeral or acromioclavicular joint)
	OA (glenohumeral or acromioclavicular joint)
	Glenohumeral instability (e.g., labral tears)
	Adhesive capsulitis ("frozen shoulder")
Neurologic	Cervical nerve root and radicular referred pain
	Neuralgic amyotrophy
	Spinal cord lesions: tumors, syringomyelia
Neurovascular	Complex regional pain syndrome (see Chapter 18)
Thoracic conditions (referred pain)	Mediastinal tumors
	Angina
Systemic and diffuse conditions	Polymyalgia rheumatica (see Chapter 14)
	Myositis (see Chapter 13)
	Chronic pain disorders (see Chapter 18)
	Polyarticular synovitis
Bone disorders	Tumors
	Osteonecrosis (see Chapter 16)
	Paget's disease (see Chapter 16)
Subdiaphragmatic (referred pain)	Gallbladder disease
	Subphrenic abscess

injury, however, is not always obtained. Subsequent calcification in the tendon following a supraspinatus injury can be asymptomatic or present with acute pain.

- Manual labor is a risk factor for rotator cuff lesions. There is typically no acute injury; instead, there is a history of repetitive movements over years that lead to injury.
- Athletes involved in throwing and racket sports are at risk of rotator cuff tendinopathy and labral tears. Football players are at risk of clavicle fracture, shoulder dislocation (which may lead to long-term instability), and disruption of the acromioclavicular (AC) joint.

- Pain from degenerative glenohumeral or AC joint arthritis might be a long-term sequelae of a bone or joint injury.
- The shoulder girdle is one of the most common sites for a chronic pain syndrome.
- Myofascial pain of the shoulder girdle is common and may mimic the symptoms of cervical radiculopathy, reflux esophagitis, or ischemic heart disease.
- Severe, persistent, sleep-disturbing pain of recent onset may be indicative of avascular necrosis, osteomyelitis, or bony tumors. Although uncommon in the shoulder region, these conditions should not be missed.

Where is the pain?

- Pain from the shoulder may be referred to the deltoid insertion.
- Well-localized pain may occur with AC joint arthritis—the patient will have no trouble pointing out the affected joint— but remember that referred C4 nerve root pain and pain from bone lesions of the distal clavicle is maximal in the same area.
- Glenohumeral articular and capsulitis pain are not well localized (e.g., the patient covers his shoulder with his hand).
- Pericapsular pain may be associated with SAI syndromes but may also be myofascial (typically) or referred from the cervicothoracic spine.
- Bilateral shoulder pain should increase suspicion of the presence of an inflammatory polyarthritis such as RA (see Chapter 5), juvenile idiopathic arthritis (JIA, Chapter 7), psoriatic arthritis (see Chapter 8) or CPPD arthritis (see Chapter 15)—but these would be rare without other joint symptoms.
- Diffuse pain across the shoulder girdle muscles in those over 55 years of age raises the possibility of PMR (see Chapter 14). This pain is often associated with immobility and stiffness, particularly early in the day.
- A deep aching pain associated with stiffness is characteristic of adhesive capsulitis (frozen shoulder). The use of the term *frozen shoulder* is popular, but often incorrectly applied. It is a condition that is rare in patients under 40 years of age. The condition occurs in three phase: a painful phase, an adhesive ("frozen") phase, and a resolution phase. Phases often overlap and the duration varies, but long-term limitation of shoulder movement remains in up to 15% of patients. It is associated with diabetes.

Does the pain vary?

Movement- or posture-related pain may be a clue to its cause:

- Rotator cuff lesions often present to rheumatologists with an SAI pattern of pain—that is, pain reproducibly aggravated by specific movements during each day such as reaching up (overhead) with the arm. Articular, bone, and adhesive capsulitis pain is more likely to be persistent.
- A history of recurrent bouts of shoulder pain in children and adolescents may suggest glenohumeral instability due to hypermobility

or previous trauma, e.g., a labral tear. In an unstable shoulder, pain may result from synovitis, subchondral bone damage, or an SAI disorder. The frequency of recurrent anterior subluxation is inversely proportional to the age at which the initial dislocation occurs.

Are there spinal symptoms?

There is an association between neck conditions and shoulder pain. C4 nerve root pain is referred to the shoulder, while adhesive capsulitis is associated with cervical nerve root symptoms (the nature of the link is unknown). Inflammatory neck lesions caused by CPPD and psoriatic spondylitis can lead to pain referred to the shoulders, mimicking PMR.

Examination

Visual inspection

Inspect the neck, shoulders, and arms from the front, side, and back with the patient standing.

- Abnormality of the contour of the cervicothoracic spine could indicate muscle imbalance/spasm or might be associated with a nerve root origin of pain.
- Scapular asymmetry at rest is especially relevant when examining children and may indicate a congenital bony deformity. Subtle degrees of asymmetry are common and are not usually due to specific pathology.
- Diffuse swelling of the whole shoulder may suggest a shoulder effusion/hemarthrosis or subacromial bursitis. In the elderly, Milwaukee shoulder should be considered. Swelling of the AC joint occurs with joint diastasis, arthritis, and distal clavicular bone lesions.
- Arm swelling and skin changes distally could indicate a complex regional pain syndrome (see Chapter 18).

Elicit any tenderness

Eliciting tenderness of discrete shoulder structures is often unrewarding:
- Tenderness of the AC joint, humeral insertion of the supraspinatus tendon, and the long head of biceps tendon may be clues to pathology, but palpation may not yield a specific diagnosis.
- An appreciation of trigger points associated with myofascial pain and tender points in fibromyalgia (see Chapter 18) is important in the interpretation of regional soft tissue tenderness.

Document bilateral shoulder movements

This aids diagnosis but also gives an indication of the level of functional impairment and can help in monitoring changes over time (see Table 2.3). The movements are first tested actively (the patient does the movement) and then passively (the clinician supports the limb). Muscle strength can also be assessed while testing active movement.

- Observe arm elevation in the scapular plane from behind, noting symmetry of scapular movement, the pattern of pain during elevation, and the range of elevation. Hunching of the shoulder at the outset of arm elevation often occurs with an impingement problem. A painful arc may suggest a rotator cuff lesion. Inability to lift the arm suggests a rotator cuff tear or weakness, capsulitis, or severe pain, e.g., acute calcific supraspinatus tendonitis.

- Observe and compare internal rotation of shoulders, which can be judged by how far up the back the hand can reach. Poor performance may be due to rotator cuff weakness, weakness of the scapular stabilizing muscles, or pain (generally from shoulder impingement syndrome). This maneuver assumes normal elbow function.
- Observe the range of external rotation of the humerus from the front. Ask patients to flex their elbows as if they were holding a tray, and then rotate the arms outwards. Minor degrees of restriction caused by pain are not specific, but severe restriction is characteristic of adhesive capsulitis.
- Passive range of motion should be tested with two hands: one hand guides the movement while the second rests on the shoulder. Many patients will subconsciously flex the spine to compensate for restricted range of motion at the shoulder; using both hands can help detect this and other abnormalities in movement at the joint.

Test for subacromial impingement
- Always compare the affected with the asymptomatic side and make conservative judgments about muscle weakness if there is pain impeding voluntary effort.
- Most tests rely on their ability to narrow the distance between the humeral head and the CA arch, by driving the greater tuberosity under the CA arch as the humerus rotates (see Figure 2.5).
- Whether the tests are specific for lesions of the subacromial structures or for the site of impingement are unknown.

Movement of the glenohumeral joint
Move the glenohumeral joint passively in all directions by moving the upper arm with one hand and placing the other over the shoulder to feel for "clunks", crepitus, and resistance to movement:
- If the humeral head can slide anteriorly (often with a "clunk") without rotation in the glenoid it suggests instability.
- Grossly reduced passive shoulder movement (notably external rotation, with or without pain) is the hallmark of adhesive capsulitis.
- Pull down on both (hanging) arms. If the humeral head moves inferiorly (sulcus sign), there may be glenohumeral instability.

Stress the acromioclavicular joint
Stressing the AC joint may reproduce the pain. This is conventionally done by compression or shear tests:
- These tests should not normally be painful. Although painful tests have not proved to be specific for AC pathology (pain from SAI may also be present), a positive test may provide a clue that the AC joint is arthritic or dynamically unstable, or that impingement of structures in the subacromial space under the AC joint is occurring.
- Hold the patient's arm in forward flexion (90°) and draw it across the top of the patient's chest. The resulting compression of the AC joint may produce pain. AC joint pain can also be elicited by passively

Table 2.3 Isolated muscle testing of shoulder girdle muscles

Muscle: nerve root, peripheral nerve supply and muscle action	Muscle position	Isolated muscle test	Common pathology affecting muscle strength/bulk
Supraspinatus: C5/C6. Suprascapular nerve. Initial humeral abduction and stability of raised upper arm	From behind, seen and felt above the scapular spine at rest and when activated	Abduct arm from neutral against resistance	Tear or disuse following damage, e.g., after a fall, chronic overuse stress, or in athletes (throwing arm)
Infraspinatus: C5/C6. Suprascapular nerve. External rotation and stability of humeral head	From behind, seen and felt arising from medial scapular border passing laterally (below the scapular spine)	External rotation of arm in neutral, elbow supported and flexed at 90°	Tear or disuse following chronic damage
Serratus anterior: C5–C7. Long-thoracic nerve. Pulls the scapula forward on the thoracic wall (extends forward reach of arm)	Appreciated from behind when patient is pushing against a wall with arms outstretched in front, in that scapula remains fixed	Test by pushing wall with an outstretched arm or push-up. If paralyzed there will be lifting and lateral excursion of the scapula	Damage to long-thoracic nerve from trauma. Patient may also have SAI
Deltoid: C5/C6. Axillary nerve. Flexion, extension but mainly abduction of humerus	Arises from the scapular spine and acromion, then swathes the shoulder inserting into the humerus laterally	Wasting may be obvious. Weakness in isometric strength of an arm abducted to 90°	Lesions of axillary nerve damaged by anterior shoulder dislocation (external rotation may also be weak from denervation of teres minor)

elevating the arm through 180°, bringing the hand to the ceiling. Pain is experienced in the upper 10° or so of movement.

Shoulder examination with the patient supine

Examine the shoulders with the patient supine to test whether there is anterior cuff deficiency, glenohumeral joint laxity, or a labral tear: this is especially important in young adults and adolescents to identify an "unstable shoulder." Hold and support the upper arm held in slight abduction and external rotation (the elbow is flexed). Move the arm gently (cranially in the coronal plane) and apply gradual degrees of external rotation.

(a)

Painful arc
(active)

Action: Patient standing.
Slow arm abduction
(scapular plane).

Positive test: Pain onset (maximal)
at (variable) angular
range.

(b)

Neer test
(passive)

Action: Patient sitting/standing.
Passive forward flexion.
Scapula fixed.

Positive test: Pain at (variable) angle
of flexion.

(c)

Empty can
(active)

Action: Patient sitting/standing.
Active forward flexion
to 90° then internal
rotation—'can empties'.

Positive test: Pain with flexion or
rotation of arm.

(d)

Kennedy–Hawkins
(passive)

FIX

Action: Patient sitting/standing.
Passive forward flexion (90°).
Fix elbow with hand.
Passive internal rotation.

Positive test: Pain at some stage of
elevation or rotation.

Fig. 2.5 Tests useful for eliciting subacromial impingement.

- Deficiency of anterior structures is suggested by patient apprehension
  that pain is imminent or that the shoulder will slip forward ("the
  apprehension test"). With a labral tear there may be an audible or
  palpable "clunk."
- Pressure downward on the upper arm (taking the pressure off anterior
  shoulder structures by an anteriorly translocated humeral head) may
  relieve this apprehension or the pain associated with it ("the positive
  relocation test.")

- An unstable shoulder identified with the tests just described may denote previous traumatic injury (e.g., shoulder dislocation) or a hypermobility disorder.

Diagnosis and management

The optimum initial imaging for investigating undiagnosed shoulder pain is disputed. Some clinicians advocate management of shoulder problems based on history and examination alone. This is a practical approach to a common problem because many problems get better in the short term. The long-term sequelae of such management strategies, however, are unknown. Studies of shoulder pain in primary are suggest that chronic shoulder problems are common, often despite initial improvement.

Radiographs

- The standard projection for screening purposes is anteroposterior (AP), although the AP axial-lateral view taken with the arm abducted may add information about the relationship of the glenoid and humeral head. Look for calcific deposits in soft tissue (such as the basic calcium/ phosphate crystals seen in Milwaukee shoulder—see Chapter 7).
- Supraspinatus outlet views are often used to assess acromial configuration and identify inferior acromial osteophytes in patients with SAI.
- If recurrent dislocation is suspected, associated humeral head defects may be identified by an AP film with internal humeral rotation or a Stryker view. Bilateral films distinguish anomaly (invariably bilateral) from abnormality.
- Bilateral AP AC joint views with the patient holding weights may identify and grade degrees of AC joint diastasis (separation). Distal clavicular erosion may be due to RA, hyperparathyroidism, myeloma, metastases, or posttraumatic osteolysis.
- Although characteristic patterns of abnormality are associated with SAI (see Plate 2), minor age-related radiographic abnormalities are normal.

Other imaging: ultrasound, arthrography, CT arthrography, MR, bone scan

- Ultrasound scoring systems for locating and grading rotator cuff tears now exist. The technique permits examination of the rotator cuff with the shoulder in different positions, but is highly operator dependent.
- Patterns of rotator cuff abnormality and subacromial impingement are well recognized with both arthrography and MR. However, there is no consensus about whether ultrasound, MR, or arthrography is most accurate for detecting rotator cuff tears.
- Children, adolescents, and young adults suspected of having unstable shoulders should have an MR examination, because detailed views of the humeral head, glenoid labrum, periarticular glenohumeral soft tissues, and subacromial area are important.
- MR is the modality of choice in young adults when instability is diagnosed. Rotator cuff lesions and labral abnormalities are best assessed with MR. Enhancement with IV contrast may increase the chance of detecting a labral tear.

- No specific patterns of bone scan abnormality have been consistently recognized for isolated shoulder lesions, although a triple phase bone scan may be diagnostic for complex regional pain syndrome in the upper limb.

Other diagnostic procedures
- Local anesthetic injection may help disclose the site of shoulder pain, although it is possible that by the time anesthesia occurs the injected anesthetic has spread to areas not intended as a target.
- Joint aspiration is essential if infection is possible. Fluid is usually aspirated easily from a grossly distended shoulder capsule. Hemarthrosis can occur in shoulders with degenerative joint disease (often in association with chondrocalcinosis), hemophilia, trauma, and pigmented villonodular synovitis.
- Electrophysiological tests (EMG/NCV) may confirm muscle weakness and help establish the presence of neuromuscular disease, e.g., myositis or neuralgic amyotrophy.
- Blood tests are required if looking for infection, inflammatory disease, etc.
  - A normal creatine kinase (CK) and aldolase will rule out myositis in the majority of cases.
  - Blood urea, electrolytes, creatinine, alkaline phosphatase, calcium, phosphate, thyroid function tests, and myeloma screen should be considered if metabolic bone or myopathic disease is considered.

Treatment (see Chapter 19)
- Physical therapy should play a focal part in encouraging mobilization of the joint, and early assessment is prudent. The following principles are recommended:
  - Know whether there is an additional neck/spinal generated pain component (physical therapists are independent diagnosticians and some may erroneously aim therapy at cervicothoracic segments for individual shoulder lesions).
  - Do not refer to physical therapy without knowledge of who will see the patient, and the approach that will be taken for instability and rotator cuff weakness.
- Simple analgesics are often necessary.
- Local steroid injections (see Plates 12 and 13) can be considered in the following situations:
  - tendonitis of the rotator cuff
  - adhesive capsulitis (see Plate 12)
  - AC joint pain
  - subacromial bursitis (see Plate 13).
- The principles of steroid injection and rehabilitation are dealt with in the last two sections of this chapter.
- There are several situations where local steroids should be avoided:
  - bicipital tendonitis (which should be treated with rest, analgesia, and physical therapy);
  - the first 6 weeks of an acute rotator cuff tear;

- when symptoms have become chronic and conservative therapy has not helped for a presumptive clinical diagnosis. This requires reassessment, imaging, and a decision about whether surgery may be required.
- Surgical intervention may take the form of subacromial decompression arthroscopy, synovectomy of the SC joint and AC joint, or excision of the distal end of the clavicle:
  - subacromial decompression may be necessary for chronic rotator cuff tendonitis especially when imaging has shown inferior acromial osteophytes;
  - other interventions include repair of a rotator cuff or biceps tendon rupture and joint replacement (mainly for pain relief rather than improvement in function).
- Lithotripsy does not offer advantages over steroid injection and physical therapy for calcific supraspinatus tendonitis.

Pain around the elbow

Functional anatomy

- The humeroulnar articulation is the prime (hinge) joint at the elbow. The radius also articulates with the humerus and, to allow forearm and hand supination/pronation, with the ulna at the elbow (see Figure 2.6).
- Normal extension results in a straight arm, but some muscular people lack the last 5–10° of extension and some (especially women) have up to an extra 10° of extension (hyperextension).
- Normal flexion is to 150–160° and forearm supination/pronation range is around 180°.
- Owing to obliquity of the trochlea, extension is associated with a slight valgus that can be accentuated in women (up to 15°).
- Unilateral acute traumatic or chronic overuse lesions of the elbow are common. Bilateral symptoms may occur in these situations, but also consider the possibility of an inflammatory arthritis affecting the elbows or referred pain from the neck.
- Pain may also be referred from proximal neurologic lesions in the arm, the shoulder or even from distal lesions such as carpal tunnel syndrome (CTS).

Taking a history

Is the pain exclusively located in the elbow or referred from elsewhere?

Establish whether the pain is associated with neck pain and whether it has neurogenic qualities or is associated with paresthesias or numbness. There may be referral of pain from C6 or C7 nerve roots, shoulder lesions, or even from compression of the median nerve in the wrist.

Is there a history of acute or chronic (overuse) trauma?

- Pain at the lateral epicondyle 1–2 weeks after a weekend of "home maintenance" might suggest lateral epicondylitis (tennis elbow) following excessive use of a screwdriver, for example.
- Other common sites of pain, where characteristic conditions related to overuse are recognized, include the medial humeral epicondyle ("golfer's elbow") and the olecranon bursa (repetitive pressure/friction). Although typically acute in onset, these conditions may develop insidiously.
- Fractures around the elbow and fractures/dislocations in the forearm are common. Dislocation of the radial head alone is rare and is usually associated with concurrent fracture of the ulna (radiographs may not easily identify the fracture). If not associated with fracture (and especially if recurrent), the condition may be associated with generalized hypermobility (see Chapter 16) or shortening of the ulna owing to bone dysplasia.
- In children, a strong pull of the forearm or wrist (occurring primarily in preschool children) can lead to a partial dislocation of the elbow ("nursemaid's elbow"), which can be corrected by supinating and flexing the forearm while supporting the radial head.

Fig. 2.6 Bony configuration at the (right) elbow (anterior view)

- In children, osteochondritis of the humeral capitellum can occur in mid to late childhood (Panner's disease), typically following repeated trauma.

Does the pain radiate distally?

- Forearm pain may be an additional clue to C6 or C7 radicular pain, but may also be due to the spread of musculoskeletal pain along the extensor group of muscles from lateral epicondylitis or from entrapment of the median nerve in the elbow region.
- Peritendinitis crepitans is pain, tenderness, and swelling in the forearm associated with occupational overuse. It is thought to be due to damage of the long wrist/hand flexors and extensors at the muscle–tendon junction.
- Diffuse pain in the forearm can occur as a result of overuse injury, particularly in musicians and typists, although there is overlap with regional pain syndromes.
- Pain around the forearm may also arise from inflammation at the wrist (see the next section) particularly in De Quervain's tenosynovitis.

Is there prominent stiffness with the pain?

- Stiffness is often nonspecific but may denote inflammation such as synovitis of the joint or olecranon bursa and, therefore, raises the possibility of an autoimmune rheumatic or crystal deposition disease.
- In the middle aged and elderly, gout (see Chapter 15) of the olecranon bursa and surrounding soft tissues, particularly overlying the border of the ulna, is not uncommon and is often misdiagnosed as a cellulitis.

Ask about locking

Locking of the elbow in either flexion or supination/pronation may be due to loose intra-articular bodies. A single loose body is most commonly due to osteochondritis dissecans of the capitellum (e.g., in children with overuse throwing injury—"Little League elbow") and multiple loose bodies are associated with OA or synovial chondromatosis.

Is the pain unremitting and severe?

This type of pain suggests bony pathology:

- Although nonfracture bone pathology is rare in the elbow region, local bony pain might suggest osteochondritis or avascular necrosis, or, if part of a wider pattern of bony pain, metabolic bone disease.
- In the elderly and others at high risk for osteoporosis, supracondylar and other fractures may occur with surprisingly little trauma.

Are there symptoms in other joints?

Ask about other joints, low back (sacroiliac) pains, and risks for gout:

- Elbow synovitis alone is an uncommon presenting feature of adult RA.
- Elbow synovitis occurs in children presenting with JIA (see Chapter 7) but is rare (3%).
- Periarticular enthesitis is a recognized feature of spondyloarthropathy (SpA) (see Chapter 8) and may mimic tennis elbow.
- The periarticular tissue around the elbow is a moderately common site for gout.

Examination

Look for abnormalities, then palpate with the thumb. Observe the active, passive, and resisted active range of joint and related tendon movements and consider examining for local nerve lesions. A complete assessment should include examination of the neck, shoulder, and wrist.

Visual inspection

Look for obvious deformity or asymmetry in the anatomical position:

- Up to 10° of extension from a straight arm is normal. More extension might suggest a hypermobility disorder.
- A child with an elbow lesion typically holds the extended arm close to the body, often in pronation.

Look for swelling or nodules:

- Swelling due to joint synovitis is difficult to see in the antecubital fossa unless it is florid: it is most easily seen (and more easily felt) adjacent to the triceps tendon insertion.
- The olecranon bursa, which may be inflamed, overlies the olecranon and does not as a rule communicate with the joint. Overlying erythema, although nonspecific, may be associated with infection or gout.
- Nodules over the extensor surface or ulna border may be associated with RA (see Chapter 5).
- Psoriatic plaques are commonly found at the elbow extensor surface.

Observe active flexion and supination/pronation with the elbows held in 90° of flexion:

- Although the range of movement may be affected by extra-articular pain, loss of range usually implies an intra-articular disorder.

Palpate the lateral epicondyle of the humerus

- In lateral epicondylitis ("tennis elbow") there is tenderness, which may extend a little distally. Wrist and finger extension against resistance with the elbow in extension or passively stretching the tendons (by having the patient make fist, flex wrist, pronate forearm, then extend elbow) may reproduce the pain.
- Lateral epicondyle tenderness may be due to inflammation of the radiohumeral bursa that lies under the extensor tendon aponeurosis.
- Note that tenderness of lateral and sometimes medial epicondyles can occur in chronic pain syndromes. In these cases, however, the relevant extensor or flexor tendon provocation tests are likely to be negative.

Palpate the medial humeral epicondyle

- Tenderness suggests traumatic medial epicondylitis ("golfer's elbow"), a regional or chronic pain syndrome, or enthesitis. Confirm the site of the pain by stretching the wrist flexors—supinate the forearm, then passively extend both the wrist and elbow simultaneously. Resisted palmar flexion of the wrist or forearm pronation with elbow extension may also cause pain. Tasks that rely on this repetitive movement are often the provoking cause.
- Consider osteochondritis of the medial humeral epicondyle as a cause of persistent pain following an injury. The 8–15-year-old age group is at particular risk as this is a site of secondary ossification.

Passively flex and extend the elbow joint

Passively flex and extend the joint and note the range of movement and "end-feel" (the feel of resistance at the end of the range of passive joint movement):

- "End-feel" may tell you whether there is a block to full flexion or extension from a bony spur or osteophyte (solid end-feel) or from soft tissue thickening/fibrosis (springy, often painful).
- Note any crepitus (often associated with intra-articular pathology) and locking (caused by loose bodies in the joint).

Supinate and pronate the forearm

Passively supinate and pronate the forearm supporting the elbow in 90° of flexion with your thumb over the radioulnar articulation:

- There may be crepitus or instability/subluxation associated with pain. Instability might suggest a tear or damage to the annular ligament (due to trauma or chronic/aggressive intra-articular inflammation).

Test peripheral nerve function if there are distal arm symptoms

- Given its course around the lateral epicondyle, the integrity of the radial nerve should always be tested when a lateral elbow lesion is suspected.
- The median nerve runs in the antecubital fossa and may be affected in traumatic elbow lesions. It is particularly susceptible where it runs between the two heads of pronator teres (from medial epicondyle and the coronoid process of the ulna) and separates into anterior interosseous and terminal median nerve branches.

- The ulnar nerve lies in the groove behind the medial epicondyle. Bony or soft tissue abnormality in this area may affect nerve function and lead to reduced sensation in the little finger and weakness in the small muscles of the hand, the flexor carpi ulnaris (FCU), the extensor carpi ulnaris (ECU), or the abductor digiti minimi (ADM). The median and ulnar nerves are dealt with in more detail in the later sections, Wrist Pain and Symptoms in the Hand.

Diagnostic procedures

Radiographs and other imaging

- Standard AP and lateral radiographs are the most straightforward way of imaging the elbow initially. CT or MR may then be needed if the diagnosis is still obscure and referred pain can be ruled out.
- Look for periosteal lesions and enthesophytes (new bone spurs at clear entheses like the triceps insertion). Periosteal apposition and enthesophytes are typical in psoriatic arthritis (see Chapter 8).
- A lateral radiograph may show displacement of the anterior fat pad caused by a joint effusion or hemorrhage (the "sail sign").
- Dislocations of the radial head and associated ulna fractures in children are easily missed. To make this diagnosis, a high degree of suspicion and further imaging are often needed.

Needle arthrocentesis/olecranon bursocentesis

- Arthrocentesis/bursocentesis with fluid sent for microscopy and culture should always be done in suspected cases of sepsis. Fluid should be sent for polarized light microscopy in cases of bursitis that may be due to gout. Serum urate is worth requesting but may not be raised in acute gout.
- Examination of fluid for crystals should always be considered in cases of monoarthritis in the elderly or patients on dialysis.

Electrophysiology

If nerve entrapment is suspected and there is some uncertainty after clinical examination, then electrophysiological tests may provide useful information. Testing can help identify the degree and likely site of nerve damage and can help to discriminate between a peripheral and nerve root lesion.

Treatment

- The management of fractures is beyond the scope of this text.
- Epicondylitis is best managed early on with rest, splinting, analgesia, and local steroid injections. The efficacy of physical manipulation has not been proven, although there are theoretical reasons why ultrasound therapy could be of value (because it passes through the myofascial planes and concentrates near bone). Resistant cases may benefit from surgery—a "lateral release."
- Steroid injections may be of value in the following situations:
  - lateral or medial epicondylitis (hydrocortisone)
  - inflammatory arthritis (usually long-acting steroid)
  - olecranon bursitis
  - ulnar nerve entrapment.

See Corticosteroid Injection Therapy and Principles of Rehabilitation at the end of this chapter; also see Plates 12–15.

- Surgical procedures include excision of nodules and bursae, transposition of the ulnar nerve, synovectomy, excision of the head of the radius, and arthroplasty.
- Arthroplasty in inflammatory arthritis is best reserved for intractable pain and should be undertaken by an experienced surgeon. Lesser procedures such as proximal radial head excision can be effective to improve pain and function if forearm pronation and supination are poor.

Wrist pain

Functional anatomy of the wrist

- The wrist includes radiocarpal (scaphoid and lunate) and intercarpal articulations. The ulna does not truly articulate with the lunate but is joined to it, the triquetrum, and the radius (ulnar side of distal aspect), by the triangular fibrocartilage complex.
- The intercarpal joints are joined by intercarpal ligaments and are most stable when the wrist is in full extension. The anterior carpal ligaments are stronger than the posterior ones and are reinforced by the flexor retinaculum. Wrist and finger flexor tendons, the radial artery, and the median nerve enter the hand in a tunnel formed by the carpal bones and the flexor retinaculum (carpal tunnel).
- Flexion (70°), extension (70°), radial and ulnar deviation (about 20° and 30° from midline, respectively) occur at the wrist but supination/pronation of the wrist and hand is due to radiohumeral movement at the elbow.
- The flexor carpi radialis (FCR) and ulnaris (FCU) are the main flexors of the wrist, although the palmaris longus (pl) also helps (see Figure 2.6). All arise from the medial humeral epicondyle.
- All carpal extensors arise from the lateral humeral epicondyle (see Figure 2.7).
- Radial deviation (abduction) occurs primarily when radial flexors and extensors act together. Ulnar deviation (adduction) occurs primarily when ulnar flexors and extensors act together.

Taking a history

Table 2.4 details the major diagnoses for painful conditions of the wrist and hand.

Determine the exact location of the pain

- Pain localizing only to the wrist most likely comes from local tissue pathology. Cervical nerve root pain as a result of a C6, C7, or C8 lesion and pain from peripheral nerve lesions is likely to be located chiefly in the hand.
- Pain at the base of the thumb, aggravated by thumb movements, in middle and old age is typical of OA (see Chapter 6) of the trapezium-first metacarpal joint. Pain in this area might also be due to tenosynovitis of thumb tendons.

Trauma history

- Injury/post-injury conditions are common. A history of trauma is important.
- Common fractures in adults are: scaphoid and base of the first metacarpal (Bennett's), and head of the radius (Colles').
- Distal radioulnar physeal injuries may occur in children.
- Posttraumatic chronic wrist pain following injuries may be due to ligamentous injury and chronic carpal instability or osteonecrosis (lunate).

(a)

Digital flexor tendon sheaths

Flexor pollicis longus tendon sheath

Common flexor tendon sheath

Flexor retinaculum

Flexor carpi radialis tendon sheath

Flexor digitorum superficialis and flexor digitorum profundus tendons

(b)

Extensor digitorum communis and extensor indicis propius (fourth compartment)

Extensor pollicis longus (third compartment)

Extensor digiti minimi (fifth compartment)

Extensor pollicis brevis and abductor pollicis longus (first compartment)

Extensor carpi ulnaris (sixth compartment)

Extensor carpi radialis longus et brevis (second compartment)

Extensor retinaculum

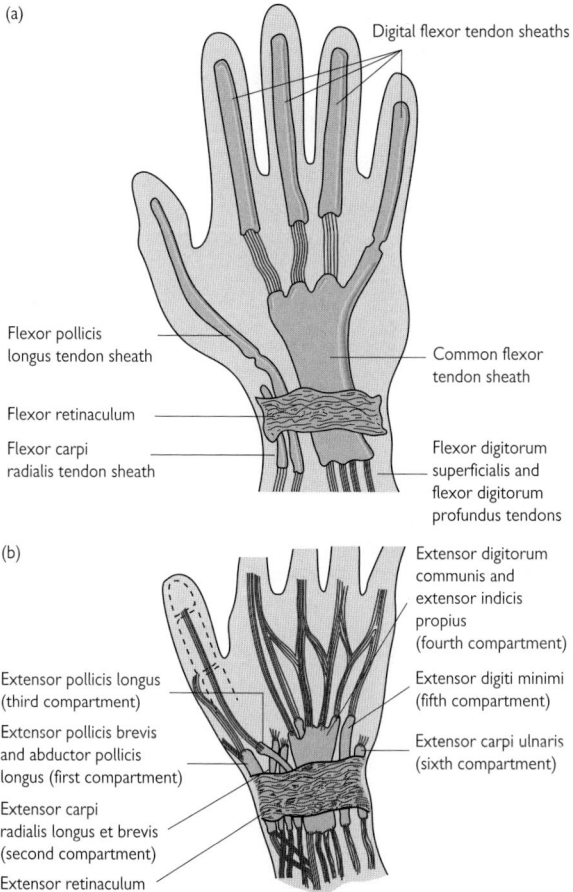

Fig. 2.7 Flexor (a) and extensor (b) tendon sheaths crossing the wrist. Flexor carpi radialis (FCR) inserts into the second and third metacarpals. Flexor carpi ulnaris (FCU) inserts into the pisiform, hamate, and fifth metacarpal. Extensor carpi radialis longus (ECRL) inserts into the base of the second, extensor carpi radialis brevis (ECRB) into the third, and extensor carpi ulnaris (ECU) into the fifth metacarpal, respectively.

Table 2.4 Painful conditions of the wrist and hand: major diagnoses

Articular disorders	Inflammatory arthritis (e.g., RA, JIA)
	Degenerative arthritis*
	Crystal arthritis
	Ligamentous lesions*
	Carpal instability (e.g., lunate dislocation)
Periarticular disorders	De Quervain's tenosynovitis
	Tenosynovitis of common flexor/extensor tendon sheath
	Flexor pollicis tenosynovitis
	Distal flexor stenosing tenosynovitis (trigger finger or thumb)*
	Ganglia*, subcutaneous nodules, tophi
	Diabetic cheiroarthropathy
	Dupuytren's contracture*
Bone pathology	Fracture*
	Neoplasia
	Infection
	Osteochondritis (lunate—Kienböck's; scaphoid— Prieser's) (see Chapter 16)
Neurologic	Median nerve entrapment (carpal tunnel* or at pronator teres)
	Anterior interosseous nerve syndrome
	Ulnar nerve entrapment (cubital tunnel or in Guyon's canal in wrist)
	Posterior interosseous nerve entrapment
	Radial nerve palsy
	Brachial plexopathy
	Thoracic outlet syndrome
	Cervical nerve root irritation or entrapment*
	Complex regional pain syndrome (see Chapter 18)
	Spinal cord lesions, e.g., syringomyelia

* Common conditions.

- Unusual or florid pain descriptors suggest a regional pain syndrome (e.g., reflex sympathetic dystrophy). Following trauma, regional pain syndromes are not uncommon in children, adolescents, or young adults.

Are there features to suggest synovitis?

- Pain due to wrist joint synovitis may be associated with stiffness and be worse at night or in the early morning. Stiffness in the hand may have various causes, but these will include multiple tendon/small joint synovitis, diabetic cheiroarthropathy, or even scleroderma (see Chapter 12).

- Wrist synovitis occurs commonly in adult RA and in children with both systemic and rheumatoid factor positive JIA. It occurs in 5% of oligoarticular JIA cases (see Chapter 7).
- In the elderly, wrist synovitis may be due to calcium pyrophosphate dihydrate (CPPD) crystals (see Chapter 15).

The quality of the pain

- Although primary bone pathology is rare, local bony pain (unremitting, severe, preventing sleep) might suggest avascular necrosis in those at risk or, if part of a wider pattern of bony pain, metabolic bone disease (e.g., physeal pain in children with rickets).
- Radicular pain may be burning in quality and is typically associated with numbness and paresthesias. Such neurogenic pain is commonly due to nerve root irritation or compression.

Other joint/musculoskeletal symptoms

- Wrist and extensor tendon sheath synovitis is a common presenting feature of adult RA. Other joints may be affected.
- CPPD arthritis commonly involves the wrist and can mimic RA in its joint distribution and presentation in the elderly.
- Wrist synovitis and enthesitis occur in SpA. Pain may be considerable, although swelling is minimal. There may be inflammatory-type symptoms of spinal pain and enthesitis elsewhere.

Ask specifically about job/leisure activities

- Repetitive lateral and medial wrist movements with thumb adducted can cause tenosynovitis of the abductor pollicis longus (APL) or the extensor pollicis brevis (EPB), commonly called De Quervain's tenosynovitis.
- If there is no obvious history of trauma, tendonitis may be a presenting feature of a systemic autoimmune rheumatic disease or even gonococcal infection in adolescents and young adults.
- Overuse pain syndromes may occur as a result of repetitive activity. The term *repetitive strain injury* is controversial. Objective assessment of pain, location of swelling, etc., from the outset is invaluable in assessing the response to treatment. Lack of objective findings (if imaging is normal) suggests a regional pain disorder.

Examination

Visual inspection

Inspect the dorsal surface of both wrists looking for swelling, deformity, or loss of muscle bulk.

- Diffuse swelling may be due to wrist or extensor tendon sheath synovitis.
- A prominent ulna styloid may result from subluxation at the distal radioulnar joint due to synovitis or radioulnar ligament damage.
- Prominence ("squaring") of the trapezoid–first metacarpal joint commonly occurs in OA of this joint.

- Loss of muscle bulk in the forearm may be due to a chronic T1 nerve root lesion or disuse atrophy.

Flexion/extension range tests for major wrist lesions
- The normal range of both flexion and extension in Caucasian adults is about 70°. Synovitis invariably reduces this range.
- When wrist synovitis is present, swelling on the dorsum of the wrist may become more apparent. Substantial common flexor or extensor tendon swelling will probably also block the full range of wrist movement (soft tissue approximation "end-feel").
- There is normally an additional 20° of flexion and extension to the active range with passive movement.
- Elicited pain and crepitus are unlikely to be specific for any type of lesion but may draw your attention to the anatomical site of the lesion.

Examine the dorsum of the wrist in detail
- Note any abnormal excursion of the ulnar styloid associated with pain and/or crepitus suggesting synovitis.
- Posttraumatic carpal instability, particularly scapulolunate dissociation, is relatively common. The latter is demonstrated by eliciting dorsal subluxation of the proximal scaphoid pole by firm pressure on its distal pole as the wrist is deviated radially from a starting position with the forearm pronated and the wrist in ulnar deviation. Note any gap between the scaphoid and lunate and any associated tenderness.
- Note any tenderness or thickening of the common extensor tendon sheath and tendon sheath of APL and EPB.
- Tenderness at the base of the thumb may be due to wrist synovitis, carpal or carpometacarpal OA, tenosynovitis, a ganglion, or a ligament lesion.
- Finkelstein's test for De Quervain's tenosynovitis may be used to elicit APL/EPB tendon pain. With the thumb adducted and opposed, the fingers are curled to form a fist. Passive ulnar deviation at the wrist stretches the abnormal tendons and elicits pain. Although it is a sensitive test, it is not specific for tendon pain.
- In adults, protrusion of the thumb out of the fist on the ulnar side of the hand during the first part of this test is unusual and suggests hypermobility.

Test the integrity of the tendons
Many muscles/tendons that move both the wrist and digits originate at the elbow; therefore, the quality of information gained from isolated tendon resistance tests (for either pain or strength) may be affected by pain elsewhere around the wrist, wrist deformity, or elbow lesions.

Interpret findings cautiously. Useful information might be obtained by passive movement of a tendon rather than by resisted active movement, and also by feeling for thickening or crepitus of the tendons.

Diagnosis and treatment
The diagnosis and treatment of wrist conditions is covered in the following section on symptoms in the hand.

Symptoms in the hand

Symptoms in the hand are a common presenting feature of some systemic conditions, and localized neurologic and musculoskeletal lesions are common, especially in adults. Detailed knowledge of anatomy is beyond the scope of this text. Functional anatomy is important and the more common abnormalities are summarized in the subsections that follow.

Functional anatomy of the hand

The long tendons

- Digital power is provided primarily by flexor and extensor muscles arising in the forearm. Their action is supplemented and modified by small muscles in the hand. Precise movements of the hand are mainly due to small muscles.
- Powerful digital flexors (see Figure 2.7): flexor digitorum superficialis (FDS), flexor digitorum profundus (FDP), and flexor pollicis longus (FPL).
- fds flexes proximal interphalangeal joints (PIPs) and, more weakly, metacarpophalangeal joints (MCPs)/wrist.
- fdp flexes distal interphalangeal joints (DIPs) and, increasingly weakly, PIPs, MCPs/wrist.
- FPL flexes (at 90° to other digits) mainly the PIP but also the whole thumb in a power grip (see below).
- Powerful digital extensors (see Figure 2.7): the extensor digitorum (ED) arises from the lateral epicondyle splitting at the wrist to insert into each digital dorsal expansion (digits two to five) that attaches to all three phalanges (see Figure 2.8). The fifth digit has an additional tendon, extensor digiti minimi (EDM) that also arises at the lateral epicondyle.
- APL abducts the thumb at the mcp provided the wrist is stable.
- EPB and EPL extend the thumb.
- Extensor indicis (EI) arises from the ulna posterior border distal to EPL and joins the index finger ed tendon.
- The muscles of the thenar eminence (see Table 2.5) act synchronously. All except adductor pollicis (ulnar nerve, C8/T1) are supplied by the median nerve from C8/T1 nerve roots. All three muscles are supplied by the ulnar nerve (C8/T1).

The intrinsic muscles

- The longitudinal muscles of the palm (four dorsal and four palmar interossei and four lumbricals) all insert into digits.
- Palmar interossei, from metacarpals 1, 2, 4, and 5, insert into dorsal tendons.
- Each dorsal interosseous arises from origins on two adjacent metacarpals. The muscles abduct the second and fourth fingers and move the middle finger either medially or laterally.
- The four lumbricals (see Figure 2.7, Table 2.6) arise from tendons of FDP in the palm passing to the lateral side of each MCP inserting into the dorsal expansions.
- The interossei combine with lumbricals to facilitate fine control of flexion and extension of MCPs and PIPs.

Fig. 2.8 Extensor expansion of a finger.

Table 2.5 Muscles of the thenar eminence

Muscle	Origin	Insertion
Abductor pollicis brevis	Flexor retinaculum, scaphoid, and trapezium	Thumb proximal phalanx and dorsal expansion
Flexor pollicis brevis	Flexor retinaculum, trapezium, trapezoid, and capitate	Thumb proximal phalanx (base of radial side)
Opponens pollicis	Flexor retinaculum and tubercle of the trapezium	First metacarpal (lateral border)
Adductor pollicis	Capitate, bases of second/ third metacarpals and distal third metacarpal	Thumb proximal phalanx (medial side)

(a)

Third lumbrical

First lumbrical

Opponens pollicis

Abductor pollicis

Lexor pollicis brevi

Abductor pollicis brevis

Abductor digiti minimi

Flexor digiti minimi

Flexor retinaculum

(b)

Second dorsal interosseus

First dorsal interosseus

Third dorsal interosseus

Forth dorsal interosseus

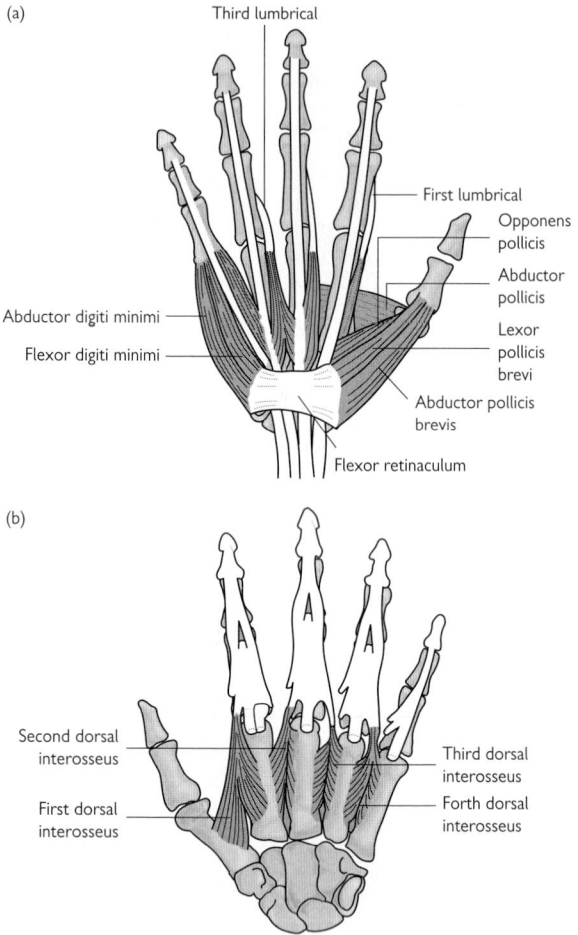

Fig. 2.9 (a) Lumbrical muscles and muscles of the thenar and hypothenar eminences. (b) Dorsal interossei.

Table 2.6 Muscles of the hypothenar eminence

Muscle	Origin	Insertion
Abductor digiti minimi	Flexor retinaculum (FR), pisiform, and pisohamate Ligament	Base of the fifth proximal phalanx and dorsal expansion
Flexor digiti minimi brevis	Flexor retinaculum and hook of hamate	Base of the fifth proximal phalanx
Opponens digiti minimi	Flexor retinaculum and hook of hamate	Medial side of the fifth Metacarpal

Grip
- For power, the wrist extends and adducts slightly, and the long digital flexors contract.
- A modified power grip, the hook grip, is used to carry heavy objects like a suitcase. The thumb is extended out of the way and extension at MCPs accompanies flexion at PIPs/DIPs.
- More precision in the grip can be obtained using varying degrees of thumb adduction, abduction, and flexion. The thumb can be opposed with any of the four other digits depending on the shape of the object to be held and the type of manipulation required.

Taking a history
A history of acute or overuse trauma with subsequent localized symptoms requires a straightforward application of anatomical knowledge, precise examination, and judicious choice of imaging techniques for diagnosis. However, there are more subtle or less easily delineated patterns of symptoms in the hand, particularly when pain is diffuse or poorly localized.

Is the pain associated with immobility or stiffness?
- Stiffness may be associated with joint or tendon synovitis but is not specific. Prompting may provide more accurate localization of symptoms.
- If unilateral, especially on the dominant hand, remember that diffuse hand pain may be due to a regional pain syndrome.

Is stiffness local or diffuse?
- Patterns of joint involvement in autoimmune rheumatic disease and polyarticular arthritis are summarized in Chapter 3.
- If localized in the palm, look for evidence of a Dupuytren's contracture (associated with diabetes). If diffuse, there may be thickening of soft tissue from a systemic process, e.g., hypothyroidism, scleroderma, diabetic cheiroarthropathy, or disorders of mucopolysaccharide metabolism (the latter especially in infants, although Fabry's syndrome can present in adulthood, and is associated with acroparesthesias and palmar telangiectasias).

- Stiffness due to an upper motor neuron lesion (an interpretation of increased tone) is unlikely to be confined to the hand and is likely to be associated with weakness. The pattern of symptoms over time should give a clue to its etiology.

Are there neurologic qualities to the pain or characteristics typical of a common nerve lesion?
- "Burning" or "deep" episodic pain varying with head, neck, and upper spinal position is typical of cervical nerve root pain. Ask about occupation and other activities that are associated with neck problems, the relationship with sleep posture, and frequent headaches.
- Pain on the radial side of the hand waking the patient at night and often relieved, at least partially, by shaking the hand is typical of median nerve entrapment in the wrist. However, pain in this condition is often poorly localized at initial presentation, and may be described as "hand swelling". Remember other lesions that produce pain in the area around the thumb base: trapezoid–first metacarpal joint OA, tenosynovitis of APL/EPB (De Quervain's) or EPL, referred pain from a C6 nerve root lesion, and ligament lesions (e.g., ulnar collateral ligament of first MCP—"skier's thumb").

Tingling/pins and needles/numbness
Make sure both you and the patient understand what you each mean by these terms.
- Symptoms usually denote cervical nerve root or peripheral nerve irritation/compression, although they can reflect underlying ischemia.
- Tingling in the fingertips of both hands, however, is recognized to occur commonly in patients diagnosed with fibromyalgia.
- Symptoms associated primarily with specific positions of the whole arm may be due to thoracic outlet compression of neurovascular structures.

Pain arising from bone
Pain in the hands arising from bones may be difficult to discriminate. Radiographs will often lead to confirmation of the diagnosis.
- The most common tumor in the hand is an enchondroma. It is usually painless. If they are painful, then one should suspect infarction or malignant change.
- Secondary metastases and malignant bone tumors in the hand are rare but must be ruled out in children, adolescents, and young adults with persistent localized bone pain.
- Paget's disease of hand bones can occur but is relatively rare.
- Digital bone pain from osteomalacia/rickets occurs but is unusual at presentation.
- Digital pain may rarely be due to sarcoidosis, hyperparathyroid bone disease, thyroid acropachy, hypertrophic pulmonary osteoarthropathy (HPOA), or pachydermoperiostitis. Look for clubbing.

Ischemic pain?
A history suggestive of ischemic pain in the hands is rare in rheumatologic practice. Persistent ischemic digital pain is a medical emergency.

- Digital vasomotor instability (e.g., Raynaud's phenomenon [RP]) is episodic and triggered by cold and emotion, and characterized by digital color changes: white/blue then red.
- Pain from vasculitis is likely to be persistent and associated with a purpuric rash, nail-fold infarcts, or splinter hemorrhages.
- Ischemic pain associated with cervicothoracic posture or prolonged arm elevation maneuvers may be due to thoracic outlet syndrome.
- Pain may be due to thromboembolism (e.g., antiphospholipid syndrome), infective endocarditis, or thromboangiitis obliterans (Buerger's disease).

Swelling
Examination is more reliable than a history.

- Apart from isolated lesions such as ganglia, patients' description of soft tissue or joint swelling may be unreliable and should be substantiated by examination. Nerve lesions can give the impression that swelling is present (think what a dentist's local anesthetic does for your lip!). Patients with carpal tunnel syndrome, for example, frequently complain of hand swelling at night.

Weakness
Ask about trauma, neck, and median nerve entrapment symptoms.

- Acute tendon injuries are common industrial accidents. Chronic occupational overuse may also lead to rupture.
- If weakness is profound and there has been no obvious trauma, the cause is likely to be neuromuscular.
- If not associated with pain, weakness is more likely to be neurologic than musculoskeletal in origin.
- Weakness associated with pain may be due to a neurologic or musculoskeletal lesion, the latter situation often due to an inability to use the hand (or part of it) because of pain or an alteration in biomechanical function as a result of deformity, which may only be slight.
- True weakness associated with stiffness is associated with myelopathy or even motor neuron disease. A detailed history of the progression of symptoms is important and neurologic examination should be thorough.

Trigger finger
This may denote stenosing tenosynovitis of a digital flexor tendon. Damage to the tendon and its sheath can result in a fibrous nodule attached to the tendon that moves and catches under the proximal annular ligament just distal to the MCP. It may not be painful. This most commonly affects middle and ring fingers and is prevalent among professional drivers and cyclists, and those in occupations requiring repeated use of hand-held heavy machinery.

Examination
The sequence described here is comprehensive but should be considered if a general condition is suspected. Often an examination only needs to be more specifically directed.

Inspection of the nails and fingers

- Pits/ridges are associated with psoriatic arthritis (see Plate 3).
- Splinter hemorrhages may be traumatic but are associated with infective endocarditis or vasculitis.
- Obvious cuticle damage and punctate cuticle erythema (dilated capillary loops) are features of secondary Raynaud's phenomenon, scleroderma, or myositis (see Plates 4, 20, 21).
- Periungual erythema is associated with a number of autoimmune rheumatic and connective tissue diseases.
- Multiple telangiectasias are associated with limited cutaneous scleroderma (see Chapter 13).
- Diffuse finger thickening (dactylitis) may be due to gross tendon thickening (e.g., SpA or sarcoid, see Plate 19), or connective tissue fibrosis/thickening (scleroderma, cheiroarthropathy). Bony or soft-tissue DIP or PIP swelling should be discriminated.
- A shiny/waxy skin appearance, often pale, may indicate scleroderma.
- Scattered, tiny, nonblanching dark red punctate lesions are typical of cutaneous skin vasculitis.
- Erythematous or violaceous scaly papules/plaques over MCPs or PIPs may suggest dermatomyositis.

Note any diffuse swelling of the hand

- Diffuse soft-tissue or skin swelling may occur in association with RA, RS₃PE syndrome, JIA, complex regional pain syndrome (see Plate 5), and scleroderma.
- RS₃PE (remitting seronegative symmetric synovitis with pitting edema), which presents mainly in adults in their 70s, may be a distinct type of nonerosive polyarticular/tendon synovitis but may be associated with other, often hematologic, conditions.
- Swelling associated with complex regional pain syndrome may be localized or diffuse (see Plate 5). Skin may be shiny, and later there is often a dark red or blue mottled appearance.
- Typical skin appearances are critical to making a clinical diagnosis of scleroderma. The skin may be initially puffy but later shiny and tight and, with progression, atrophic with contractures.

Note any muscle wasting

Wasting may be due to a degree of chronic denervation (e.g., the thenar eminence in CTS), disuse atrophy (e.g., painful polyarthropathy, joint hypomobility), or catabolism of muscle (e.g., polymyositis, RA). In the elderly there may be age-related muscle loss ("sarcopenia").

Note any deformity of digits

- Deformities tend to occur with long-standing polyarticular joint disease, e.g., OA, severe RA, and psoriatic arthritis.
- Isolated deformities may be due to previous bone or tendon trauma, severe neurologic lesions and Dupuytren's contracture. A mallet finger (loss of active DIP extension) is due to rupture of the distal extensor tendon expansion usually due to direct trauma.

Inspect the palm and dorsum of the hand
- Palmar erythema is not specific but is associated with autoimmune disorders of connective tissue and joints.
- Check for Dupuytren's contracture (fascial thickening on ulnar side).
- On the dorsum of the hand, ganglia and swelling of the common extensor tendon sheath are usually easily noted. Swelling of the extensor tendon sheath is commonly associated with RA in adults.

Palpation of joints and nodules
Palpation of joints and nodules is best done using thumb pads with the patient's wrist supported.
- Swelling should be noted for site, consistency, tenderness, and mobility. Osteophytes and exostosis are periarticular or at sites of pressure, may be tender, but are always fixed (see Plate 16d).
- Ganglia are hard and usually quite mobile (can occur anywhere).
- Rheumatoid nodules occur anywhere but typically are found on the dorsum of the hand and the extensor surface of the elbow; tophi (usually distal) are rubbery, hard, relatively fixed, but may be moved (see Plate 16a).
- Synovitis is often represented by soft ("boggy"), often springy, swelling around a joint. It may be tender and warm but this is not invariable.
- Synovitis in a single joint may be due to autoimmune rheumatic disease, oa, infection, or foreign-body synovitis (e.g., rose thorn synovitis).

Palpate tendons in the palm or on the volar aspect of the phalanges
- Thickening, tenderness, and crepitus suggest tenosynovitis but tenosynovitis can be hard to spot if it is mild. Tethering and thickening of tendons in the palm associated with excessive digital flexion when the hand is at rest and a block to passive finger extension suggests chronic flexor tenosynovitis (take care to note any contributory joint damage).
- Passive tendon movement by gently flexing/extending a proximal phalanx may disclose palpable tendon nodules, crepitus, and tenderness.

Discriminate Dupuytren's contracture from flexor tendonopathy
Dupuytren's contracture typically involves the fourth and fifth fingers (40% bilateral). It is common in males aged 50 to 70. The fascia extends to the second phalanx, thus, if severe, the condition causes fixed flexion of MCPs and PIPs. It is associated with epilepsy, diabetes, and alcoholism, and usually is not painful.

Diagnostic tests for hand and wrist disorders

Radiographs
- An AP view of the hand and wrist is a useful screening tool to characterize a polyarthropathy and diagnose traumatic or metabolic bone lesions (see Table 2.7).
- Radiographs may reveal soft tissue swelling around joints compatible with a diagnosis of synovitis.

Table 2.7 Some conditions/features that may be diagnosed on simple AP hand/wrist radiographs

Bone conditions	Fractures (e.g., scaphoid, base of first metacarpal)
	Tumors
	Metabolic bone diseases (e.g., rickets, hyperparathyroidism)
	Avascular necrosis (e.g., posttraumatic—lunate, sickle cell disease)
	Sarcoidosis (may also have arthropathy)
Specific features	Cartilage damage (joint space loss and subchondral bone changes)
	Articular erosions
	Osteophytes
	Infection (cortex loss, patchy osteolysis)
	Calcium deposition in joint (e.g., triangular ligament chondrocalcinosis)
	Soft tissue swelling (e.g., over ulnar styloid in wrist synovitis)
	Periarticular osteoporosis (associated with joint inflammation)
	Carpal dislocation (e.g., lunate displacement in chronic carpal pain)
Polyarticular/ overall patterns of radiological abnormality	OA (distribution of osteophytes and subchondral bone changes)
	RA, JIA (e.g., deformities, erosion appearance/distribution)
	Psoriatic arthritis (e.g., deformities, erosion appearance—DIPs)
	CPPD arthritis/gout (e.g., erosion appearance in gout)

- Radiographs are insensitive for identifying erosions in early autoimmune joint disease.
- An oblique view of the hand may add information about joint erosions if an erosive MCP arthritis is considered.
- Lateral and carpal tunnel views of the carpus can be obtained by varying the degree of X-ray projection angle; however, unless searching for evidence of fracture these views are rarely needed.

Further imaging: US, MR, and bone scan
- In experienced hands, US can be a useful way of looking for early synovitis and patterns of abnormality in association with median nerve entrapment.
- MR may demonstrate a torn or avulsed triangular cartilage in patients with a posttraumatic painful wrist or with carpal instability.

- MR images of the carpal tunnel are especially useful in confirming median nerve compression/tethering and soft tissue wrist pathology, particularly when symptoms recur after carpal tunnel release surgery.
- MR can provide valuable information about the degree and distribution of inflammatory disease in joints and tendons, particularly in children and patients with whom history and examination are difficult.
- MR is more sensitive than radiography in identifying joint erosions in RA. Choosing MR over US depends on availability and sonographer experience.
- Bone scan is not specific for any single condition, but in young adults (after closure of epiphyses and before OA is likely) it may be useful for disclosing patterns of inflammation at and around joints. ^{99m}Tc-labeled human immunoglobulin may be more specific for detecting patterns of synovitis in children and adults.

Laboratory tests

- CBC, ESR, CRP. The characteristic, though nonspecific, picture in patients with a systemic inflammatory condition such as RA or polyarticular JIA, is mild anemia with normal red cell indices, high or high-normal platelets, and increased acute phase response. Lymphopenia frequently accompanies autoimmune disease. Neutrophils are raised in infection, with steroids, and in systemic JIA or adult onset Still's disease.
- Blood urea, electrolytes, creatinine, and urate will detect hyperuricemia and renal impairment associated with gout (see Chapter 15). Blood calcium, phosphate, albumin, vitamin D, and alkaline phosphatase (± PTH) will screen for metabolic bone disease.
- Rheumatoid factor (RF) and anti-citrullinated protein antibody (ACPA) tests such as anti-cyclic citrullinated peptide (CCP) may be useful for diagnosing rheumatoid arthritis. Antinuclear antibody (ANA) and a screen of extractable nuclear antibodies (ENAs) may be helpful for the evaluation of a number of disorders, including systemic lupus erythematosus (SLE), Sjogren's, and scleroderma.
- In children with JIA, a positive ANA is associated with an increased risk of uveitis.
- Other investigations to consider: serum angiotensin converting enzyme (sACE) for sarcoidosis, glycosylated hemoglobin in diabetics, serum and urinary protein electrophoresis for myeloma.

Other diagnostic procedures

- Nerve conduction studies are useful to evaluate upper limb neuropathies.
- Joint/bursa fluid aspiration is mandatory in suspected cases of sepsis and should be sent for culture and microscopy. Crystal arthropathy should also be considered.

Treatment of wrist and hand disorders

Treatment for specific diseases is considered in Part 2. Management of the soft tissue lesions in the hand and wrist, like elsewhere, combines periods of rest and splinting with active physical therapy, avoidance of repetitive activity, and analgesia. In most cases, the condition will resolve spontaneously, but severe or persistent pain and disability may warrant input from a hand occupational therapist, local steroid injections, or occasionally surgical soft tissue decompression.

- Conditions that respond to local steroid therapy include:
  - tenosynovitis, e.g., De Quervain's
  - tendon nodules and ganglia
  - flexor tenosynovitis (and trigger finger)
  - Dupuytren's contracture
  - carpal tunnel syndrome
  - synovitis: radiocarpal and radioulnar at the wrist, MCPs and PIPs, first carpometacarpal (CMC).
- The accuracy of needle placement is likely to be improved by US guidance; however, greater efficacy from such an approach over blind injection has not yet been shown.
- See Corticosteroid Injection Therapy and Principles of Rehabilitation at the end of this chapter.
- Functional evaluation (from a physical and occupational therapist) is likely to be of use in cases of polyarthropathy. Early use of splints, orthotics, and exercises may lead to greater functional ability and a decrease in symptoms.
- Surgical options for the hand and wrist may include:
  - fusion or resection of the carpal bones
  - ulna styloidectomy and wrist synovectomy (RA)
  - tendon repair and transfer operations (RA)
  - synovectomy of joints and/or tendons (RA)
  - fusion of small joints
  - PIP/MCP replacements
  - Dupuytren's release/fasciectomy
  - carpal tunnel release
  - trapeziectomy for thumb CMC joint OA

Many of these procedures primarily reduce pain; function may not be restored.

Upper limb peripheral nerve lesions

Background

- Upper limb peripheral nerve lesions are common. Most are entrapment neuropathies. Occasionally, nerve trauma may present to primary care providers or rheumatologists with (primarily) regional muscle weakness.
- Although not specific for its diagnosis, the triad of pain, paresthesias, and weakness is suggestive of nerve entrapment. Features may be considered more specific for nerve entrapment if there is a history of acute or overuse trauma proximal to the distribution of the symptoms.
- Lesions may characteristically occur in association with specific activities, occupations, or sports (e.g., ulnar neuropathy in cyclists).
- Accurate diagnosis relies on demonstration of the anatomic lesion. Useful in this respect is knowledge of likely sites of entrapment or damage and, in the case of entrapment, the ability to elicit a positive Tinel sign (i.e., percussion over the site of entrapment eliciting sensory symptoms in the appropriate nerve distribution).
- Always compare examination findings in both upper limbs.
- Nerve conduction studies are an adjunct to clinical diagnosis. They should not be relied on to make a diagnosis in the absence of good clinical data.
- MR techniques and their interpretation are becoming increasingly more sophisticated in identifying patterns of abnormality in these disorders.

The long thoracic nerve

- Entrapment is in the differential diagnosis of painless shoulder weakness. The nerve origin is at C5–C7, and its course runs beneath the subscapularis and into the serratus anterior.
- Muscle paralysis is often painless and implies loss of the last 30° of overhead arm extension, disrupted scapular rhythm, and scapula winging. Winging is demonstrated by inspection from behind with the patient pressing against a wall with an outstretched arm.
- Damage to the nerve occurs typically from an anterior direct blow or brachial plexus injury. Damage sometimes occurs after carrying heavy backpacks (e.g., army recruits) or after surgical resection of a cervical rib.
- It can also occur spontaneously after infection. There is no specific treatment.

The suprascapular nerve

- The nerve origin is at roots C4–C6; its course is lateral and deep to the trapezius, through the suprascapular notch, terminating in the supraspinatus and posteriorly in the infraspinatus. It carries pain fibers from the glenohumeral joint and AC joint.
- Impingement of the nerve at the suprascapular notch should be considered in a patient complaining of shoulder pain despite a normal examination and imaging tests.
- Injury to the nerve often gives diffuse shoulder pain, although painless paralysis of the muscles can occur.

- Injury is often thought to occur from repeated stretching of the nerve at the notch. Weightlifters are prone to bilateral injury and volleyball players prone to dominant side injury.
- Compression by ganglia or tumors occurs and can be confirmed by MR.

Ulnar nerve

The ulnar nerve originates from C8 and T1. It lies along the medial side of the brachial artery in the upper arm, then above the medial humeral epicondyle where it passes posteriorly, piercing the medial intermuscular septum. It then runs behind the elbow in a groove between the olecranon and medial epicondyle, covered by a fibrous sheath and arcuate ligament (cubital tunnel). Following the line of the ulna in the flexor compartment of the forearm, branches supply the flexor digitorum profundus (FDP) and the flexor carpi ulnaris (FCU). The nerve enters the hand on the ulnar side dividing into superficial (palmaris brevis and skin over the medial one and a half digits) and deep (small muscles of the hand) branches.

- Lesions are usually due to entrapment.
- The ulnar nerve is occasionally damaged in the relatively exposed cubital tunnel (cubital tunnel syndrome) resulting in pain and paresthesias along the medial forearm, wrist, and fourth/fifth digits. Damage may occur from direct trauma, compression, or recurrent subluxation. The Tinel test at the elbow may be positive and there might be sensory loss over the palmar aspect of the fifth digit.
- There are a number of sites where entrapment of the ulnar nerve may occur around the wrist, either proximal to the volar carpal ligament or beneath it or the pisohamate ligament. External compression, acute or recurrent trauma, and ganglia are the usual causes. Symptoms have been noted in cyclists, users of jack hammers or vibrating tools, and in avid videogame players. Entrapment of the purely sensory cutaneous branch can occur from excessive computer mouse use.
- Motor weakness may be most evident by observing general muscle wasting in the hand (hypothenar eminence, interossei, adductor pollicis) and flexion deformity of the fourth and fifth digits—the latter caused by third and fourth lumbrical weakness (see Plate 6).
- Flexion of the wrist with ulnar deviation (FCU) and thumb adduction may be weak (adductor pollicis weakness will be evident if you ask the patient to run the thumb across the base of the fingers as normally it can sweep across smoothly).
- "Froment's sign" also signifies weakness of the adductor pollicis and is demonstrated by a weakness in holding paper between the thumb and the index finger when both are in the sagittal plane.
- Discrimination of a wrist site from an elbow site of nerve entrapment is helped by the site of a positive Tinel test, preservation of power of wrist flexion/medial deviation (FCU) in a wrist lesion, and electrophysiology.
- Rest, analgesia, and occasionally local steroids are helpful. A review of posture, repetitive activity, and a biomechanical assessment with changes in activities and technique are recommended. Surgical decompression may also be necessary.

Radial nerve

The nerve origin is at roots C5–C8, and its course runs anterior to subscapularis, and then passes behind the humerus in a groove that runs between the long and medial heads of triceps. It then winds anteriorly around the humeral shaft to lie between brachialis and brachioradialis. In the flexor compartment of the arm it divides at the level of the lateral epicondyle into superficial branch (cutaneous/sensory) and the posterior interosseous nerve (PIN), which runs through the supinator muscle into the forearm to supply the extensor compartment muscles.

- Entrapment needs to be considered in those cases of shoulder or upper arm trauma where subsequent presentation includes arm and wrist weakness.
- Compression of the radial nerve in the upper arm causes stiffness in the dorsal arm and forearm, weakness of the wrist, and little finger extension. The triceps is usually unaffected as nerve supply to the muscle leaves the radial nerve proximally.
- Transient compression of the nerve at the site of the medial head of triceps has been described in tennis players.
- Compression can occur as the nerve pierces the lateral intermuscular septum just distal to the radial head and also where the PIN pierces the supinator.
- At this lower site, compression is often a consequence of trauma, may be associated with a positive Tinel test and local tenderness, and the pain may be reproduced by extreme passive forearm pronation combined with wrist flexion. Symptoms may mimic those of lateral epicondylitis. Surgical exploration may be necessary to confirm a diagnosis.

Median nerve

The nerve origin is from the C6–T1 nerve roots. Starting at the brachial plexus, it runs together with the brachial artery in the upper arm (supplying nothing), then enters the forearm between the two heads of pronator teres (from the medial humeral epicondyle and coronoid process of the ulna). It runs deep in the forearm, dividing into median and anterior interosseous branches. The median branch enters the hand beneath the flexor retinaculum on the radial side of the wrist. All pronator and flexor muscles in the forearm (except FCU and the medial half of FDP) are supplied by the two branches. The median nerve supplies sensory nerves to the radial side of the hand.

- Entrapment syndrome at the wrist is very common.
- In the rare pronator syndrome, trauma, swelling, or masses between the two pronator heads can cause entrapment, giving lower arm pain, paresthesias, and weakness of forearm pronation. There is local tenderness and reproduction of pain from resisted forearm pronation or wrist flexion.
- Pain in CTS is often present at night and relieved by exercising the hand. Daytime symptoms can persist. Pain can be referred up the arm, even to the shoulder. Sensory symptoms are confined to the radial three and a half digits.

- Clumsiness is a common early feature of CTS.
- Symptoms reproduced by a positive Tinel's sign (percussion over the volar aspect of the wrist, with the wrist hyperextended) and Phalen's maneuver (volar aspect of the wrist rested on the back of a chair and the hand allowed to fall loosely under gravity, held for one minute) indicates nerve compression.
- A severe or chronic lesion is associated with sensory testing abnormality (see Figure 2.10) and motor weakness of the abductor pollicis brevis (APB), opponens pollicis, and the first and second lumbricals.
- Nerve conduction studies are indicated if the diagnosis is uncertain, the condition is progressive, motor neuron disease is suspected (thenar muscle wasting marked/progressive with minimal sensory symptoms), dual pathology is suspected, surgical decompression is being considered, and in cases of surgical failure. False negative results occur in 10% of cases.
- MR appears to be more sensitive than US for detecting abnormalities involving the median nerve in or around the carpal tunnel.
- Etiology of CTS is debated but probably multifactorial. The following are associated: Colles' fracture, trauma, carpal OA, diabetes, inflammatory joint/tendon disease (e.g., RA, scleroderma), ganglia, menopause and pregnancy. Hypothyroidism, acromegaly, amyloid, and benign tumors are also associated with CTS.

Treatment of carpal tunnel syndrome
- Night splinting may be curative, especially early in the condition.
- NSAIDs are helpful if there is underlying inflammatory disease.
- Local steroid injections are of value. If partial remission is achieved, consider repeating the injection (see Plate 15).
- Surgical decompression is indicated when there is failure of conservative therapy, progressive/persistent neurologic changes, or muscle atrophy/weakness.
- Failure of surgical release of the carpal tunnel requires further consideration of underlying causes such as a ganglion or other soft tissue lesion. Reconsider also whether there really is a mechanical/local or perhaps a more subtle cause (e.g., mononeuritis or peripheral neuropathy, entrapment at the pronator or nerve root lesion).

Fig. 2.10 Approximate distribution of dermatomes on the anterior (a) and posterior (b) aspects of the (right) upper limb. Approximate area of sensory change in lesions of the median (c) and ulnar (d) nerves.

Thoracic back and chest pain

Background

- The typical thoracic spine (T1–T12) moves less than the lumbar and cervical vertebrae. Segmental movement in any direction is about 6°. However, given the number of segments, this can add up to appreciable mobility overall. Less segmental movement results in reduced frequency of problems overall (only 6% of patients attending a spinal clinic have thoracic spine problems).
- Ribs (1–10) articulate posteriorly with vertebrae at two points: the articular facet of the rib head with the costovertebral facet on each vertebral body and the articular facet of the rib tubercle with the costotransverse facet on each vertebral lateral process. These are both synovial joints. Ribs 11 and 12 do not have costotransverse joints.
- The ribs, each continuous with its costal cartilage, articulate anteriorly by a synovial joint with the manubrium (1–2), sternum (2–7), each costal cartilage above (8–10), or do not articulate (11/12—floating ribs).
- A massive block of spinal extensor muscles is responsible for maintaining the body against gravity. Some extend over some distance (e.g., the spinalis thoracis from the upper thoracic to the mid-lumbar spinous processes).
- Dermatomes are circumferential and extend from T2 at the clavicles to T10 at the umbilicus. However, up to five nerve roots may contribute innervation of any one point in a truncal dermatome.

Taking a history

The interpretation of cardiac, esophageal, or pleural chest pain as musculoskeletal in origin is a common occurrence. It may result in missing a serious condition (see Tables 2.8 and 2.9).

- A review of the patterns of quality and radiation of cardiac and esophageal pain in the clinical context should always be considered.
- Pleuritic pain is common. Chronic pulmonary emboli may be underdiagnosed, and have serious consequences. Any inflammatory, infective, or infiltrative pleural lesion will be painful.
- Lesions confined to pulmonary parenchyma do not produce pain.
- Pericardial pain can be misinterpreted as musculoskeletal or pleuritic.
- Mediastinal abnormalities can produce pain that is often referred.

The interpretation of neurogenic or musculoskeletal chest pains as cardiogenic, esophageal, or pleural is a common occurrence and may lead to unnecessary investigations. Take a good history (see Table 2.10).

- Thoracic spine lesions can result in referred anterolateral chest pain.
- Costovertebral and costotransverse joint dysfunction is relatively common and is generally age-related but can occur in anyone with spinal deformity. It may produce thoracic spine pain alone or result in an extensive pattern of radiation of pain over the back, lateral, and anterior chest wall.
- Lower cervical spine lesions can refer pain to the anterior chest wall.

Table 2.8 Characteristics of chest pain from non-neurologic and nonmusculoskeletal pathology

Process	Characteristics of pain
Angina	Gradual onset often related to exercise, a heavy meal, or emotion. Squeezing, strangling, or constriction in chest, can be aching or burning in nature. Commonly substernal but radiates to any of anterior chest, interscapular area, arms (mainly left), shoulders, teeth, and abdomen. Reduces with rest and sublingual nitrates
Myocardial infarction	Similar to above regarding quality and distribution. Longer duration. Less easily relieved
Pericardial inflammation	Sharp or steady substernal pain. Can be referred to shoulder tip, anterior chest, upper abdomen, or back. Often has a pleural component and is altered by change in position—sharper more left-sided when supine but eased by leaning forward
Aortic dissection	Acute onset with extremely severe peak. Felt in center of chest or back. Lasts for hours
Pleuritic inflammation	Common. Sharp, knifelike, superficial. Aggravated by deep inspiration, sneezing, or coughing. If accompanied by hemoptysis consider pulmonary embolism
Mediastinal conditions	Empyema or surgical emphysema may be intense and sharp and radiate from substernal to shoulder area. Associated with crepitus. Mediastinitis and tumor pain resembles pleural pain. May have constant feeling of constriction/oppression
Peptic disease	Penetrating duodenal ulcers can cause intense, persistent midthoracic back pain
Esophageal reflux	Persistent retrosternal burning is typical. Often postprandial, when lying or at night/early morning. Esophageal spasm can be similar to angina and can cause midthoracic back pain but reflux symptoms often coexist

- Many painful chest conditions are associated with radiation of the pain down the left arm. This pattern is not specific for myocardial ischemia.
- Lower cervical pain may be referred to the interscapular region.
- Interscapular pain may also be associated with mechanical lumbar disorders. Unlike infection, tumors, and fracture, referred pain is eased or abolished by changes in position or posture.

If there is thoracic back pain alone and it is acute and/or severe, consider osteoporotic fracture, tumors, and infection.

- Osteoporotic vertebral collapse is common in postmenopausal women. An acute, nonminimal-trauma-associated severe pain is typical.

Table 2.9 Painful neurologic and musculoskeletal conditions of the thoracic spine and chest wall

Thoracic vertebral disease	Osteoporotic or pathological fracture
	Tumors, e.g., osteoid osteoma, metastasis
	Osteomyelitis
	Paget's disease
	Osteomalacia, rickets
	Costovertebral joint dysfunction
Nerve irritation	Root irritation/compression from disc prolapse or osteophyte at exit foramen, from structure distal to exit foramen, or from neuroma
Biomechanical/ degenerative	Scoliosis (nonstructural compensatory, structural)
	Diffuse idiopathic skeletal hyperostosis (DISH)
	Calcium pyrophosphate dihydrate disease (of ligamentum flavum)
Herpes-zoster of intercostal nerve	
Chest wall/superficial lesions	Rib fracture
	Other rib lesions, e.g., tumors, fibrous dysplasia, osteomalacia
	Costochondritis/Enthesitis
	Intercostal muscle tear/strain
	Mastitis or fibrocystic disease of the breast
	Myofascial pain and fibromyalgia
	Parietal pleural inflammation/infection/ infiltration
Spondyloarthropathy (e.g., ankylosing spondylitis)	Spinal inflammation
	Acute discitis
	Chronic indolent discitis
Scheuermann's osteochondritis	In adolescents only

Fractures occur in many other situations, e.g., AS or a neoplastic bone lesion.

- Spinal infections should not be missed. The most common are *Staphylococcus aureus*, *Brucella*, and *Mycobacterium tuberculosis* (see Chapter 17).

Ask about the quality of pain

- Musculoskeletal pain (local or referred) generally associates with specific movements, positions, or postures, and it is reproducible.
- Pain that increases with coughing, sneezing, or deep inspiration, is suggestive of pleural lesions. Rib and intercostal lesions or costovertebral joint dysfunction may also cause this sort of pain.

Ask about other symptoms and risk factors

- The pain from a fracture/lesion (osteoporotic, malignancy, infection) is often localized and extreme, waking the patient at night.
- Acute or chronic thoracic spine lesions may be associated with cord compression. Ask about recent change in sphincter function and progressive lower limb stiffness or heaviness.
- Risks for osteoporosis (see Chapter 16).
- Systemic symptoms of fever (osteomyelitis).
- Bone pain elsewhere (metastases, osteomalacia, Paget's disease).
- Spinal pain in adolescence (for an adult with kyphosis/spinal pain).
- A positive family history is recognized in idiopathic juvenile scoliosis, osteoporosis, and generalized osteoarthritis (see Chapter 6).
- Depression and anxiety are important modulators of pain. However, although thoracic back and chest pains may be psychogenic, it is imprudent to settle on this diagnosis without excluding musculoskeletal conditions and diseases of viscera that can cause referred pain.

Examination

Visual inspection

Observe the patient (who has undressed down to his or her underwear) from the back and front. Look for deformity, asymmetry, swellings, and note the respiratory pattern.

- Any scoliosis should be noted. Nonstructural scoliosis is frequently due to posture, severe back or abdominal pain, leg length discrepancy, and, rarely, can be psychogenic. Structural scoliosis may be due to various lesions at any age.
- There is a normal mild thoracic kyphosis; however, marked kyphosis in adults (particularly postmenopausal women) might suggest multiple osteoporotic vertebral fractures or degenerative disc disease. A loss of normal kyphosis (flat spine) may be seen in spondylitis or possibly severe muscle spasm.
- Loose folds of skin on the back might denote multiple vertebral fractures.
- Costochondral swelling occurs in some cases of costochondritis or rickets (referred to as a "rickety rosary" due to the large "beads" that appear below the surface of the skin) in children. Look for synovitis of costosternal or sternoclavicular joints (which is found with spondyloarthropathy).

Palpation

Palpate over the vertebrae, paravertebral joints, and back musculature with the patient prone. Palpate the anterior chest wall.

- Spinal osteomyelitis may be associated with obvious skin swelling and erythema, exquisite focal tenderness, and extensor spasm. Tumors may give similar signs, though skin erythema is not likely.
- Costotransverse joints may be tender (4–5 cm from midline). Discomfort at any costovertebral joint and its referred pain can be elicited by individual rib manipulation (downward pressure on the rib lateral to its vertebral joints when the patient is prone).
- Identify any trigger points that reproduce myofascial pain in back muscles.
- Tender swelling of the sternoclavicular, costomanubrial, or sternocostal joints may suggest spondyloarthropathy or SAPHO (synovitis, acne, pustulosis (palmoplantar), hyperostosis and (aseptic) osteomyelitis).
- Inflammation of costal cartilages is often associated with painful swelling and tenderness. Rib and intercostal lesions should be easily discriminated from referred pain by eliciting local tenderness.

Check thoracic spinal movement

Movements of the thoracic spine should be checked. Ask the patient to sit on the couch with their arms folded in front of them. Guided by movements of the spinous processes, gauge the range of thoracic spine movement.

- Approximate normal ranges of movement in the aforementioned position are extension 30°, lateral flexion 30°, flexion 90°, and rotation 60°.
- Scoliosis is often associated with rotation that is accentuated on flexion.
- Abnormal mobility will not be specific for any underlying condition, but may draw attention to the major affected spinal segment. Painful segments are guarded and may appear hypomobile.
- Spondylitis may become obvious if there is extensive spinal hypomobility.
- Chest expansion should be measured from forced expiration to complete inspiration measuring at expansion, with a tape, at the level of the xiphisternum. Normal young adult chest expansion should measure at least 3 cm.

Other examination

- Given the range of serious conditions causing chest pains, a full medical examination is important and should always be considered.
- Neurologic examination of the legs should be considered in anyone who is at risk of spinal cord compression. Look for increased tone, weakness, and brisk reflexes.
- Breast and axillary lymph node examination should be performed.

Diagnostic procedures

Radiographs

- Lateral view radiographs generally provide more information about thoracic spine lesions than anteroposterior views; however, together, both views can confirm osteoporosis, degenerative disease

(e.g., previous Scheuermann's osteochondritis, ochronosis, DISH), and Paget's disease (see Chapter 16).
- Look for vertebral squaring (in AS) and either marginal or nonmarginal syndesmophytes as in psoriatic spondylitis (See Plate 7) or other SpA (see Chapter 8).
- Discriminate enthesitis from DISH at the corners of vertebrae by the presence of erosions with bone reaction (enthesitis) compared with bone proliferation alone (DISH). Enthesitis, associated with chronic spondylodiscitis, is part of the SpA spectrum of diseases.
- Normal radiographs do not exclude malignancy.
- Bone lesions can be well characterized by CT (e.g., osteoid osteoma).

MR
- MR is important in discriminating tumor from infection.
- Disc lesions, spinal canal, and cord are well visualized with MR.
- Fat suppressed or gadolinium-enhanced MR sequences may be necessary to detect enthesitis or spondylodiscitis associated with SpA.

Bone scan
- A bone scan is a sensitive test for infection and malignancy.
- In suspected cases of (previously undiagnosed) malignancy, it is more sensitive than radiographs, can often confirm the lytic or sclerotic nature of a lesion, and will identify any other skeletal sites of disease.
- It is a useful investigation in patients with malignancy who present with back pain. A lack of additional lesions strongly suggests against a single spinal abnormality being malignancy related.
- Tomography can detect abnormality in the pars interarticularis, facet joint, and disc/vertebral body.
- Bone scan sensitively identifies rib and, in most cases, inflammatory intercostal lesions. If solitary, the differential diagnosis is of a metastasis, primary malignant or benign bone tumor, healed rib fracture, fibrous dysplasia, Paget's bone disease, hyperparathyroidism, or infection.

Other procedures to consider in patients with chest pain
- CXR, then consider pulmonary ventilation/perfusion scan and spiral CT to evaluate for pulmonary embolism.
- CT of the chest in patients with unexplained pleural pain.
- ECG and an exercise stress test for patients with possible cardiac ischemia.
- Transthoracic echocardiography to show thickened pericardium or an effusion associated with pericarditis.
- Upper gastrointestinal endoscopy in suspected cases of peptic ulceration.
- Diagnostic trial of a proton pump inhibitor in cases of reflux esophagitis.

Treatment
For treatment of thoracic and chest-wall lesions, see the following section on Low Back Pain and Disorders in Adults and also Chapter 20.

Low back pain and disorders in adults

Epidemiology

- The lifetime prevalence of back pain is 58%, and the greatest prevalence is between 45 and 64 years of age.
- Low back pain is the fifth most common reason for all physician visits in the United States.
- Two percent of the workforce in the United States is compensated for back injuries every year.
- The financial health care and indirect employment costs of low back pain in the United States are estimated to be more than $24 billion.

Lumbar and sacral spine anatomy

- There are normally five lumbar vertebrae. Anomalies are not uncommon at the lumbosacral junction.
- The transition between the mobile lumbar spine (flexion, extension, and lateral flexion) and fixed sacrum together with high weight-loading combine to make the region highly prone to damage.
- The facet joints are sharply angled, effectively reducing rotation in lumbar segments.
- The sacroiliac joints (synovial) are held firmly by a strong fibrous capsule and tough ligaments. The amount of normal movement (essentially rotation) is normally inversely proportional to age.
- The spinal cord ends at L1/L2. Nerves then run individually, are normally mobile in the spinal canal, and together are termed the cauda equina.
- Each nerve exits its appropriate lateral intervertebral exit foramen, passing initially superior and then laterally to the disc, e.g., L4 from L4/L5 exit foramen. However, in the spinal canal each nerve descends immediately posterior to the more proximal intervertebral disc before it exits. Thus, for example, L4 root symptoms can occur from either lateral herniation of the L4/5 disc or posterior herniation of the L3/L4 disc (or from both).
- Facet joint innervation is from posterior primary rami, each of which supplies the corresponding joint at its level, one higher and one lower.

Basic principles of assessment

- Low back pain can arise from damage or inflammation of the thoracic or lumbar spines or from the posterior pelvis. Pathology in retroperitoneal abdominal and pelvic viscera can result in referred pain to the low back.
- A simple way of categorizing back pain is to consider its cause to be mechanical, inflammatory, neurologic, or referred, or due to bone pathology (see Table 2.10).
- Over 90% of episodes of low back pain in adults are mechanical, self-limiting, and do not require investigation.
- Indicators for further investigation include age > 55 years, stiffness, focal pain, pain that disturbs sleep, nerve root symptoms, and chronic persistent (> 6 weeks) pain.

Table 2.10 Common and/or serious causes of low back pain in adults

Mechanical/ degenerative (very common)	Hypermobility (see Chapter 16)
	Facet joint arthritis
	Disc disease (annular tear, internal disruption, prolapse)
	Scoliosis/kyphosis
	Spinal stenosis
	Sacroiliitis
Inflammatory (uncommon)	AS (Chapter 8)
	Sacroiliitis (e.g., AS, brucellosis)
Infection (rare)	Osteomyelitis (e.g., Staphylococcus aureus, TB, brucellosis) (see Chapter 17)
Bone disease (common)	Osteoporotic fracture (see Chapter 16)
	Paget's disease
	Osteomalacia
Neoplasia (rare)	Secondary metastases
	Multiple myeloma
Other	Sickle cell crisis
	Renal disease (e.g., tumors, infection)
	Gynecologic disease
	Fibromyalgia (see Chapter 18)

- The low back is often a focus for those who may use pain (consciously or unconsciously) as a protective device in the face of domestic, emotional, or occupational stress. These stresses commonly influence the description and impact of pain but rarely act alone in causing pain—there is usually some underlying organic pathology.

Taking a history

Differentiate whether the pain is likely to be primarily mechanical or inflammatory, due to bone pathology or referred

- The site and extent of the pain does not easily discriminate the cause. All disorders may be associated with mechanical deformity and/or muscle spasm that may cause pain in a more diffuse distribution.
- Generally, pain due to mechanical lesions is acute in onset, while patients with pain from inflammatory lesions present after symptoms have been present for some time.
- Inflammatory pain is often associated with morning stiffness that can last for several hours and is eased by movement. Mechanical lesions tend to worsen with use. Many mechanical or degenerative lesions may have an inflammatory component, e.g., internal disc disruption causing discogenic pain.

- Intrinsic bone pathology often causes severe, unremitting, focal pain. Sleep is disturbed. Pain does not ease substantially with movement.
- About 3% of patients presenting with back pain have nonmusculoskeletal causes. A significant proportion of women have pelvic conditions such as ovarian cysts or endometriosis. Pain may be cyclical.
- For those aged over 55 with no previous similar episodes of pain, a search for an underlying neoplastic lesion is required.
- Associated systemic symptoms are common in osteomyelitis and may be present if a malignancy has disseminated.

Ask about pain radiation and symptoms in the legs

- Progressive neurologic leg symptoms suggest a worsening/expanding lesion such as a tumor, infection/vertebral collapse, Paget's disease, or lumbosacral spinal stenosis.
- Pressure on nerves below the spinal cord (i.e., the cauda equina) sufficient to cause a disturbance in perineal sensation and/or bowel/bladder paralysis is a neurosurgical emergency (i.e., cauda equina syndrome).
- Leg pain caused by nerve root irritation/compression is often clearly defined and sharp, often accompanied by numbness or paresthesias. The most commonly involved nerve roots are L4, L5, or S1. Pain generally radiates to below the knee and often, but not always, to the heel and big toe.
- Sciatic nerve entrapment at the level of the piriformis muscle can produce identical radicular symptoms to L5 or S1 nerve root entrapment.
- Neurologic symptoms in the distribution of the femoral nerve (primarily anterior thigh musculature) might suggest a high lumbar nerve root lesion (L1–L3 for example).
- Disc prolapse is the most common cause of nerve root pain, but bony encroachment at the nerve root exit foramen by vertebral end plate or facet joint osteophytes and/or soft tissue thickening or fibrosis can also lead to foraminal stenosis, which can also cause nerve root pain.
- Discs do not need to prolapse to cause pain. Annular tears and internal disruption (i.e., microfractures in vertebral end plates) can cause a pattern of pain, termed discogenic pain, characterized by low back and referred buttock/posterior thigh pain aggravated by movement.
- Generally, all mechanical lesions of the lumbar spine can result in referred pain around the pelvis and anterior thighs. However, pain from lumbar facet joints and probably other segmental structures can be referred to the lower leg.
- Aching in the back and posterior thighs after standing is typical of, but not specific for, spondylolisthesis. There are often added spasms of acute pain, especially if there is segmental instability.
- The symptoms of spinal stenosis are often relieved by sitting bent slightly forward, since the spinal canal dimensions increase in this position.

- Sacroiliitis often causes referred pain to the buttocks and back of thighs. It occurs commonly in spondyloarthropathy (see Chapter 8).
- Sacroiliac pain can occur in multiparous women—the condition may be associated with hypermobility.

Note the description of the pain

- Pain may be severe, whatever the cause; however, note whether the patient's descriptors of it suggest nonorganic influences.
- Sharp, lancinating leg pains suggest nerve root irritation/compression (radicular pain) whereas leg pain referred from other structures within a lumbar segment is generally deep and aching. The distribution may be similar. More persistent, rather than episodic, radicular pain may denote stenosis of the nerve root exit foramen.
- A description of bilateral buttock/leg pain that worsens on walking is consistent with spinal stenosis, especially in those with normal peripheral pulses and no bruits.
- A change in the description of pain in someone who has an established diagnosis may be important, e.g., subacute, severe, unremitting localized pain in a patient with AS who normally has mild inflammatory pain might reflect a superimposed discitis; or, acute severe unremitting sleep-disturbing pain in an elderly woman with known chronic mechanical pain associated with OA might suggest osteoporotic fracture.
- Florid descriptions of the pain and its severity are associated with psychological modulators of pain.

Previous back pain and trauma, occupation, and family history

- Scheuermann's disease (which is associated with irregular vertebral endplates) causes spinal pain in adolescence. It is a risk for spinal degeneration and kyphosis in adults.
- Previous trauma may have caused pars interarticularis fractures (an antecedent of spondylolisthesis), vertebral fracture (risk of further mechanical damage), or ligament rupture (subsequent segmental instability).
- It is generally accepted that the high prevalence of disc disease among manual workers at a relatively young age provides some evidence for a causal relationship.
- It is often the case that patients with chronic pain following (sometimes trivial) trauma may be dissatisfied with the quality of care received at the time of the injury. Be aware that many believe that the way in which spinal pain is handled at its onset significantly influences its subsequent course.
- Sacroiliitis is an early part of brucellar arthritis (20–51% of patients). Poor animal- or carcass-handling hygiene or ingestion of infected foodstuffs or milk can lead to infection. Spondylitis is a late feature and is characterized by erosions, disc infection, and abscesses.
- A positive family history of low back pain might, in context, suggest SpA (sacroiliitis), hypermobility (see Chapter 16), or generalized osteoarthritis (see Chapter 6).

Examination

Inspect the undressed patient from the side and behind

- Note the fluidity of movement when the patient is undressing.
- Check the skin for redness, local swelling, and skin markings. Redness and swelling occasionally accompany osteomyelitis.
- Lipoma, hairy patches, café-au-lait patches, or skin tags often reflect underlying structural nerve or bone abnormality, e.g., spina bifida, diastematomyelia, or neurofibromatosis.
- Skin folds often suggest an underlying significant structural change such as osteoporotic fracture or spondylolisthesis.
- Note any deformity: hyperlordosis (associated with L5/S1 damage and weak abdominal musculature), prominent thoracolumbar kyphosis (multiple disc degeneration or vertebral fractures), scoliosis (degenerative, compensatory muscle spasm for unilateral pain).
- Look from the side. A gentle lordotic curve is normal. Flattening suggests muscle spasm or fusion in SpA. With major spondylolisthesis, a step between spinous processes can sometimes be seen.

Observe active movements while the patient is standing

Lumbar forward flexion ("…with your legs straight, slowly reach down to try and touch your ankles…"), lateral flexion ("…with your legs and back straight, tip sideways and run your hand down your leg toward your knee…") and extension ("…with your legs straight, slowly bend backwards…"). Note: flexion can be mediated by the hip joints; extension can be affected by slight pelvic tilt and body sway. Ask what can be achieved normally and what is painful.

- Abnormal movements are not specific for any condition, although they may help to localize a problem.
- Pain in extension is characteristic of retrospondylolisthesis, facet joint arthritis, or impinging spinous processes. All may be relieved by flexion.
- Failure of the spinous processes to separate in a patient who manages good forward flexion would be consistent with permanent spinal stiffness, e.g., AS, with flexion mediated by the hip joints.
- Forward flexion can be measured using the modified Schöber's test. When erect, mark the skin at the point midway between the posterior superior iliac spines (Venus' dimples) and again 10 cm above and 5 cm below. Measure the increase in distance between the outer marks at full forward flexion—in a young adult this is normally more than 6 cm.
- Ask the patient to stand on one foot then lift onto their toes a few times. Weakness might imply an L5 nerve root entrapment (gastrocnemius/soleus).

Observe the gait pattern

An abnormality of gait may reflect any spinal or lower limb problem:
- An antalgic gait.
- A wide-based gait suggests unsteadiness (due to dizziness, muscular weakness, proprioceptive, or cerebellar deficit etc.).
- Leaning forward/stiff legged—although not specific, in older people this may denote spinal stenosis.

Examiner straightens leg to elicit nerve root pain down leg. Look for difference between R and L leg response

Fig. 2.11 The slump test identifies pain from lumbar disc and nerve root irritation or compression (see text).

- Shuffling, which could suggest Parkinsonism (back pain/stiffness is a recognized early sign).
- Foot drop, which could suggest L5 or S1 nerve root compression.
- Flat feet, hind feet valgus, and genu recurvatum on stance phase, might suggest general hypermobility—associated with various low back lesions.

Check extension and lumbar rotation (patient seated)
With the patient seated on the couch, check lumbar extension and rotation (the pelvis is now fixed).
- Typically, combined rotation and extension can elicit pain from arthritic facet joints. It is a sensitive though not specific test.
- Slumping forward (see Figure 2.11) stretches the dura. Increased lumbar pain may be elicited in cases of disc prolapse but, more importantly, leg pain can be elicited in cases of nerve root entrapment. A more provocative test can be done by gently extending each knee in turn in the slump position. Look for asymmetry.

Examine the sacroiliac joints and hips (patient supine)
With the patient supine, examination of the sacroiliac joints and an examination of the hips should be done to exclude pain arising from these structures.
- Test flexion and the rotational range of each hip by lifting the leg, flexed at the knee, so that the upper leg is vertical. Passive movement should normally be pain free.
- No SI joint stress test is specific. Tests are designed to reproduce pain in cases of SI joint dysfunction or sacroiliitis. Here are two:
  - Press down and out firmly over both anterior superior iliac spines at the same time.

- Lift one leg, flex, and abduct the hip slightly. Exert an axial force into the acetabulum at two or three different angles. This test is considered by many to be more useful, and probably stresses both the joint and many of the sacral ligaments, but is less specific if the hip joint is abnormal.

Straight leg raise (Lasegue's test)

The normal variation in straight leg raise ranges from 60° to more than 90° in adults. Compare sides.

- Discomfort from normal tightening of the posterior thigh or calf muscles must be discriminated from a positive test. A positive test (leg raising restricted to 40° or less by radicular pain) is most specific in patients aged <30 years and for L5 or S1 nerve root lesions.
- A crossed straight leg raise (pain elicited by raising the unaffected leg) is even more specific for nerve root entrapment.
- To identify more subtle cases of nerve root entrapment, apply additional foot dorsiflexion at the maximum possible angle of (pain-free) leg raise.
- Lasegue's test does not always reproduce pain in every patient who has sciatica. It is also often negative in older patients with the condition when it is chiefly due to foraminal stenosis and when central posterior disc prolapse occurs (giving bilateral sciatica but no root compression).

Neurologic examination

- Neurologic examination of the legs is essential in suspected cases of nerve root entrapment, cord compression, spinal stenosis, and cauda equina syndrome.

Examination of the prone patient

Ask the patient to turn to lie prone. Palpate low back and over sacrum.

- Diffuse tenderness may be due to muscle spasm.
- Superficial tenderness over the spinous processes or interspinous interval might suggest interspinous ligament disruption or impinging processes.
- Paravertebral bony tenderness may suggest facet joint arthritis.
- Costovertebral angle (CVA) tenderness could indicate renal pathology.
- Tenderness over the SI joints is not specific for sacroiliitis.
- A positive femoral stretch test reproduces L1–L4 (especially L3) radicular pain in the anterior or medial part of the thigh. Flex the patient's knee to 90° and passively extend the hip.

Other examination

- In suspected cases of spinal stenosis or cauda equina syndrome, it is essential to check for sensory loss in the sacral nerve dermatomes. It is also important to check anal sphincter tone by rectal examination (S5).
- In suspected cases of spinal stenosis, the patient can be asked to walk until limited by pain, then re-examined. If there is any ischemia of the cauda equina or of a nerve root (from foraminal stenosis), nerve root signs may become more obvious.

Table 2.11 Testing muscle strength in the lower limbs (patient supine unless otherwise stated). Weakness may denote nerve root entrapment

Muscle or muscle group	Nerve roots	Test*
Hamstrings (knee flexion)	L5, S1, S2	Ask patient to flex the knee to 45°, hold patient's ankle and ask them to bend the knee further against your hold
Iliopsoas (hip flexion/internal rotation)	L1, L2, L3	Ask patient to lift the leg with a bent knee, hold up the upper leg and resist your push. Try to push the leg down and slightly outwards
Quadriceps femoris (hip flexion, knee extension)	L2, L3, L4	1. Hold the patient's relaxed upper leg above the couch (grasped underneath above the knee). The lower leg should drop loosely. Ask them to straighten the lower leg against your resistance
		2. From patient standing test repetitive squatting for more subtle weakness
Tibialis anterior (ankle dorsiflexion).Tibialis posterior (ankle inversion and dorsiflexion)	L4, L5	1. With the knee straight ask the patient to pull back their foot (show them first) against your pull. Resist dorsiflexion
		2. Standing or walking on heels tests for more subtle weakness. Note: if the hind foot rests in valgus or the patient significantly everts the foot during dorsiflexion, the test may also recruit peroneal muscles (L5, S1)
Extensor hallucis longus	L5, S1	Ask the patient to pull their big toe back against your finger (at the base)
Gastrocnemius and soleus(ankle plantar flexion)	S1, S2	1. Ask the patient to point their toes. Resist the movement by pressing against the ball of the foot
		2. Standing or walking on the toes tests for more subtle weakness

* Compare sides. Score according to scale, for example: 0 = no muscle contraction; 1 = contraction visible; 2 = active movement, gravity eliminated; 3 = active movement against gravity; 4–/4/4+ = active movement against slight/moderate/strong resistance; 5 = normal power.

Table 2.12 A mnemonic: principal combinations of signs used for identifying lumbar nerve root lesions

Nerve root	Paresthesias and sensory change	Muscle weakness	Tendon reflex changes
L2	Upper thigh: anterior, medial + lateral surfaces	Hip flexion and adduction	None
L3	Anterior surface of lower thigh	Hip adduction + knee extension	Knee jerk possibly reduced
L4	Anteromedial surface of lower leg	Knee extension, foot dorsiflexion +inversion	Knee jerk decreased
L5	Anterolateral surface of lower leg + dorsum/medial side of foot/toe 1	Hip extension and abduction. Kneeflexion. Foot/toe 1 dorsiflexion	None
S1	Lateral border + sole of foot. Back of heel + calf	Knee flexion. Plantar flexion andeversion of foot	Ankle jerk decreased

Diagnostic procedures

- There are two important initial steps in investigating low back pain. First deciding whether radiographs will help. Second, although relatively rare in practice, the possibility of infection, malignancy, and cauda equina compression always needs to be considered. Simple radiographic views are insensitive indicators of these conditions and, in most cases, are not specific although most radiologists would agree they are desirable in addition to CT or MR. Laboratory tests are mandatory in all suspected cases of inflammation, infection, and malignancy.

Radiographs—decision-making in requesting them (see Table 2.13)
- Lumbar spine radiographs are not always helpful. Remember that nine out of ten cases of back pain in the primary care setting are mechanical and self-limiting. Features on a plain radiograph of the lumbar spine correlate poorly with the presence or pattern of pain.
- Spondylosis is common, age related, and often not symptomatic.
- Children, athletes, and young adults with back pain need prompt radiographic investigation. Failure to detect and treat a pars interarticularis fracture may lead on to a spondylolysis. Abnormalities are more readily appreciated in these age groups as the frequency of age-related degenerative changes in the spine is low.
- Obtaining radiographs to help in the management of patients is a different issue than obtaining them to aid diagnosis and one that requires careful thought, e.g., is the patient likely to perceive that they have received suboptimal care if a radiograph is not requested?

- Spondylolysis may be seen on a lateral view but is more easily seen on oblique views. Oblique views will also show pedicle stress fractures in athletes.
- Spondylolisthesis may be identified and graded by a lateral film. Flexion and extension views may be helpful in delineating subtle cases and instability (spondylolytic).
- General osteopenia is a risk factor for low bone mass; however, it is not a sensitive indicator of low bone mass.
- Look for vertebral squaring (in AS), non-marginal syndesmophytes (in other SpA, such as psoriatic), or flowing syndesmophytes (in DISH).
- Consider obtaining an AP view of the pelvis. Established (but not early) sacroiliitis can be ruled-out. A further "coned" view is often helpful.
- Sacroiliitis (periarticular osteoporosis, erosion, sclerosis of bone, widening joint space) occurs in all types of SpA. It can be unilateral.
- Sclerosis of the SI joint on the lower iliac side alone suggests osteitis condensans ilii, which may be associated with back pain in multiparous women. Joint space is normal and joint margin well defined.
- Patterns of metabolic bone disease, Paget's disease and hip pathology are usually readily identifiable on a pelvic film.

Bone scan
- A bone scan is an extremely sensitive test for infection or malignancy. It is a useful investigation in patients with previously diagnosed malignancy who present with back pain, especially in those who have had no previous skeletal metastases. A lack of additional lesions strongly suggests against a single spinal abnormality being malignancy related.
- It is not specific for the various degenerative lesions but can help localize the site of a lesion.
- Bone scan SI joint appearances in sacroiliitis can be unreliable.

CT or MR?
The choice of imaging depends largely on likely clinical and radiographic differential diagnosis:
- For spondylolytic spondylolisthesis, CT shows the exact site of pars' defects. The usual appearance is of sclerotic irregular edges.
- Nerve impingement can be shown by CT or MR.
- Intervertebral disc prolapse, both posterior and posterolateral, can be shown by either technique. Prolapse material is of similar CT density and MR signal to the disc and well defined against epidural fat.
- Changes in the normal disc signal pattern are associated with age-related disc degeneration. Discogenic pain has been associated with MRI abnormalities classified according to Modic.
- On $T2$-weighted MR, disc material is usually of higher signal than "scar" (e.g., fibrosis from a previous lesion), in which signal decreases with aging. Recent scarring enhances immediately but old scarring does so only slowly. This discrimination requires gadolinium-enhanced MR.
- CT or MR shows early sacroiliitis in AS when X-rays are normal.
- The shape and outline of the spinal canal are ideally shown on CT but are also seen with MR. It is difficult to distinguish fibrous structures

Table 2.13 Commonly reported patterns of radiographic abnormality in adults, the interpretation, and suggested reaction

Radiographic abnormalities	Lesion suggested	Sensible further action
Lumbosacral anomalies	Risk for future back pain	May not be clinically significant. Risk for low back pain (esp. if hypermobile)
Generalized osteopenia	Osteoporosis	Measurement of bone density. Rule out secondary causes, e.g., myeloma
Narrowed disc space, marginal vertebral end-plate osteophytes or both	Intervertebral disc disruption	MR if persistent symptoms or signs of same level nerve root entrapment, spinal or nerve root exit foramen stenosis
Localized lucent or sclerotic lesion, loss of cortex	Tumor, infection, or fracture	Discuss case with radiologist. MR or CT may be advised. A bone scan may be helpful. Initiate appropriate laboratory tests immediately
Facet joint OA	Facet joint syndrome	Consider whether there is associated spinal/nerve root exit foramen stenosis (?radicular symptoms) or symptoms suggestive of spondylolisthesis. CT or MR is then likely to be appropriate
Pars interarticularis defect	Spondylolysis/ ?spondylolytic	Probable prior fracture. Further oblique film centered on suspected level or CT should confirm. Association with symptoms or signs of disc disease or spondylolisthesis suggests an unstable segment. Flexion and extension lateral view radiographs may show instability. MR helpful for imaging soft-tissues including nerves
Short lumbar pedicles	Spinal stenosis	Consider MR if symptoms suggest spinal stenosis
Mixed patchy sclerosis and lucency in entire (enlarged) vertebra(e)	Paget's disease	Neurologic leg symptoms suggest spinal/exit foramen stenosis or vascular '''steal'''

from sclerotic or cortical bone on MR, but it discerns intrathecal contents more readily, which is an advantage in identifying intradural tumors.

- Spondylodiscitis (part of SpA), if chronic, may be difficult to discriminate from degenerative disc/vertebral end-plate disease. Fat-suppressed or gadolinium-enhanced sequences may show high signal at the anterior disc vertebral end-plate junctions.

Screening for infection, malignancy, or metabolic bone disease
- In cases where the history and examination suggest a mechanical condition, but where the clinician wishes to be more confident of excluding an inflammatory condition, an ESR and CRP are suggested.
- An elevated ESR/CRP might indicate a need for further laboratory investigation.
- An infection screen should include a CBC (with differential), ESR, CRP, and blood and urine cultures. If spinal tuberculosis (Pott's disease) is suspected, imaging studies and appropriate microbiological testing should be performed, although radiographic changes occur late in the course of disease. Traditionally, three, early morning urine samples are sent for culture, but the diagnostic yield is quite low.
- Serum and urine protein electrophoresis (with immunofixation) are essential tests in the work-up for myeloma. CMP is also important since hypercalcemia and acute renal impairment have prognostic significance in this condition.
- Routine blood tests may point to an underlying metabolic bone disorder such as Paget's disease or osteomalacia. These tests are normal in postmenopausal osteoporosis.
- If osteoporosis is diagnosed (see Chapter 16) a screen for secondary causes should include ESR (and if raised, serum and urine protein electrophoresis), calcium, phosphate, and sex hormones, and also serum 25-hydroxyvitamin D, iPTH, TFTs, LFTs, and Cr.

Treatment (also see Chapter 20 for greater detail)
- An important therapeutic intervention in the case of acute pain is to take the patient seriously, take a positive view, and in the absence of bad prognostic signs (e.g., nerve root pain), urge early mobility.
- Analgesics and muscle relaxants can be used in the short term, initially regularly, then as required.
- Physical therapy with graded-activity programs may be of value, certainly early in disc disease or spondylosis.
- Cord compression due to bone collapse from a tumor is an acute emergency and should be discussed immediately with an oncologist or radiation oncologist, and a spine-orthopedic or neurosurgeon.
- Cases with disc prolapse failing to respond to conservative therapy, or cases where there is ongoing or rapidly progressive neurologic deficit, should be referred for surgery.
- Available surgical techniques for acute or persistent disc disease include decompression procedures (e.g., nerve root decompression and partial facetectomy), prosthetic intervertebral disc replacement, intradiscal thermocoagulation, and intradiscal steroid injections,

although evidence for long-term efficacy is lacking for all these procedures.
- Surgery for spinal stenosis is useful for relieving leg neurogenic features but not indicated if there is no significant neurologic compromise. Surgery is not usually done if the only effect of spinal stenosis is back pain.
- In chronic back pain, aerobic exercises combined with behavioral methods may be more effective than exercise alone and can help motivate the patient. Methods may also incorporate psychological and social assessment and management.
- The common treatments available for chronic back pain include:
  - analgesics and muscle relaxants
  - antiepileptics/antidepressants for neuropathic pain
  - local anesthetic/steroid injections
  - acupuncture
  - transcutaneous electrical nerve stimulation (TENS)
  - physical therapy
  - ergonomic advice
  - multidisciplinary programs:
    - counseling
    - cognitive therapy
    - education
    - relaxation
    - corsets and belts.
- Timely surgery for structural scoliosis (more common in JIA than the general population) can lessen spinal curvature.

Spinal disorders in children and adolescents

(See also Chapter 20.)

Background

- Common conditions in adults such as degenerative back pain and intervertebral disc disease are rare in childhood or adolescence.
- In hospital series, up to 85% of referred children have identifiable causes (see Table 2.14) although spinal hypermobility in the context of generalized hypermobility and fibromyalgia has not been adequately addressed.
- Not all presentations are with pain. Some children present with either deformity or neurologic symptoms.
- A diagnosis must be firmly established (or at least rigorously sought) because serious disease can present with few symptoms.

Taking a history

Keep an open mind about whether a history from the child, parents, or primary caregiver provides the most useful information. There are merits in consulting all of them, although this process may be time-consuming.

Table 2.14 Cause of childhood back pain. Experience of an orthopedic clinic (a review of 233 referrals)

Cause of back pain	Frequency (%)
Nonspecific (i.e., no cause found)	32
Scoliosis	21
Spondylolysis/Spondylolisthesis (nontrauma)	11
Scheuermann's disease	7
Infection	6
Tumors, e.g., osteoid osteoma	4
Psychogenic	4
Disc prolapse	3
Inflammatory, e.g., spondyloarthropathy	3
Trauma (excluding strains)	2
Limb length inequality/biomechanical	2
Renal pain	<1
Rickets	<1
Congenital anomalies	<1

Severity, distribution, and quality of pain

- Pain may be mild even in the presence of a serious underlying disorder.
- If the pain occurs (or initially occurred) during sports, consider pars interarticularis fractures, spondylolytic spondylolisthesis or Scheuermann's disease (vertebral epiphyseal osteochondritis).
- Persistent pain, unrelieved by rest and disturbing sleep, requires consideration of a bone, bone and/or disc infection, or osteoporotic fracture (steroid-related or juvenile idiopathic osteoporosis (JIO)).
- JIO is rare, occurs between 6 and 13 years of age and is more common in boys. The main differential diagnosis is osteogenesis imperfecta (see Chapter 16).
- Although uncommon, neurologic symptoms such as burning pain, paresthesias, and weakness in the legs suggests nerve root irritation.
- Spinal stiffness in a child (typically between 2 and 6 years of age) associated with irritability and a diffusely tender back may be due to infectious discitis (though organisms are only found in 50%). In an older child or adolescent (typically 10–15 years of age) and with a less striking history, immobility-related stiffness could represent juvenile enthesitis related arthritis (ERA).

If pain is absent …

Spinal conditions are not always associated with pain. Occasionally a child may present with back deformity or neurologic symptoms in the legs alone.

- The history may be nonspecific and, for example in a very young child, nothing more than a refusal to walk.
- Scheuermann's disease commonly presents in teenagers with a painless thoracic kyphosis. Pain is more likely to be present if the chondritis is thoracolumbar rather than thoracic. The condition is often asymptomatic.
- Spinal dysraphism (bony abnormality—usually spina bifida, associated with neural anomaly—invariably cord tethering) and spinal cord tumors can often present with neurologic leg symptoms/signs alone without back pain. Symptoms may be mild initially.
- Scoliosis is usually pain free. Pain with scoliosis usually indicates significant underlying pathology. The differential is wide (see Table 2.15).
- The most frequent single cause of a scoliosis in schoolchildren (40%), found from radiographic screening, is pelvic tilt due to leg length inequality.

Past developmental, medical, family, and social history

- Ask about milestones in musculoskeletal development. Abnormality or delay might suggest spinal dysraphism or neuromuscular conditions.
- Osteoporosis may be evident from previous fragility fracture— axial or appendicular—or may be intimated from risk factors, e.g., steroid use.
- Previous low back trauma may have been pars interarticularis fractures preceding (the current) vertebral slip or disc prolapse.
- Irradiation (e.g., of previous Wilms') is a cause of scoliosis.

Table 2.15 Causes of scoliosis in children and adolescents

Structural scolioses (vertebral rotation, vertebral structural change, and loss of normal spinal flexibility)	Idiopathic: infantile (0–3 years); juvenile (3–10 years); adolescent (> 10 years)
	Neuromuscular
	Congenital: failure of vertebral formation, segmentation, or both
	Neurofibromatosis
	Heritable disorders of connective tissue, e.g., osteogenesis imperfecta
	Trauma: fracture; surgical (e.g., post-laminectomy); irradiation
	Spondyloepiphyseal dysplasia
	Metabolic bone disease
	Lumbosacral anomalies (e.g., spondylolytic spondylolisthesis)
	Cervicothoracic anomalies (e.g., cervical fusion (Klippel–Feil))
	Rheumatoid arthritis
	Extraspinal contractures (e.g., postempyema, postburns)
Nonstructural scolioses (lateral spinal curvature but no vertebral rotation)*	Postural
	Nerve root irritation associated
	Abdominal pain associated (e.g., appendicitis, renal pain)
	Associated with local inflammation Spinal infection
	Spinal tumors
	Secondary to leg length discrepancy
	Related to soft-tissue contractures around the hip
	Psychogenic

* It is characteristic of nonstructural scolioses that if the underlying cause is successfully dealt with, the scoliosis resolves.

- Ask about previous TB or risk factors for TB in patients you think are at risk of TB osteomyelitis.
- Torticollis may be associated with chronic squint, previous trauma (which may be associated with a psychogenic component), and neuroleptic drugs. It can be a sign of an underlying neurologic or inflammatory lesion or occurs because of an underlying structural anomaly.

- A history of a heritable disease of connective tissue can often be elicited from the family of a child with structural scoliosis.
- A history of back pain is sometimes elicited from families of children with nonspecific back pain. Joint dislocation and multiple soft-tissue musculoskeletal injury (especially overuse) in family members raises the possibility of general hypermobility—either joint hypermobility syndrome or a heritable connective tissue disease, e.g., Marfan syndrome (see Chapter 16).
- The existence, or child's perception, of social disharmony at home or school is likely to be more important in influencing the impact of back pain rather than a cause of it. Nevertheless, in children with nonspecific spinal pain or fibromyalgia, social conflict resulting in stress and anxiety may be very important in generating symptoms.

Examination

It is best, and certainly ultimately more informative, to undertake the examination only when the child is comfortable with the situation, with their modesty and dignity preserved, and with consent to go ahead after a reassurance that the examination will be stopped if it is painful. With younger children there may be "an examinable moment", usually after the child has gained confidence in the surroundings and with the situation. Observing a young child while playing is a considerate way of starting the examination.

Age-related variations in biomechanical development and gait patterns
- Walking while holding a hand or furniture develops by 12 months and normally independent walking by 18 months.
- Until 3 years the stance is broad-based in relation to pelvic width, the knee may not fully extend, and the ankle may be plantar flexed at foot-strike.
- Climbing stairs is usually done using alternate feet by age of 3 years.
- Tiptoe walking is not abnormal at first but should disappear by 2 years. If this pattern remains, consider spasticity, tethered cord, or muscle weakness.
- Flat feet up to age 5 are normal (a consequence of the distribution of fat and paucity of muscle development). Only investigate if symptomatic.
- Leg alignment often concerns parents. Up until 2 years of age it is normal to have genu varum. From 2 to 5 years, mild genu valgum may occur. Angles of >10° or asymmetry may be associated with underlying disease.
- Regression of motor development is a clue to the presence of disease.

Observation
Observe children unclothed to underwear if possible. Look for weakness, scoliosis, kyphosis, and swellings.
- The main cause of spinal asymmetry will be scoliosis (see Table 2.15).
- Localized soft tissue swelling may denote soft tissue extension of a spinal though an apparent kyphosis associated with scoliosis is usually a result of spinal rotation.

- In children with neck pain, look for a short neck (rule out Klippel-Feil) or asymmetric scapulae (Sprengel's deformity: a congential abnormality associated with a higher, hypoplastic scapula).
- Adolescent kyphosis may be due to Scheuermann's disease or fractures. Unless there has been steroid use, the former is more likely.
- Note any skin markings such as café-au-lait spots, skin indents (lumbar area) and lumbosacral hair. They may be markers of bony abnormality.
- Note any muscular weakness. With truncal weakness (e.g., DM, (see Chapter 13)) the child may have to roll over before getting up from a supine position. Hip girdle weakness may be present in a child unwilling to squat and unable to stand from squatting without exhibiting Gower's sign (unable to stand up from the floor without using hands to push off).

Examine the gait pattern

- Look for asymmetry and a limp.
- Back or leg pain from any cause can give rise to a limp. Also, limp may be the only feature of a serious underlying neurologic or bony deformity.
- Asymmetry of shoulder height, transverse posterior skin folds, pelvic tilt, and arm swing may be a clue to spinal pathology.

Spinal examination with the child standing

Examine the whole spine while the child is standing. The immature spine is usually far more flexible than an adult's.

- Ask about the presence and site of neck or low back pain during forward flexion, extension, and lateral flexion (and rotation for neck). Experienced examiners should be able to detect significantly limited movements.
- Palpate along the line of (lumbar) spinous processes. An inward step may be caused by spondylolisthesis.
- Palpate any swellings. Lipomas are painless. Soft tissue tumors may be, but are not necessarily, tender and fixed.

Examine the sitting patient

Examine the child who is sitting on the couch, legs hanging over the side.

- This is the best way to elicit pain from posterior vertebral structure pathology in thoracic or lumbar segments (e.g., pars osteoid osteoma, pars fracture). Combine extension and rotation movements. Ask if the pain is worse on one side than the other.

Examine the supine patient

Examine the child or adolescent when supine. Look for leg length discrepancy, lower leg asymmetry, and do a neurologic examination.

- Measure and determine actual or apparent leg length discrepancy. True leg length discrepancy is a cause of nonstructural scoliosis. Apparent leg length discrepancy/pelvic tilts can occur to compensate for scoliosis caused by spinal lesions.
- Different foot or leg sizes/appearances are a nonspecific sign of spinal dysraphism.
- Hip and sacroiliac examination should be done routinely in children with low back pain. Tests for dural irritation and neurologic

examination are essential (see section Low Back Pain and Disorders in Adults).

- Though limb pain, weakness and other neurologic symptoms occur, the majority of children with intradural tumors have none of these features. A normal examination does not rule out serious pathology.

Examine the prone patient

- Palpate over the spinous processes, interspinous spaces, paracentrally between spinous processes (over facet joints) and in the sacroiliac area.
- Diffuse tenderness may only be a reflection of muscle spasm and its extensive mechanical effect. Where there are isolated areas of tenderness, feel for skin warmth, as this may be a site of infection.

Diagnostic procedures

Radiographs

- Radiographs have a characteristic appearance in certain cases of bone tumor but may also, in some cases, be normal (see Table 2.16).
- A normal bone scan rules out most serious pathology.
- A widened interpedicular distance on an AP film is a sign of meningomyelocele, spinal dysraphism, or an intraspinal mass.
- Posterior vertebral scalloping on a lateral radiograph is seen in lumbar or cervical spines, and is most commonly associated with lesions occurring in childhood and most commonly due to spinal tumors, neurofibromatosis, osteogenesis imperfecta, Ehlers–Danlos, and Marfan syndrome.
- Spondylolysis/pars fractures may be visible on lateral X-rays but are best characterized by oblique films (see Plate 8). Associated internal disc derangement or radiculopathy is best characterized using MR.
- Appearances of Scheuermann's disease (juvenile kyphosis, associated with multiple irregular vertebral endplates, with anterior ring epiphyseal fragmentation and vertebral wedging) are an occasional incidental X-ray finding.
- Radiographs of the neck may show a degree of cervical spine fusion (Klippel–Feil syndrome). Suspect hypermobility in nonaffected segments and investigate C1/C2 with MR if there are high cervical pain or myelopathic symptoms.
- Bone scan can detect spinal bony abnormalities; a negative test rules out most subtle lesions e.g., osteoid osteomas.
- Consider SI joint radiographs and MR in patients with prominent immobility-related low back pain and stiffness (commonly due to spondyloarthropathy-related conditions).

Diagnosing scoliosis

- The cause of painful scoliosis must be determined. Consider MR or CT of any localized area of pain. Idiopathic scoliosis is asymptomatic and is a diagnosis of exclusion.
- Mild idiopathic scoliosis (5–10°) can be determined on a posteroanterior thoracolumbar radiograph and is relatively common in the school population (7%). A scoliosis of >20° occurs in 1 in 500 people and is three to four times more common in girls than boys.
- In 10–20% of those with a trunk inclination of >5°, the scoliosis progresses at least a further 5°. Most have a nonprogressive scoliosis.

Table 2.16 Radiographic features of spinal tumors in children (see also Table 20.7)

Tumor type	Notable clinical features and radiological appearances
Osteochondroma	Has the appearance of an exostosis
Osteoid osteoma	Radiographs often normal. Bone scan will localize lesion and CT sharply define it
Osteoblastoma	Lytic with central ossification on radiograph. Can metastasize
Aneurysmal bone cyst	Lucent lesion with central trabeculae on radiographs. MR important to document soft-tissue expansion
Langerhans cell histiocytosis (eosinophilic granuloma)	Either solitary, polyostotic, or associated with systemic illness. Lytic lesion can cause solitary vertebral collapse, even collapse of adjacent bones. Used to be called histiocytosis X
Myeloma	Rare in children. Lytic lesions on radiographs. Distribution of lesions can be shown with bone scan but use as adjunct to radiographs
Ewing's sarcoma	Age 5–20 usually. "Moth-eaten" destruction of bone on radiograph
Lymphoma	Sclerotic ("ivory") vertebra on film
Osteosarcoma	Mixed lytic/sclerotic appearance on radiographs
Metastases	Most likely are from leukemia or neuroblastoma
Intra- and extramedullary tumors	Delay in diagnosis common. Up to 50% have abnormal films: widened spinal canal, pedicle erosions, scalloping of vertebral bodies. MR usually characterizes the lesion

Laboratory tests

Laboratory tests should be sought if infection, inflammation, or malignancy is considered (see section Low Back Pain and Disorders in Adults).

The management of various spinal disorders in adults and children is included in Chapter 20.

Pelvic, groin, and thigh pain

Anatomy

Anatomy of the pelvis and hip region

- The bony pelvis consists of two innominate bones (ilium above the acetabulum and ischium below it) that articulate with each other at the anterior symphysis pubis and posteriorly with the sacrum at the SI joints.
- SI joints are initially synovial but become fibrous with age. A few degrees of rotation can be demonstrated in children and young adults.
- Strong ligaments stabilize the posterior pelvis through sacroinnominate, lumbo(L5)–sacral, and lumbo(L5)–iliac attachments.
- The symphysis pubis is a cartilaginous joint and normally does not move.
- When standing, weight is transferred through the head of the femur. The femoral head is stabilized in the acetabulum by the acetabular labrum and strong pericapsular ligaments.
- The ligamentum teres crosses the hip joint and carries blood vessels to the head of the femur in children and young adults. In old age, blood supply is largely via vessels that enter the femoral neck.
- Two bursae are found at the insertion of the gluteus maximus: one separates it from the greater trochanter, the other separates it from the vastus lateralis.
- The ischial bursa separates gluteus maximus from the ischial tuberosity and can become inflamed from overuse.

Anatomy of pelvic musculature

- Three groups of muscles move the hip joint: the gluteals, the flexor muscles, and the adductor group.
- The major gluteal group muscles are:
  - gluteus maximus (L5, S1/2): arises mainly from ilium and sacrum, projects down posterolaterally and inserts into the posterior femur and the lateral tensor fasciae latae. It extends and externally rotates the hip (the hamstrings also extend the hip).
  - gluteus medius (L4/5, S1): lies deeper and more lateral. It inserts into the lateral greater trochanter and abducts and internally rotates the hip.
  - piriformis, obturator internus, and quadratus femoris arise deep in the pelvis and insert into the posterior greater trochanter. All externally rotate the hip.
- The major hip flexor, the psoas major (L2/3), is a massive muscle that arises from the lateral part of the vertebrae and intervertebral discs (T12–L5) and lateral processes of the lumbar vertebrae. It runs anteriorly over the iliac rim, across the pelvis, under the inguinal ligament, and inserts into the lesser trochanter. The iliacus (L2–L4) arises from the "inside" of the iliac blade, passes under the inguinal ligament medially to the lesser trochanter. Both flex, but the psoas also internally rotates the hip.

- The psoas is enveloped in a fascial sheath. Retroperitoneal or spinal infections that track along soft tissue planes sometimes involves the psoas sheath and can cause inflammation in the psoas bursa, which separates the muscle from the hip joint.
- All adductor muscles arise from the pubis or ischiopubic rami. The adductor longus and gracilis are the most superficial; they arise from the pubis and insert into the femoral shaft and pes anserinus ("goose's foot") below the knee, respectively. The adductor magnus (L4/5) is the largest of the deeper adductors; it inserts into the medial femoral shaft.
- Adductors stabilize movement around the hip toward the end of the stance phase of the gait. Body weight is transferred onto one leg during this action; therefore, adductors need to be strong, especially for running.

Functional anatomy of the hip

- With a flexed knee the limit of hip flexion is about 135°.
- Hip extension (at 30°), internal rotation (at 30–35°), and external rotation (at 45–55°) is limited by strong, pericapsular ligaments.
- Abduction is limited to 45–50° by contact between the greater trochanter and acetabular labrum rim. Adduction is limited to 20–30° with a fixed pelvis (see Plate 9). These are adult ranges.
- Greater femoral neck anteversion (angle of the neck compared to the distal femur) allows greater internal rotation of the hip (and reduced external rotation). Tibial torsion can compensate but this and hip anteversion results in a toe-in gait. Femoral neck retroversion (if the angle is posterior to the femoral intercondylar plane) allows greater external rotation of the hip, usually resulting in a toe-out gait (see Figure. 2.22).
- Normally, infants have more anteversion than older children or adults (30–40° at age 2 compared with 8–15° at age >18).

Neuroanatomy

- The femoral nerve is formed from L2–L4 nerve roots and supplies mainly muscles of the quadriceps group and some deeper hip adductors.
- With contributions from L4–S3 roots, nerves from the plexus converge at the inferior border of the piriformis to form the sciatic nerve. This is at a foramen formed by the ilium (above and lateral), sacrum (medial), sacrospinous ligament (below), and the sacrotuberous ligament (posteromedial).
- In about 10% of people, the sciatic nerve divides before exiting the pelvis. In some, a branch exits above the piriformis muscle. Piriformis syndrome is entrapment of the sciatic nerve by the piriformis muscle, and may benefit from physical therapy.

Taking a history

Age

Age is a risk factor for some conditions:

- Congenital hip dislocation is common (prevalence 1:500), more so in girls than boys (8:1). It should be considered in toddlers if there is delay in motor milestones or pain on weight bearing.
- The most common cause of hip pain in children aged 2–12 years is transient synovitis (which is unilateral and self-limiting). The differential diagnosis includes Legg–Calvé–Perthes disease (osteonecrosis of the femoral head) and Lyme or poststreptococcal arthritis.
- Legg–Calvé–Perthes disease (age 3–12 years) is four to five times more common in boys, and bilateral in 10–20% of cases.
- Slipped capital epiphysis is rare in children younger than 8 or older than 16 years old. It is associated with obesity and endocrine disorders (4% are hypothyroid).
- Unless there has been previous hip disease (e.g., osteonecrosis, synovitis), trauma, or a long-standing biomechanical abnormality (e.g., epiphyseal dysplasia, heritable disease of connective tissue), hip osteoarthritis (OA) is uncommon in adults less than 55 years old
- Paget's disease of bone is rare in adults over 50 years old.

Distribution and type of bone and soft tissue pain

- All mechanical lesions of the lumbar spine can result in referred pain around the pelvis and thighs. It is often bilateral, localizes poorly, and is aching in nature.
- Lateral pelvic pain is often referred from the lumbosacral spine. If pain localizes (i.e., the patient points) to the greater trochanter, it may be due to trochanteric bursitis, enthesitis, or meralgia paresthetica (lateral femoral cutaneous nerve syndrome, see Table 2.17).
- Hip joint pain is felt in the groin, but it can be located deep in the buttock when ischial bursitis and sacroiliac pain should also be considered. It may be referred distally to the anteromedial thigh and knee.
- Groin pain on weight-bearing suggests hip pathology such as synovitis, osteonecrosis or OA, but it is not specific. Tendonitis of the adductor longus, osteitis pubis, a femoral neck stress fracture (4% of all stress fractures), osteoid osteoma, or psoas bursitis can give similar symptoms.
- Bone pathology typically gives unremitting pain. Sleep is often disturbed.
- Pain from deep musculoskeletal pelvic structures is typically poorly localized, although can be severe. If the pain appears to be "catastrophic," consider pelvic bone disease (tumors, infection, Paget's disease, osteomalacia, osteoporotic fracture) (see Chapters 16 and 17), or an unstable pelvis (chronic osteitis pubis with diastasis/laxity of the symphysis pubis and sacroiliac joints).
- Enthesitis and osteitis pubis associated with spondyloarthropathy (SpA) (see Chapter 8) are probably under-recognized.
- Aching in the back of the legs after standing is found with spondylolisthesis (i.e., anterior displacement of a vertebra).

Table 2.17 Patterns of pain around the proximal leg and their major causes

Pattern of pain	Causes
Pain in buttock and posterior thighs	Referred pain from: lumbar spine e.g., facet, OA, spondylolisthesis; SI joint inflammation; lower lumbar nerve root irritation; sciatic nerve entrapment (piriformis syndrome)
	Localized pain: ischial bursitis/enthesitis or fracture; coccydynia
	Diffuse muscular pain/stiffness: myositis or PMR
	Paget's or other bone lesion of sacrum
Lateral pelvic pain	Referred from lumbosacral spine
	Trochanteric bursitis/enthesitis
	Gluteus medius tear
	Lateral hip joint pain, e.g., osteophyte
Groin pain	Hip disease, e.g., OA, osteonecrosis, synovitis
	Psoas bursitis
	Adductor tendonitis, osteitis pubis
	Pelvic enthesitis
	Paget's disease (pelvis or femur)
	Femoral neck or pubic ramus fracture
	Hernia
Anterior or medial pain	Referred from: lumbar spine, e.g., facet OA, thigh spondylolisthesis; upper lumbar nerve root; hip joint, femoral neck, psoas bursa
	Myositis, PMR, diabetic amyotrophy
	Meralgia paresthetica (anterolateral)
	Adductor tendonitis, osteitis pubis
	Ischemia (claudication)
	Lymph nodes

- Sacroiliac pain and stiffness radiates to the buttocks and posterior thighs.

Pain in a muscular distribution
- Diffuse pain in the buttocks and thighs occurs in polymyalgia rheumatica (PMR). It is often sudden or subacute in onset, associated with stiffness, and may give similar symptoms to those caused by sacroiliitis but invariably occurs for the first time in a much older age group.

- Pain is not characteristic of an autoimmune myositis (see Chapter 14). When it does occur, it is unlikely to be confined to pelvic musculature or to be unilateral, but should be considered where acute or subacute onset diffuse pelvic girdle/thigh pain accompanies weakness.

Quality and distribution of nerve pain

- Nerve root pain is often clearly defined and sharp. It may be burning in quality and is often accompanied by numbness or paresthesias. L5 or S1 lesions generally cause pain below the knee, but can also cause posterior thigh pain. L1–L3 root lesions can cause pain in the anteromedial thigh.
- Pain with paresthesias on the anterolateral part of the thigh may be due to entrapment of the lateral cutaneous nerve of the thigh under the lateral part of the inguinal ligament (i.e., meralgia paresthetica). Symptoms may be referred to this area with L2 or L3 nerve root lesions, since this is where the nerve originates (see Figure 2.12).
- Diabetics with uncontrolled hyperglycemia are at risk of diabetic amyotrophy. Acute unilateral or bilateral thigh pain with muscle wasting occurs. It should not be misdiagnosed as PMR (in which weakness or wasting do not occur) or inflammatory myopathy.
- Soccer players are at risk of adductor tendonitis (often an adductor apophysitis) and osteitis pubis due to substantial mechanical forces placed on pelvic structures during running and kicking.
- Although hip fractures are usually obvious, they can also present subacutely in a patient who continues to walk; this is particularly common among the elderly, who may develop stress fractures of the hip.

Previous trauma, low back, and musculoskeletal problems

- Previous trauma or disease causing permanent deformity of any lumbosacral or hip joint structure can be considered a risk factor for further trouble (see Table 2.18).
- Multiparity is a risk factor for osteitis pubis, sacroiliac, and pelvic pain.
- Trochanteric bursitis may coexist with referred back pain.
- Tears of the gluteus medius can occur at its greater trochanter insertion and give similar symptoms to those caused by bursitis.
- Historically, tailors were at risk of ischial bursitis because of sitting on the floor continually crossing and uncrossing their legs, which causes friction irritation of soft tissues overlying the ischial tuberosity.

Examination

The reader is referred to the sequence of examination for the low back, including the sacroiliac and lower limb neurologic examination (see pp. 80–83). Always consider lower spinal, muscle, or neurologic pathology when assessing weakness and pain around the pelvis.

Observation and palpation

For observation and palpation the patient should be supine on a couch:

- Look for leg length discrepancy (hip disease, scoliosis) and a leg resting in external rotation (hip fracture).
- Psoriasis over the knees may be associated with sacroiliitis.

Fig. 2.12 The approximate areas within which sensory changes may be found in lesions of the lateral cutaneous nerve of the thigh (hatched area) and high lumbar radiculopathy (broken line). The shaded areas denote the distribution of sensory symptoms associated with meralgia paresthetica.

- Swelling in the groin may be a hernia (reducible, moves with cough), lipoma (soft/nontender/diffuse), a saphenous varix, or lymphadenopathy (hard/rubbery and mobile). A hip joint effusion cannot be felt.
- Tenderness over the hip joint in the groin is not specific for joint pathology: the joint is deep, muscles and psoas bursa overlie it.
- If the groin is very tender with slight touch, consider hip fracture or infection. Hyperpathia (and allodynia) is consistent with complex regional pain syndrome (see Chapter 18).
- Numbness over the anterolateral thigh suggests meralgia paresthetica (see Figure 2.12).
- The adductor longus tendon can be palpated at its insertion at the pubic tubercle and distally along the upper medial thigh. The pubic tubercle is found by palpating slowly and lightly downwards from umbilicus over the bladder until bone is reached.
- Pain from osteitis pubis or adductor apophysitis is often significant, with abdominal rectus contraction (ask the patient to slowly lift his or

Table 2.18 Risk factors for painful pelvic or hip lesions

Risk factor	Pelvic/hip pathology
Mechanical abnormality of the low back	Referred pain
	Trochanteric bursitis
Mechanical abnormality of the hip (e.g., Perthes', slipped epiphysis, epiphyseal dysplasia, Paget's)	Hip OA
Corticosteroid use	Osteoporotic fracture
	Osteonecrosis of the femoral head
Autoimmune rheumatic disease (e.g., RA, JIA, AS)	Synovitis hip
	Secondary OA of the hip
	Pyogenic arthritis of the hip
	Osteoporotic fracture
Maternal history of hip fracture; low body mass index; low bone mass; falls	Osteoporotic hip fracture
Multiple pregnancies	Osteitis pubis (± pelvic instability)
Soccer players	Adductor tendonitis/apophysitis
	Osteitis pubis

her head and shoulders off the couch, keeping your finger on the pubic tubercle).

Hip examination

The hip should be examined while the patient is supine. Tests generally help to discriminate articular and extra-articular disease, but not the causes of articular disease:

- Measure and determine actual or apparent leg length discrepancy: measure from the anterior superior iliac spine to the medial tibial malleolus; by flexing hips and knees, the site of shortening should become apparent.
- A fixed loss of extension is a sign of intra-articular hip disease. The patient flexes the hip and knee on one side until normal lumbar lordosis flattens out (confirmed by feeling pressure on your hand placed under their lumbar spine during the maneuver). If the other hip flexes simultaneously, it suggests hip extension loss on that side (Thomas' test).
- Using the patella or tibial tubercle as pointers, test the rotational hip range in extension by rotating the straightened legs by holding the heels.
- Rotational movements are also tested by lifting the leg, flexed 90° at the knee, and swinging the foot out (internal rotation) or in (external rotation). Hip flexion can be tested in this position too (see Plate 9). Patients without intra-articular pathology should have a pain-free range of movement.

- Rotational ranges in hip flexion and extension may differ between left and right in an individual. Also, variations in femoral neck anteversion contribute to variations in rotation range.
- To test hip abduction/adduction, fix the pelvis to avoid pelvic tilt by placing one hand firmly over the iliac crest (see Plate 9). Occasionally, pain at the end of abduction or internal rotation occurs with a bony block (solid "end-feel"). In an older patient this might suggest impingement of a marginal joint osteophyte.
- Barlow's maneuver checks for congenital dislocation of the hips in babies. Flex and adduct the hips exerting an axial force into the posterior acetabulum to demonstrate posterior dislocation.
- Greater retroversion (allowing excessive hip external rotation) usually occurs in cases of slipped femoral epiphysis. External rotation is accentuated when the hip is flexed. The slip (usually inferoposterior) is thought to occur in association with a period of rapid growth.

Muscle activation tests

Specific muscle activation against resistance can be used to elicit pain, but results need to be interpreted cautiously in the context of known hip disease:

- Hip adduction against resistance (sliding their leg inward toward the other against your hand) reproducing pain is a sensitive test for adductor longus tendonitis, but may be positive in osteitis pubis, hip joint lesions, and other soft tissue lesions in the adductor muscles.
- Test the psoas by resisted hip flexion while in slight internal rotation. Psoas bursitis or infection tracking along the psoas sheath is likely to give intense pain with minimal resistance.
- Hip abduction (sliding the leg outwards against your hand) may be particularly painful in cases of gluteus medius tears but also in trochanteric bursitis or intra-articular pathology.

Palpate posterolateral structures

Ask the patient to lie on their side and palpate the posterolateral structures (see Figure 2.13):

- Tenderness over the greater trochanter is usually well-localized although it may be anterior or posterolateral to the trochanter and refers a small way down the leg.
- The ischial tuberosity and its overlying bursa lie at the apex of the buttock.
- The soft tissues overlying the point where the sciatic nerve exits the pelvis is found midway between the ischial spine and the greater trochanter. There may be tenderness as a result of soft tissue lesions or trauma causing sciatic nerve entrapment (piriformis syndrome), which can lead to foot drop.
- A tender coccyx (coccydynia) can be palpated in this position. It can also be palpated (and the sacrococcygeal joint moved) from a bidigital examination, though this requires the index finger to be placed inside the rectum, the thumb outside, the two digits then holding the joint.

Diagnostic procedures

Radiographs

An AP radiograph of the pelvis is a good initial screening test in patients with pelvic, hip, or thigh pain. AP and lateral lumbar spine films may be warranted.

- The pelvis is a common site of involvement in myeloma, metastatic malignancy, and Paget's disease of bone (see Chapter 16).
- Established, but not early, sacroiliitis can be ruled out. The main differential diagnoses of the causes of sacroiliitis are: AS, psoriatic or reactive arthritis, enteric arthropathy including Whipple's disease, brucellosis and other infections, hyperparathyroidism and osteitis condensans ilii (sclerosis of the SI joint on the lower iliac side).
- Widening of the symphysis in children may be a sign of congenital disorders of development (e.g., epispadias, achondrogenesis, chondrodysplasias, hypophosphatasia), trauma and hyperparathyroidism (see Chapter 16).
- Widening of the symphysis pubis, osteitis pubis (bone resorption and sclerosis) and osteitis condensans ilii are signs associated with chronic pelvic pain in multiparous women.
- General osteopenia is a risk factor for general low bone mass measured by densitometry; however, it is not a sensitive or specific indicator of osteoporosis (i.e., may be osteomalacia or rickets).
- Regional osteoporosis confined to the femur is nonspecific but may reflect hip synovitis, infection, or transient osteoporosis of the hip (rare).

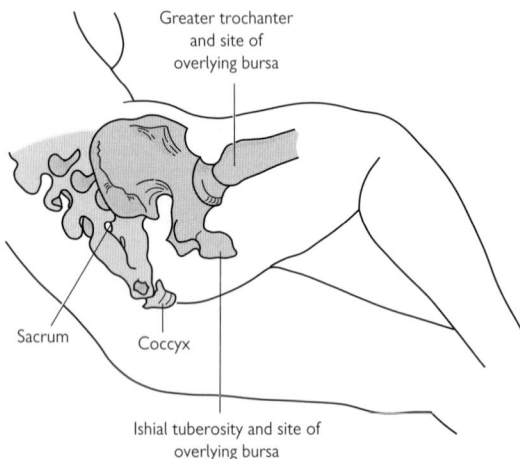

Greater trochanter and site of overlying bursa

Sacrum

Coccyx

Ischial tuberosity and site of overlying bursa

Fig. 2.13 Bony anatomy of the posterior hip and pelvis, showing the position in which lesions around the greater trochanter and ischial bursa can be palpated.

- Early synovitis and infection may be demonstrated through subtle radiological signs such as joint space widening and change in soft tissue fat planes.
- A "frog leg" (lateral) view of the hip shows the anterior and posterior femoral head more clearly than an AP view (useful in early osteonecrosis/Perthes', slipped epiphysis).
- The acetabulae are best visualized on 45° oblique views (acetabular fractures can be missed on a conventional AP view).
- "Stork" views of the symphysis pubis (standing on one leg) are useful for confirming diastasis of the joint.

Diagnostic ultrasound

- US is a sensitive and simple way of confirming a hip joint effusion. Using US, fluid can be aspirated for culture and an assessment of the extent of synovial thickening can be made.
- Tendon damage in the groin area should be identifiable with US alone (guided steroid injection can then be done if necessary) but MR may be needed either to characterize pathology further or rule out joint pathology.

Bone scan

Bone scan is a useful screening test, but it is nonspecific:

- Characteristic, though nonspecific, patterns of bone scan abnormality are recognized in the hip/pelvic area. The following conditions can be recognized: sacroiliitis, bone malignancy, myeloma, Paget's disease, hip fracture, femoral head osteonecrosis (see Plate 10), osteoid osteoma, OA and synovitis of the hip, osteitis pubis/adductor apophysitis (requires special seated "ring" view), and bursitis/enthesitis at the greater trochanter.
- Bone scan is a useful investigation in children and adolescents as a screening investigation if other radiology tests are normal.

CT and MR

- CT/MR of the high lumbar region should be considered to confirm a nerve root lesion, causing groin or thigh pain.
- Specific patterns of X-ray attenuation or signal change around the SI joints occur in sacroiliitis with CT/MR, although active and previous inflammation cannot easily be distinguished.
- A suspicion of bony malignancy from radiographs of the pelvis requires further characterization. CT is the technique of choice for characterizing bone lesions around the hip such as femoral neck stress fracture, osteoid osteoma, or other bone tumors. CT may give more information about the lesion (and is valuable for "guided biopsy") but MR is useful in checking for pelvic visceral lesions.
- MR is the technique of choice if hip infection or osteonecrosis is suspected. In adults, patterns of signal change have been correlated with prognosis.

- During a single examination the pattern of hip synovitis (vascularity and thickness), cartilage loss, and subchondral bone erosion can be documented. This is particularly useful in children with JIA.

Laboratory tests
- ESR and CRP may be normal in inflammatory SI joints, lumbar vertebral disc, and pelvic enthesis disorders.
- PMR is almost always associated with an elevated ESR/CRP.
- Myeloma is unlikely if the ESR is normal.
- A high alkaline phosphatase is typically associated with an acute phase response, although in the elderly, it might suggest Paget's disease.
- ANA and RF are unlikely to help diagnostically.
- Major metabolic bone disease such as osteomalacia and hyperparathyroidism is usually excluded by a normal serum calcium and phosphate.

Treatment

Treatment of spinal and neuropathic pain is covered in the section Low Back Pain and Disorders in Adults.
- NSAIDs may be required for a number of the conditions just described, particularly OA, hip synovitis, and tendon inflammation.
- Physical therapy and rehabilitation play a vital and early part in management, maintaining mobility, preventing tissue contracture, and restrengthening/stabilizing the lower back, pelvis, and hip.
- Either physical therapists or podiatrists may help in accurately evaluating back and lower limb biomechanics. Asymmetry and muscular imbalance may be modifiable relatively simply with foot orthotics, for example.
- Steroid injections may be important in the following conditions:
  - meralgia paresthetica
  - osteitis pubis
  - trochanteric bursitis/enthesitis
  - ischial bursitis/enthesitis
  - adductor tendonitis
  - coccydynia
  - hip synovitis (under imaging guidance)
  - sacroiliitis—in intractable pain and under X-ray or US guidance.
- Injection techniques are covered in Corticosteroid Injection Therapy at the end of this chapter.

Surgery
- When the hip has been damaged by an inflammatory arthritis or OA, the principal surgical intervention is joint replacement. Osteotomy has been mainly superseded by more reliable replacement.
- Surgical synovectomy of the hip is a difficult procedure and opening the hip carries a risk of avascular necrosis. This procedure is very rarely done.

- Excision arthroplasty is only really necessary where infection or poor bone stock make reconstruction unwise. Power is often greatly reduced and even the previously fit young patient will not be able to ambulate without crutches.
- In children in particular, it is important to assess spinal and knee disease, especially contractures, before embarking on hip surgery, because the primary cause for flexion deformities or hip damage may be at these levels.

Knee pain

Anatomy of the knee

- The knee extends, flexes, and rotates.
- The main extensor quadriceps consists of four muscle segments—rectus femoris, vastus lateralis, medialis, and intermedius—which converge to form a tendon containing the patella, which then inserts into the tibia. The rectus femoris arises from the pelvis and vastus muscles from the upper femur.
- The hamstring muscles (biceps femoris, semitendinosus, semimembranosus) all arise from the ischial tuberosity and flex the knee. The biceps femoris inserts around the fibular head. The other two muscles insert into the tibia on the medial side and can externally rotate the femur.
- In the knee, the femoral condyles articulate within semicircular fibrocartilage menisci on the tibial condyles (see Figure 2.14). Only the peripheral 10–30% of the menisci is vascular and innervated and can potentially repair itself.
- As the knee approaches full extension, the femur internally rotates on the tibia (biceps femoris action), tightening each pair of ligaments relative to each other (see Figure 2.14). This configuration confers maximum stability.
- As flexion is initiated, a small amount of femoral external rotation on the tibia occurs. This "unlocking" is done by the popliteus—a muscle that arises from the posterior surface of the tibia below. It passes up obliquely across the back of the knee and inserts, via a cord-like tendon, into the lateral femoral condyle. The tendon partly lies within the knee joint capsule.
- Grooves on the femoral condyle articular surfaces allow tight congruity with the anterior horns of the menisci when the knee is extended. If full extension—and this optimal articulation configuration—is lost, then articular cartilage degeneration invariably follows. This is particularly important in inflammatory arthritis.
- The cruciate ligaments are the principal joint stabilizers. The anterior cruciate attaches above to the inside of the lateral femoral condyle and below to the tibia in front of the tibial spines though a slip attaches to the anterior horn of the lateral meniscus. Its main role is to control and contain the amount of knee rotation when the joint is flexed.
- The posterior cruciate attaches above to the inside of the medial femoral condyle. At the other end, it attaches in a posterior groove between tibial condyles. Its main role is to stabilize the joint by preventing forward displacement of the femur relative to the tibia when the knee is flexed.
- The cruciates are extra-articular and are covered by a layer of vascular synovium. Bleeding usually accompanies disruption.
- The tibial or medial collateral ligament (MCL) has superficial and deep layers (see Figure 2.15). It stabilizes the knee against valgus stresses, mostly during flexion. The superficial MCL overlies, and moves relative to, the deep part and is separated from it by a bursa. The lower part

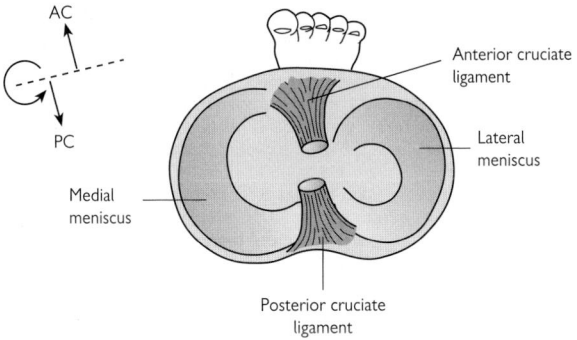

Pull of cruciates rotates femur as knee AC extends

AC

PC

Anterior cruciate ligament

Lateral meniscus

Medial meniscus

Posterior cruciate ligament

Fig. 2.14 Axial section of the right knee joint (looking down on the tibial plateau, where the foot is fixed on the floor). The femoral condyles articulate within the menisci. As the knee extends the cruciate ligaments tighten and pull the femoral condyles acting to internally rotate the femur through the last few degrees of extension. The knee therefore "locks" and is stable when the leg is straight.

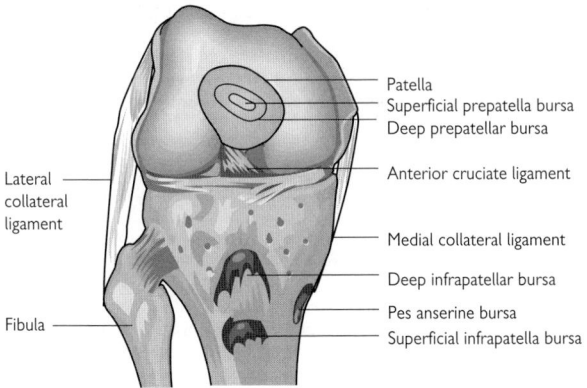

Patella
Superficial prepatella bursa
Deep prepatellar bursa

Anterior cruciate ligament

Lateral collateral ligament

Medial collateral ligament

Deep infrapatellar bursa

Pes anserine bursa

Superficial infrapatella bursa

Fibula

Fig. 2.15 Anterior knee structures.

of the superficial MCL is covered by the long adductors, gracilis, semitendinosus, and sartorius muscles, as they merge into the pes anserinus before inserting into the tibia. The MCL and pes anserinus are separated by the anserine bursa. Deeper MCL fibers attach to, and stabilize, the medial meniscus.

- The fibular or lateral collateral ligament (LCL) joins the lateral femoral condyle to the fibular head and is separated from it by a bursa. It stabilizes the knee on its lateral side. It has no meniscal attachment. A small bursa separates it from the overlapping tendon insertion of biceps femoris.
- The patella is a sesamoid bone that articulates in the femoral condylar groove and makes quadriceps action more efficient. Patella articular facet configuration can vary; congenital bi/tripartite patellae are associated with anterior knee pain.
- The strongest force on the patella is from vastus lateralis (see Figure 2.16). Mechanical factors that increase the ratio of lateral to medial forces during patella tracking such as a wide pelvis, a more lateral origin of vastus lateralis, femoral neck anteversion, external tibial torsion, and a weak vastus medialis are risk factors for patella tracking problems and anterior knee pain.
- There are bursae (see Figure 2.15) between the quadriceps tendon and the femur (suprapatellar), the patellar tendon, and tibial tubercle (deep infrapatellar), and overlying the patella (prepatellar) and patellar tendon insertion (superficial infrapatellar). The suprapatellar bursa communicates with the knee joint and large joint effusions invariably fill it.
- Posteriorly, bursae separate each of the heads of gastrocnemius (which arise from femoral condyles) from the joint capsule. The bursae communicate with the knee joint and can fill from joint effusions.

Taking a history

Ask about the site of pain

Try to establish whether pain is from articular, soft tissue, or anterior knee structures. Is it referred pain?

- Bursa, tendon, and most ligament lesions cause well-localized pain.
- Localized tibiofemoral joint line pain suggests meniscal pathology.
- Localized medial knee pain has a number of possible causes: MCL tear or chronic inflammation (calcification of MCL origin termed the Pellegrini–Stieda phenomenon), medial meniscus tear, meniscal cyst, anserine tendonitis, bursitis, or enthesitis (semimembranosus insertion).
- Enthesitis of structures at their insertion to the patella margins can result in considerable pain.
- Overuse in runners and cyclists can cause localized inflammation and pain of the iliotibial band (ITB) or its underlying bursa over the lateral femoral condyle (as the band moves across the bone as the knee flexes).
- Anterior pain in children, adolescents, and young adults invariably suggests an underlying mechanical abnormality. In older adults the most common cause is patellofemoral OA (see Table 2.19).

Fig. 2.16 (a) The iliotibial band. (b) The patella Q angle (normal values—men 10°, women 15°).

- Anterior knee pain may be referred from the hip or L3 nerve root. Hip pain is an aching pain; root pain is sharp, often with paresthesias.
- Posterior knee pain associated with "a lump" is often due to a Baker's cyst, which is caused by synovitis in the posterior knee compartment that leads to formation of a popliteal cyst.

Ask about injury

Knee injuries are common; the most significant is anterior cruciate injury. Ask about injury and whether the knee feels unstable or "gives way".

- Anterior cruciate injuries are invariably associated with a hemarthrosis, thus a painful effusion will have occurred immediately. Meniscus tears can cause immediate pain, but synovitis and swelling are delayed for about 6 hours.
- Patients may mention that the knee "keeps giving out on me". This feeling may be the pivot shift phenomenon caused by reduced anterior cruciate stability against a valgus stress as the knee is flexing.
- Anterior cruciate and MCL injuries often coexist (since they are attached). Ask about medial knee pain originally and subsequently.

Table 2.19 Causes of anterior knee pain

Commonly in adults	Patellofemoral OA (look for mechanical factors and generalized OA)
	Referred hip pain, e.g., hip OA
	Referred pain from L3 nerve root irritation
Specific to children and adolescents	Referred pain from the hip, e.g., slipped femoral epiphysis
	Bi-/tripartite patella
	Synovial plicae (synovial shelf clicking over femoral condyle on knee flexion)
	Recurrent patellar dislocation (tissue laxity, patella alta, trauma)
	Osteochondritis at patellar lower pole—overuse injury in jumping sports*
	Osteochondritis of tibial tubercle (Osgood–Schlatter's)
	Nonspecific ("chondromalacia patellae")
Causes at any age	Mechanical factors (patellar maltracking): wide pelvis, femoral anteversion, external tibial torsion; specific strengthening of lateral structures, e.g., iliotibial band syndrome; weakness or injury of vastus medialis or medial knee structures; tissue laxity, e.g., benign joint hypermobility syndrome
	Osteochondritis dissecans of patella (average age 18)
	Enthesitis at patellar margins (may be part of SpA)
	Bursitis (prepatellar, superficial/deep infrapatellar): gout (very rare in children unless inherited metabolic deficiency); autoimmune rheumatic disease; infection
	Tear/cyst of anterior meniscal horn
	Patellar fracture
	Fat pad syndrome (recurrent retropatellar tendon pain with swelling)

*Sinding–Larsen–Johansson disease.

Ask about knee locking

Knee locking is a mechanical effect of disruption of normal articulation by "loose bodies".

- Suspect meniscus damage in the middle aged or if the patient plays a lot of sports. A meniscus tear is the most common cause of the knee locking. In adolescents, locking may be due to a tear in a discoid meniscus (>98% lateral). The morphologically abnormal discs are prone to degeneration.

- Chondral fragments (from osteochondritis dissecans lesions) can cause locking; the condition is most common in the 5–20 year age group (boys > girls).
- Synovial chondromatosis is a rare cause.
- Some patients with anterior knee pain describe the knee locking or giving way. This is due to reflex quadriceps inhibition rather than true instability.

Ask about the initial onset of pain

- Acute pain is usual with injuries of cruciates and vertical meniscal tears.
- Acute onset pain without trauma (but always with swelling) suggests infection, crystal arthritis, or spontaneous hemarthrosis.
- In the very elderly, traumatic lesions may be missed, since the presentation is not always striking, e.g., intra-articular fracture with hemarthrosis.
- An insidious onset of pain is usual in cleavage tears of menisci (i.e., horizontal tears), which occur typically in adults where the disc is degenerated, in adolescents with discoid menisci, and in early osteochondritis dissecans.

Ask about the pattern and type of pain

- Pain from synovitis is often associated with stiffness and is often worse after a period of immobility. Almost without exception, knee synovitis can occur in all forms of arthritis.
- Pain from subchondral damage (e.g., OA) is almost always worse on weight bearing, but this association is not specific.
- Pain on kneeling/squatting is characteristic of anterior knee pain.
- Burning pain may be neurogenic, e.g., L3 nerve root or reflex sympathetic dystrophy pain.

Past medical, family, occupational, and leisure history

- Knee synovitis and patellar enthesitis occur in adult and juvenile enthesitis-related arthritis. Ask about previous uveitis, low back pain, urethral discharge, sexually transmitted disease, dysentery, and psoriasis.
- Gout (see Chapter 15) is not uncommon around the knee. Ask about gout risk factors and whether the patient has ever had first MTP joint pain (i.e., podagra).
- There may be a family history of generalized OA (see Chapter 6), a hereditary disease of connective tissue, or hypermobility in young adults with OA.
- Prepatellar bursitis classically occurred in housemaids, hence the nickname "housemaid's knee." Friction from repeated kneeling can cause it.
- Sports injuries are common. Anterior cruciate injury is a typical skiing injury. Meniscal injuries are common in soccer. Jumping events (e.g., high jump, basketball) can lead to patellar tendon apophysis. Cycling is associated with anterior knee pain. MCL and meniscal injuries are common in skiing and weight-bearing activities where rotation and change of direction are frequent. Cycling and running are associated with ITB/bursa pain and inflammation.

Examination

From front and behind, observe the patient standing

- Look for mechanical abnormalities that might be associated with knee lesions: patella asymmetry, prominent tibial tubercles from previous Osgood–Schlatter's (anterior knee pain), flat feet, and hypermobility (patella dislocation, hyperextension of >10°).
- Check for mechanical abnormalities, which might suggest specific pathology: genu varum (bowed leg, typical appearance with primarily medial compartment OA), obvious suprapatellar knee swelling (synovitis), psoriasis (associated synovitis or enthesitis).
- Marked genu varum occurs in the rare Blount's disease (developmental abnormality of the medial tibial physis typically in African-American boys).

Examination of the sitting patient

Ask the patient to sit on the examination table with legs hanging, knees bent. Patellar tracking and pain from medial meniscus damage can be assessed. An alternative approach is with the patient supine. Observe any muscle wasting. Palpate anterior, medial, and lateral structures.

- In patients with anterior knee pain, look for symmetric patellar alignment.
- Observe active knee extension. Patellar movement should be smooth, pain-free, and symmetric.
- Passively externally rotate each lower leg to its extreme. This is a reasonably sensitive test for conditions of the medial knee compartment (e.g., meniscus tear) and medial knee structures. Discomfort will be felt. If the MCL is totally deficient, an abnormally increased range of external rotation may occur.
- Quadriceps wasting (accentuated depression in muscle just above the patella) occurs with disuse after injuries and in chronic arthropathies.
- Sites of bursae, patellar tendon, and ligament insertions should be palpated in patients with localized pain (see Figure 2.17).
- Tibiofemoral joint line tenderness is likely to be due to either meniscus pathology or marginal osteophytes. Osteophytes give bony swelling.
- Anterior pain from patellofemoral joint disorders may be elicited by gentle pressure down on the patella. Mobilizing the patella sideways will give an impression of tissue laxity (possible underlying hypermobility).
- Factors that predispose to patellofemoral pain syndrome include: a high or lateral patella, weak vastus medialis, excessive pronation, weak ankle dorsiflexors, tight hamstrings, reduced movement at the ankle, and a wide Q-angle. The Q-angle is formed between a line from the anterior superior iliac spine to the center of the patella, and a line extended upwards from the tibial tubercle through the center of the patella. The larger the angle the greater the lateral tensile pull on the patella (see Figure 2.15).
- Localized tenderness of the femoral condyle is often the only sign of osteochondritis dissecans in adolescents. The most common site is on the inside of the medial femoral condyle (75%).

Examine for joint synovitis (synovial inflammation giving synovial thickening and/or tenderness) and an effusion

- The joint may be warm. Chronic synovitis does not always result in a warm joint, but infection, crystal arthritis, and hemarthrosis usually do.
- Gross synovitis can produce obvious effusions and/or synovial thickening most easily felt around the patellar edges.
- Effusions may be confirmed by the patellar tap test (see Plate 11).

Fig. 2.17 Position of the knee for palpation of most of its structures. Palpating for enthesitis at the patellar tendon insertion (a) Palpation over the insertion of semimembranosus and pes anserinus under the tibial plateau (b) The site of the majority of osteochondritis lesions in the knee is shown by the X.

- Small effusions can be detected by eliciting the "bulge sign". Fluid in the medial compartment is swept firmly upward and laterally into the suprapatellar pouch. Firm pressure on the lateral side of the joint may then push fluid back into the medial compartment, producing a bulge.
- Thickened synovium can be detected by experienced examiners in the absence of a detectable effusion. It is not always tender.
- Posterior compartment synovial thickening and popliteal cysts can be felt by wrapping the fingers around under the knee when it is slightly flexed.
- In contrast to adults, popliteal cysts in children are not usually associated with intra-articular pathology. Investigation is not always necessary.

Test the knee for stability
- There are many tests for instability: instability may be straight or rotational and can be graded according to consensus criteria (consult orthopedics texts).
- The Lachman test (see Figure 2.18) is arguably the most sensitive test for eliciting anterior cruciate disruption: hold the knee flexed between 20–30°, grasped above and below the joint. Attempt to move the tibia forward and backward on the femur. Ask about pain and feel for laxity or a "clunk".
- The anterior draw test is not as sensitive as the Lachmann test for detecting partial anterior cruciate tears but is easier to do. The patient lies flat, hip flexed, the knee flexed at 90°, with the foot flat on the table. Fix the foot by gently sitting on it and pull the top of the lower leg forwards in the line of the thigh. Ask about pain and feel for laxity.
- The posterior draw test identifies posterior cruciate disruption: with the knee flexed to 90°, press the top of the lower leg backward in the line of the thigh, ask about pain and feel for laxity.
- Test medial stability at 0° and 30° of flexion (MCL stabilizes maximally at 30°) by holding the upper leg still and applying a valgus force to the tibia. Laxity associated with widening of the tibiofemoral joint (with or without pain) is a positive test and suggests MCL deficiency.
- Lateral (LCL and ITB) stability is similarly tested by using a varus force on the lower leg.
- MCL tears can accompany anterior cruciate injuries and deep lesions are associated with simultaneous tears of the medial meniscus. Such complex pathology can make specific examination maneuvers difficult to interpret.

Test for meniscus damage
- McMurray's test (see Figure 2.19): Flex the knee, internally rotate the lower leg, then extend the joint. Repeat with the lower leg externally rotated. The fingers (over the joint line) may feel a "clunk" as a femoral condyle passes over a torn meniscus. Unfortunately, a false-positive McMurray's test is not uncommon, and may occur in 21–65% of cases.
- Ask the patient to turn over. Lying initially on their side allows you to do Ober's test to detect lateral soft tissue injury. When prone, look and palpate for swelling in the popliteal fossa and proximal calf that may indicate a low-lying popliteal cyst.

Anterior draw test

Lachmann test

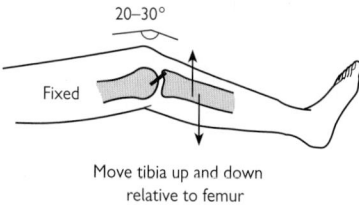

Fig. 2.18 Dynamic tests of anterior cruciate function. Patients should be relaxed lying supine on a couch. Excessive laxity is the most important sign.

McMurray's test

Action:	Hold the knee and the heel.
	Internally rotate the lower leg (1) then extend it (2)
Positive test:	(Palpable) clunk at joint line

Fig. 2.19 Dynamic test designed to elicit signs of meniscus damage. "Clunks", intra-articular pain, and coarse crepitus may indicate damage. The test is not specific and is open to misinterpretation.

- Inflammation of the bursa underlying the iliotibial band (ITB) may result in tenderness over the lateral femoral condyle. The ITB may be tight. This is demonstrated using Ober's test. The patient lies on his or her side with the lower (nonaffected) leg flexed at the hip. The (painful) knee is flexed to 90° and the thigh is extended and adducted. The test is positive if, when the examiner's hand is removed, the hip does not drop down (further stretching the ITB). Leg length inequality and foot overpronation may be causative factors.
- Detecting specific structures in the posterior fossa is often difficult because of the lack of bony landmarks and overlapping soft tissue structures. Synovial cysts may form under pressure and are often hard and tender. Diffuse thickening suggests joint synovitis.

Diagnostic procedures

Radiographs

AP and lateral weight-bearing radiographs are suitable screening views if the diagnosis is unclear after clinical assessment.

- Early synovitis may only be evident from the presence of an effusion, periarticular osteopenia, or soft tissue swelling. Patterns of bone damage in chronic arthropathies may be recognized.
- Signs of joint infection, which may not necessarily present acutely, are patchy bone osteolysis and irregular loss of bone cortex. Osteonecrosis is uncommon in the knee, but it does occur in sickle cell anemia.
- Loss of joint space, angulation deformity, osteophytes, subchondral bone sclerosis, and bone cysts are hallmark features of OA.
- In adults, linear or vague intra-articular calcification suggests chondrocalcinosis (associated with calcium pyrophosphate dihydrate (CPPD) arthritis). Gross "thumbprint" calcification is typical of synovial chondromatosis (mainly in children).
- In children, check for an osteochondral fragment (e.g., osteochondritis dissecans), normal epiphyses, epiphyseal plates and metaphyses, normal patella shape, and osteochondritis at the tibial tubercle (see Table 2.20).

Specialized radiographic views: tomographic views; "skyline" (axial with knee bent) view; or lateral view taken with at least 30° of flexion

- Tomography is useful for clarifying nonperipheral osteochondral defects.
- "Sunrise" views demonstrate anomalous patellar facet configuration and can reveal patellofemoral incongruity, but multiple views may be needed. Subchondral patellar pathology is seen more clearly with a sunrise view than on lateral views.
- Patella alta is most reliably seen on a lateral view with 30° flexion.

Further imaging

Further imaging depends on the differential diagnosis and a discussion with your radiologist:

- Periarticular soft tissue lesions can be characterized with MR, but ultrasound may be adequate (if performed by someone with expertise in this area).

Table 2.20 Interpretation of radiographic knee abnormalities in children

Radiographic abnormality	Possible conditions (most commonly)
Intra-articular calcific fragment	Osteochondritis dissecans, traumatic avulsion, synovial tumors, or chondromatosis (rare)
Epiphyseal defect/abnormality	JIA, sepsis, avulsion injury, bone dysplasias, rickets, hemophilia, hypothyroidism
Transverse radiolucent metaphyseal band or lysis	Leukemia, lymphoma, neuroblastoma metastases, infections (neonates), osteogenesis imperfecta, idiopathic juvenile osteoporosis, Cushing's disease
Joint space narrowing	JIA, sepsis, PVNS, hemophilia
Diffuse low bone density	Rickets, OI, osteoporosis, mucopolysaccharidosis
Periosteal reaction	Fracture, sepsis, infarction, tumors

- Patterns of meniscus damage are recognized on MR, give an indication of prognosis, and aid the surgeon's decision to proceed to arthroscopy.
- MR is essential if there is likely to be a combination of lesions (e.g., anterior cruciate, MCL, and medial meniscus lesions).
- In children, both US and MR will confirm synovitis.
- MR is more sensitive than radiographs or US at identifying joint erosions in RA.
- The place of CT or MR in investigating radiographically detected bone tumors depends on the nature of the lesion.

Aspiration of joint and periarticular fluid collections
- Early aspiration is essential if infection is suspected.
- The knee is a common site of monoarthritis. The principles behind management apply to all cases of single joint pathology.
- Send joint fluid for cell count, polarized light microscopy, and culture.
- In adults, the usual differential diagnosis of sepsis of knee structures is gout, so fluid should be examined by polarized light microscopy for urate crystals.
- Blood-stained fluid either suggests a traumatic tap or chondrocalcinosis. Frank blood suggests hemarthrosis, the major causes of which are cruciate tear, bleeding diathesis, intra-articular fracture, and pigmented villonodular synovitis (PVNS).
- Bursa fluid may be more successfully detected and aspirated using US guidance.

Laboratory tests
These should be directed toward suspected underlying disease:
- CBC, acute phase reactants (ESR, CRP).
- Electrolytes, BUN, creatinine, and uric acid.

- Blood calcium, phosphate, albumin, alkaline phosphatase, and 25-OH vitamin D (± iPTH) to screen for metabolic bone disease.
- Autoantibodies: rheumatoid factor (RF) and anti-citrullinated protein antibodies (ACPA) are found in rheumatoid arthritis; antinuclear (ANA), and extractable nuclear antibodies (ENAs) are found in SLE and other autoimmune diseases that may be include joint involvement.
- Serum angiotensin converting enzyme (sACE) for sarcoid.
- Infection: IgM *Borrelia burgdorferi* serology for acute arthropathy in Lyme disease, acute and convalescent streptococcal antibodies (anti-ASO titers) for reactive streptococcal arthritis.

Treatment

- In general, most soft tissue lesions will improve with rest and NSAIDs.
- Anterior knee pain may respond well to isometric exercises, adjustments to foot alignment, e.g., with sensible shoes, orthotics (support insoles), and hamstring stretching exercises.
- The acute swollen knee requires aspiration, rest for 24 h and gentle mobilization. If infection is considered, broad-spectrum antibiotics against staphylococcus (including MRSA, if relevant) and streptococcus should be started immediately while awaiting culture data. In infection, intra-articular antibiotics and steroids should be avoided (see Chapter 22). The patient should not bear weight on an acutely infected joint.
- Acute and chronic inflammation can lead to joint destruction and instability. If RA is identified, early treatment may prevent long-term morbidity (see Chapter 5).
- Physical therapy and splinting play an important role in maintaining function and preventing contractures, etc.

Address biomechanical factors

- Input from a physical therapist may be helpful in cases of anterior knee pain. Success from McConnell (patellar) taping is more likely in nonpatellofemoral OA-related anterior knee pain.
- Quadriceps strengthening exercises can be reviewed and reinforced by physical therapists in cases of knee OA.
- Knee pain, particularly anterior pain, may be linked to foot abnormalities (e.g., overpronation), and hip alignment (see Q-angle, above).
- Specific muscle strengthening exercises, foot orthotics, and knee braces should be considered.

Local steroid injection

Local steroid injections can be helpful in the following situations:
- Acute flare of non-infective inflammatory disease:
  - OA (especially where CPPD is present)—mild OA may also respond to hyaluronate injections, although this is controversial
  - autoimmune arthritis, e.g., RA, SpA
  - intra-articular gout
  - SpA, etc.
- Bursitis (may be gout):
  - pre- and infrapatella (superficial and deep) bursa (the latter may require US guidance)
  - anserine.

- Baker's cyst (note: the knee joint is injected with corticosteroids, since the joint and the cyst are connected. Direct popliteal cyst injection should be performed under US guidance only).
- Enthesopathy, e.g., semimembranosus insertion.
- Trauma, e.g., pain over the medial collateral ligament insertion.
- Other soft-tissue: ITB syndrome.

The reader is referred to Corticosteroid Injection Therapy at the end of this chapter.

Joint injection therapies

- In patients with large joint effusions, merely aspirating the effusion may provide some level of symptomatic relief
- Knee OA may respond transiently to an injectable steroid, such as triamcinolone acetate. Saline irrigation and injections with hyaluronic acid preparations are also used, but response is variable.

Note: all intra-articular injection therapies are more effective when patients' knees are immobilized for 48 hours following the procedure.

Drugs

- NSAIDs will invariably be helpful in cases of inflammatory and septic arthritis.
- Colchicine 0.6 mg BID is often useful in relieving pain from crystal arthritis in patients intolerant of NSAIDs.
- Acetaminophen may be as effective as NSAIDs for some patients
- Glucosamine and chondroitin sulfate are controversial for the treatment of osteoarthritis. Although some studies demonstrate improved pain control and function, other studies clearly indicate that these drugs are no better than placebo.

See Part 2 chapters for specific treatment of chronic autoimmune arthritides.

Surgery

- Arthroscopy is often used as a diagnostic tool in cases of undiagnosed monoarthritis and to confirm and trim cartilage tears. Synovium and synovial lesions (e.g., PVNS, synovial chondromatosis) can be biopsied or excised (synovectomy) and the joint can be irrigated.
- In appropriate cases joint replacement can be remarkably successful and is an important option to consider in OA and inflammatory arthritis where pain is severe and present at rest, and when mobility is substantially restricted.
- Arthrodesis is rarely indicated.
- Unicondylar osteotomy can aid realignment of the tibiofemoral joint, e.g., in metabolic bone disease such as Paget's disease.

Other

- In OA, capsaicin cream applied three or four times daily to the joints can ease symptoms. Response is cumulative, and may not occur for 6–8 weeks.
- Topical diclofenac gel may also be useful for the treatment of symptomatic osteoarthritis of the hands and knees.

Lower leg and foot disorders (adults)

Anatomy

Anatomy of bones and joints

- The leg absorbs six times the body's weight during weight bearing. Strong ligaments secure the ankle (formed by the tibia above/medially and fibular malleolus laterally) and talocalcaneal (subtalar) joints and bones of the midfoot (see Figure 2.20).
- Anomalous ossicles in the foot are common. Some are associated with specific pathology. There are many potential sites, but the sesamoids in flexor hallucis brevis (FHB) are invariable.
- The foot is an optimal mechanical device to support body weight when walking or running over flat, inclined, and uneven types of terrain. The configuration of bones at synovial articulations allows dorsal flexion (foot pulled up), plantar flexion (to walk on toes), inversion

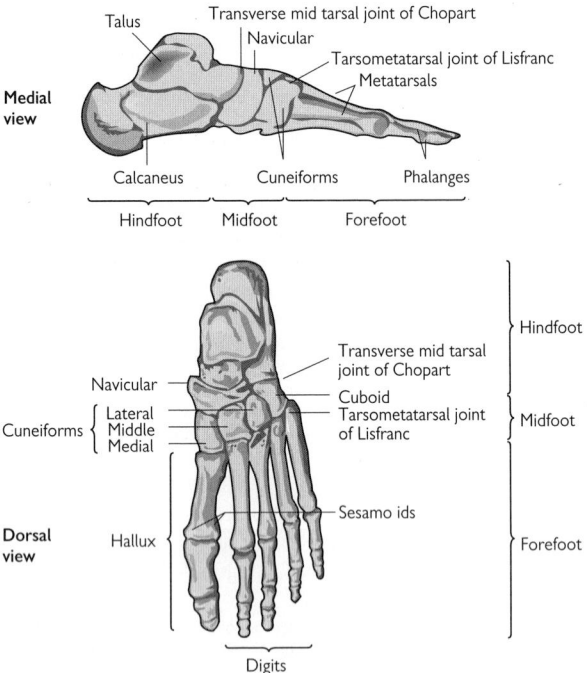

Fig. 2.20 The bones of the foot. Fracture or dislocation at Lisfranc's and Chopart's joints may occur as the result of motor vehicle accidents, falls from a height, or sports injuries (e.g., basketball).

(foot tips in), eversion (foot tips out), and small degrees of adduction and abduction. Midfoot movements allow pronation and supination.

- The normal ankle joint range is about 25° of dorsal flexion and 50° of plantar flexion from neutral (foot 90° to leg). The range of subtalar inversion–eversion is normally 10–15°.

Anatomy of the long muscles and tendons

- In the lower leg, a strong fascia connects the tibia and fibula. Lower leg muscles primarily move the foot. They are separated into compartments by fascia and are prone to pressure effects.
- The foot dorsal flexors—tibialis anterior, extensor digitorum longus (EDL), extensor hallucis longus (EHL) and peroneus tertius—lie adjacent to the anteromedial side of the tibia. Their tendons pass in front of the ankle in synovial sheaths held down by strong retinaculae (see Figure 2.21). The tibialis anterior, the bulkiest flexor, inserts into the medial midfoot (medial cuneiform).
- In the posterior lower leg, the gastrocnemius (and plantaris), which arise from the femur, plantar flexes the foot by pulling the back of

Lateral view of ankle

Common sheath of peroneus longus and brevis tendons

Superior exterior retinacula

Lateral malleolus

Inferior extensor retinacula

Retrocalcaneal bursa

Sheath of extensor digitorum longus and peroneus longus tendons

Subcutaneous calcaneal bursa

Superior and inferior peroneal retinacula

Subcalcaneal bursa

Medial view of ankle

Tibia

Sheath of flexor digitorum longus

Posterior tibial artery

Posterior tibial nerve

Flexor retinaculum

Sheath of flexor digitorum longus

Posterior tibial tendon end sheath

Fig. 2.21 Tendons, retinaculae, and bursae of the hindfoot.

the calcaneum. The soleus, which arises in the lower leg, merges with them in the Achilles tendon. This tendon has a deep and superficial bursa at its insertion site.

- Plantar flexion is assisted weakly by long muscles, which arise in the lower leg, pass behind the medial malleolus in synovial sheaths (see Figure 2.21), and insert into the sole. They mostly invert the foot. Tibialis posterior, the most bulky plantar flexor, inserts into the plantar surface of the navicular.
- The peroneus longus and brevis arise from the fibular side of the leg and pass around the lateral malleolus in a common synovial sheath held by a retinaculum. Longus passes into the sole and inserts into the medial cuneiform. Brevis inserts into the fifth metatarsal base. Both evert the foot.
- The tibial nerve and artery follow the course of the medial tendons under the flexor retinaculum (see Figure 2.21).

Anatomy of intrinsic foot structure

- Intrinsic foot structures have been greatly modified during evolution to combine provision of a flexible platform for support and a rigid lever for thrusting body weight forward when walking.
- In the sole of the foot, muscles are aligned longitudinally in four layers. The deepest layers include phalangeal interossei in the forefeet, tibialis posterior, peroneus longus, adductor hallucis, and FHB—which has two insertions into the proximal great toe phalanx, each containing a sesamoid.
- The superficial layers include flexor digitorum longus (FDL), which inserts into the lateral four distal phalanges, the phalangeal lumbricals, flexor digitorum brevis, and abductor hallucis. The latter two muscles arise from the plantar surface of the calcaneus deep to the plantar fascia.
- Flexor tendons merge with the deeper part of the plantar fascia, a swath of tissue that extends from os calcis to the metatarsal area.
- Longitudinal muscles, ligaments, and fascia contribute to stabilize the foot with a longitudinal arch—its apex at the talus but also with some effect laterally. The foot arches transversely—its apex at medial cuneiform level.

Neuroanatomy

- The sciatic nerve splits into tibial and common peroneal nerves above the knee. The common peroneal is prone to pressure neuropathy as it runs superficially around the fibular head. The nerve then divides. A deep branch runs distally with the EDL under the extensor retinaculum to the foot. It supplies tibialis anterior, EHL, and EDL. A superficial branch supplies the peroneal muscles and most of the skin over the dorsum of the foot.
- The tibial nerve runs in the posterior lower leg compartment supplying the gastrocnemius and soleus. It then passes under the medial flexor retinaculum, dividing into medial and lateral plantar nerves, which supply the intrinsic plantar muscles of the foot and skin of the sole.

Functional anatomy

- In a normal gait pattern, the foot is dorsiflexed and invertors/evertors stabilize the hindfoot for heel strike. As weight is transferred forward, the foot plantar flexes and pronates, the great toe extends (optimally between 65° and 75°), and push off occurs through the medial side of the forefoot.
- All metatarsals bear weight and can suffer weight-bearing injury.
- Ligamentous attachments around the hindfoot are strong. A fall on a pronated inverted foot without direct trauma can result in a fracture of the distal fibula. This is probably a consequence of the relative strength of the talofibular ligaments compared with bone.

Developmental factors

- Developmental characteristics often imply that different age groups are prone to a different spectrum of conditions.
- Due to ligamentous laxity, when babies begin to walk, the midfoot is flat to the floor. A longitudinal arch usually develops by 5 years.
- During growth, tendon insertions (apophyses) are often weaker than the tendons themselves. Traction strain on tendons can lead to apophysitis (osteochondritis). This is a common pattern of injury in the foot in active older children.

Conditions of the lower leg

- Patients with lower leg conditions may present with pain or deformity alone. In children, deformity may typically be due to spinal dysraphism (from birth), rickets (acquired age 1 year plus), or osteogenesis imperfecta (see Chapter 16).
- Pains in the calf may be due to local soft tissue or muscle conditions. In adults, calf pain may be due to claudication or referred lumbosacral pain ("pseudoclaudication"). These pains are often described by patients as "cramps"—suggesting a muscle problem at first. A detailed history may suggest the correct diagnosis.
- Imbalance of muscles in the foot can lead to increased tension at tendon and fascial insertions in the calf and shin, resulting in "shin splints". Shin splints usually present after activity and are relieved by rest. Conditions to consider include:
  - stress fractures of the tibia or fibula
  - tibialis posterior fasciitis—often associated with a flat, pronated foot
  - compartment syndrome (soft tissue and vascular swelling)
  - popliteal artery stenosis
  - referred nerve pain (spinal claudication)
  - peripheral vascular disease (intermittent claudication).

Taking a history

Ask about site and quality of pain in the lower leg

- Localized anterior pain occurs in bony lesions of the anterior tibia, e.g., stress fractures, periostitis, etc. (see "shin splints" in the preceding section, Condition of the Lower Leg).

- Burning pain suggests a neurogenic cause. Diffuse burning pain may be caused by peripheral neuropathy, complex regional pain syndrome (see Chapter 18), or (rarely) erythromelalgia.
- Most commonly occurring in the elderly, bilateral leg pain with "heaviness" or "stiffness" limiting walking distance is typical of spinal stenosis. An alternative would be vascular claudication where often pain is more overt, and critical ischemia can give night pain eased by hanging the legs over the side of the bed (gravity effects).
- Simultaneous knee problems may be relevant. Escape of synovial fluid from the knee into the soft tissues of the calf can present with acute pain and swelling and be misdiagnosed as a deep vein thrombosis ("pseudothrombophlebitis"). Often a history of preceding joint effusion can be elicited.
- Low-lying synovial cysts connecting with the knee can cause calf pain (with or without swelling). This invariably occurs only with chronic synovitis.

Establish possible causes of hindfoot pain (see Table 2.21)

- Establishing the cause of hindfoot pain from the history alone is difficult. There are important clues, mainly from patterns of injury or overuse.
- Posterior heel pain has a few causes. Often clinically indistinguishable from Achilles tendonitis or retrocalcaneal bursitis, enthesitis is usually associated with SpA (see Chapter 8). An os trigonum may become damaged especially in soccer players and ballerinas.
- The origin of plantar heel pain is varied. Mechanical plantar fasciitis is thought to occur more frequently in people who are on their feet for long periods of time, those who are obese, have thin heel fat pads, or poor footwear. Symptoms of arthritis and enthesopathy elsewhere, low back pain (sacroiliitis), eye inflammation (iritis), psoriasis, or previous gut or urethral infection, might suggest SpA.
- Less common causes of plantar heel pain include fracture through a calcaneal spur and lateral plantar nerve entrapment between the fascia of abductor hallucis and quadratus plantae muscles (causing pain/ paresthesias on the lateral side of the sole).
- In the elderly and postmenopausal women, calcaneal stress fractures are a recognized feature of osteoporosis (see Chapter 16) and can present with heel pain.
- Ankle and talocalcaneal synovitis, OA, ankle osteochondritis dissecans, and tendonitis around the hindfoot may be difficult to distinguish from the history alone. Synovitis or an effusion often accompanies OA of these joints.

Establish possible causes of midfoot and first MTP pain

- Gout (see Chapter 7), OA (see Chapter 6), enthesitis, and referred L5 nerve root pain are the most likely diagnoses of midfoot and first MTP pain.
- Any joint may potentially become involved in the major chronic arthropathies.
- Gout should always be considered a possible cause of painful lesions in the foot in people at risk. Gout is not always intra-articular, intrabursal,

Table 2.21 Common conditions causing localized foot pain in children, adolescents, and adults

Site of pain	Common lesions
Ankle region	Ankle or talocalcaneal joint: synovitis (e.g., gout), OA. L4/L5 root pain
Posterior heel	Achilles tendonitis. Retrocalcaneal bursitis. Achilles enthesitis. Osteonecrosis of os trigonum
Medial side of heel	As for ankle region. Calcaneal fracture. Tibialis posterior tendonitis. Plantar fasciitis.
Lateral side of heel	As for ankle region. Calcaneal fracture. Peroneal tendonitis. Fifth metatarsal base fracture*
Underneath heel	Plantar fasciitis. Calcaneal fracture. Infracalcaneal bursitis. Lateral plantar nerve entrapment
Top of foot	Midfoot joint synovitis (e.g., gout), OA. Navicular osteochondritis. Enthesitis. L5 root pain
Sole of foot	S1 root pain. Plantar fasciitis. Metatarsal stress fracture. Tibial/plantar nerve entrapment
Toes	MTP synovitis (e.g., RA, gout). MTP OA. Morton's metatarsalgia. Bursitis. Enthesitis/dactylitis

*Robert–Jones fracture from an inversion–pronation injury.

or **intratendinous**. Local or diffuse soft tissue inflammation is common and often misdiagnosed as cellulitis. Swelling is usually marked.

- L5 pain is referred to the top (dorsum) and S1 pain to the sole of the foot.
- In older adults OA of midfoot joints is common. Mild synovitis can occur with it and may be caused by CPPD crystals (see Chapter 7).

Establish possible causes of forefoot pain

- In those with forefoot pain, typically referred to as metatarsalgia, establish whether the condition is focal or due to arthropathy.
- Pain under the ball of the foot while walking is nonspecific but might suggest any MTP joint abnormality, distal metatarsal stress fracture, Freiberg's disease, plantar nerve neuroma, or bursitis.
- Patients with RA often describe pain under the MTP joints and a feeling of "walking on pebbles" (due to joint swelling and/or subluxation). Synovitis of the MTPs is a very common feature of early RA.
- Acute pain under the forefoot spreading into one or more (adjacent) toes and worse on walking suggests a plantar nerve neuroma (Morton's metatarsalgia) or intermetatarsal bursitis.
- Pain associated with paresthesias or numbness under the forefoot might be due to S1 root irritation (common) or entrapment of the tibial nerve in the hindfoot (rare). Ask about back pain and other hindfoot problems.
- Nontraumatic toe pain associated with swelling of the entire toe suggests a dactylitis (associated with SpA). Although many toes may be affected, the dactylitis may be unilateral and affect just one toe.

- The development of hallux valgus is associated with tight footwear. The established deformity is associated with altered weight bearing and a second toe (hammer) deformity. Big toe pain might be due to hallux rigidus. It is usually due to OA and important to recognize as it may prevent toe dorsiflexion sufficiently to lead to a compromised gait pattern.
- Pain specifically under the hallux may be due to damage of the sesamoids in the flexor hallucis brevis tendon and be misdiagnosed as a joint problem.

Ask for a description of the pain

- As in the hand, neurogenic pain is common and typical.
- Severe or unremitting pain when at rest suggests intrinsic bone pathology. Consider osteonecrosis, infection, fracture, and tumors, e.g., osteoid osteoma.
- Neurogenic pain may be sharp and well defined (e.g., in acute L5 or S1 root pain), deep, achy, and less well defined (e.g., chronic nerve root symptoms as in spinal or foraminal stenosis) or burning in quality. Paresthesias and numbness may accompany both.
- If swelling accompanies neurogenic pain, consider a complex regional pain syndrome. There are numerous triggers, e.g., trauma, surgery. Patients may be unwilling to walk and apparent disability may appear profound.

Weakness

If true weakness is the major problem rather than pain, the diagnosis is usually between a spinal and peripheral nerve lesion (see following section, Examination).

Examination

Observation

Observe the lower legs and feet from front and back while the patient is standing. Note any swelling, deformities, or rashes:

- Lower-leg deformities to note: tibia varum (or bow legs) in an older adult may be due to Paget's disease of the tibia. Muscle wasting might suggest disuse atrophy, old polio, or spinal stenosis (bilateral and subtle usually in older adults).
- Edema or soft tissue swelling may be relevant to an underlying condition, e.g., RA. Although it may cause discomfort, edema from cardiac failure, venous congestion, hypoproteinemia, or lymphedema is not painful unless there are ulcers or thrombophlebitis.
- Gout can cause swelling anywhere; gouty tenosynovitis can mimic the appearance of a cellulitis in the region of a joint.
- Calf swelling may be due to vein thrombosis or ruptured popliteal cyst.
- Common patterns of foot deformity are:
  - flat feet (pes planus)
  - high-arched feet (pes cavus) with high medial arch
  - hallux valgus and rigidus
  - overriding, hammer, and claw toes.
- Skin conditions from venous abnormalities are common in the elderly. Other skin lesions which may be relevant include purpura, panniculitis—which is often subtle and over the shins—and pyoderma gangrenosum.

Ask the patient to walk in bare feet

Gait patterns should be noted:

- An antalgic ("limp and wince") gait is a nonspecific indicator of pain.
- A wide-based gait (>10 cm wider than normal) suggests instability: joint instability, muscle weakness, or neurologic lesions may be the cause.
- A foot that slaps down or a high stepping gait suggests tibialis anterior weakness (L4 nerve root or common peroneal nerve lesion).
- Significant weakness of gluteus medius and gluteus maximus in L5 and S1 root lesions respectively can result in lurching during gait. In the former, as weight is taken on the affected side, gluteus medius may be weak in controlling the small 2–3 cm lateral displacement in the weight-bearing hip that normally occurs. This can be compensated for if the body center of gravity is brought over the hip by lurching the upper body over the affected side. With gluteus maximus lesions (S1) extension of the hip, which helps mediate motion through the stance phase prior to toeing-off, may be weak. Thrusting the thorax forward with an arched back (forward lurch) compensates for the weakness and helps to maintain hip extension.
- A flat-footed gait with little or weak toe-off may suggest an S1 root lesion; however, "flat-foot" (loss of the medial arch) with associated hind foot eversion and heel pain (plantar fasciitis) is extremely common. Often the arch weakness corrects when the patient is asked to walk.

Examine the lower leg

With the patient supine on the couch, examine the lower leg:

- After a ruptured popliteal (Baker's) cyst, calf tissues are often diffusely tender and swollen. Calf circumferences can be compared (e.g., 10 cm below tibial tubercle). There may also be mild skin erythema. Findings are not specific. Gout and infection (see Chapters 7 and 17) are the main alternatives if there is marked tenderness.
- Check for bruising, swelling, and tenderness around the fibula head in patients with foot drop (possible peroneal nerve palsy). Neurologic examination may be done at this point.
- Localized anterior tibial tenderness is often found in patients with stress fractures or with pseudofractures (osteomalacia—see Chapter 16).
- Tibial deformity in adults may be associated with diffuse bony tenderness and heat (arteriovenous shunting) in Paget's disease (see Chapter 16).

Examine the ankle and hindfoot

At the ankle and hindfoot, examine for joint and tendon synovitis, palpate specific structures and test passive hindfoot joint mobility:

- Synovitis of hindfoot joints is not always easily detected. With ankle joint synovitis, thickened tissue may be felt anteriorly in the ankle crease (where there may be a "springy fullness") or laterally around the malleoli.

- Posterior tibial and peroneal tendonitis are associated with soft tissue swelling of the medial and lateral hindfoot, respectively. Synovial thickening from ankle and talocalcaneal joints may also be felt here and synovitis of structures may coexist in RA or SpA. Pain from resisted movement of tendons may not be specific.
- Pathology of medial hindfoot structures may be associated with tibial nerve entrapment resulting in sensory symptoms on the sole of the foot. There may be a positive Tinel's sign.
- Posterior heel pain may be due to Achilles tendonitis, enthesitis and mechanical damage to the tendon, and retrocalcaneal bursitis. Deep tenderness may suggest an os trigonum lesion.
- The loss of passive hindfoot movements is not specific and can be associated with any cause of ankle or subtalar arthritis (20°–30° of dorsiflexion and 45°–55° of plantar flexion is average for the ankle and a 10°–20° inversion–eversion range is average for the subtalar joint). Subtalar joint movement can be difficult to test accurately.
- The pain of plantar fasciitis may be elicited by firm palpation of the medial underside of the calcaneum. A negative test does not rule out pathology, as often the history is more sensitive. Full musculoskeletal examination is required to check for features of SpA such as arthritis/enthesitis elsewhere and sacroiliitis.

Examine for midfoot lesions
Identifying specific midfoot lesions is difficult, though bony landmarks and discrete tender areas can be noted:
- Twisting the midfoot may elicit pain nonspecifically. Common lesions include gout, OA, and synovitis associated with RA and SpA.
- Bony tenderness alone without soft tissue swelling does not rule out synovitis of an adjacent joint.
- The midfoot is a typical site for neuroarthropathy in diabetes.
- Bony lumps (exostoses) that may have formed at sites of pressure are common in the foot (e.g., medial or dorsal aspect of the first MTP joint, base or head of the fifth metatarsal, distal talus, or over the midfoot). In the elderly bony pain and skin sores may form at these sites.
- Both gout and infection result in swelling, skin erythema and localized tenderness. Gout of the first MTP joint occurs at any one time in 70% of patients with the condition. It can occur anywhere in the foot.

Examine the forefoot
Check for bony or other swelling, digit separation, and examine the sole of the foot. Squeezing the whole forefoot at the line of the MTP joints is a nonspecific but useful screening test for painful forefoot lesions:
- Tender swelling of the whole toe (dactylitis) occurs in SpA (see Chapter 8), sarcoid (see Chapter 18), and HIV infection (see Chapter 17). Swelling is soft not bony. Tender bony swelling suggests a bunion and is common on the dorsal aspect of the toes and the first and fifth MTP joints.
- Forefoot splaying and interdigital separation suggests MTP synovitis or interdigital bursitis. MTP joints may be individually tender (simultaneously palpated with thumb below and finger above).

- Tenderness between metatarsal heads is typical in Morton's metatarsalgia. There may be a sensory deficit in the interdigital cleft. The differential diagnosis (in adolescents) may be osteochondritis of the second and third metatarsal head.
- Check for hallux rigidus—passive dorsiflexion should be at least 50°. Extending the big toe passively can reveal an ability to form a medial longitudinal arch in patients with flat feet (Jack's test).
- Discrete bony tenderness without swelling occurs with stress fractures.
- Uneven callus distribution under the forefoot may suggest an abnormally focused area of weight bearing and an underlying mechanical abnormality.
- Rashes on the sole of the foot are uncommon but important to consider are: pompholyx, pustular psoriasis, and keratoderma blennorrhagica (see Reactive Arthropathy in Chapter 8).
- Loss of sensation under the forefoot may be due to an S1 root lesion, peripheral neuropathy (e.g., diabetes), mononeuritis (e.g., vasculitis—see Chapter 14), Sjögren's syndrome (see Chapter 11), mixed connective tissue disease), or, rarely, tibial nerve entrapment (examine hindfoot).

Neurologic examination
Neurologic examination is essential in cases where pain is neurogenic or there is weakness, numbness, or paresthesias (see Table 2.22).

Diagnostic procedures
Imaging of the lower leg
- Suspected tibial abnormalities such as stress fractures and pseudofractures in osteomalacia and Paget's disease have characteristic radiological appearances.
- Periosteal changes occur in trauma, psoriatic arthritis (above ankle), hypertrophic pulmonary osteoarthropathy (HPOA), and pachydermal periostitis.
- In athletes with exercise-related pain, a triple-phase bone scan is part of the work-up for anterior shin pain.
- In suspected (but radiograph-negative) cases of bony disease such as cortical stress fracture, periostitis, or cortical hyperostosis, a bone scan may be useful to identify subtle pathology.

Imaging of the foot
Information available on radiographs of the hindfoot includes:
- Increased soft-tissue attenuation around the tendon insertion in cases of Achilles tendonitis or retrocalcaneal bursitis.
- Erosions or periostitis at the Achilles tendon insertion in enthesitis associated with SpA.
- Erosions in gout and RA-associated retrocalcaneal bursitis.
- Axial radiographs of the hindfoot are useful in showing talocalcaneal joint abnormalities, e.g., in RA.
- If radiographs are normal in patients with posterior heel pain, US can show patterns of tendon and bursal inflammation. MR can further characterize any discrete pattern of tendon injury.

Table 2.22 Patterns of common abnormal examination findings in lower lumbar nerve root lesions

Nerve root	Abnormal finding
L4	Weakness of ankle dorsiflexion (tibialis anterior)
	Patient finds walking on their heel difficult (strong ankle dorsiflexion needed)*
	Reduced knee reflex (L3 and L4)
L5	Weakness of big toe dorsiflexion (extensor hallucis longus)
	Weakness of foot eversion (peroneal muscles, also S1)
	Sensory deficit over dorsum of foot
	Reduced ankle reflex (L5 and S1)
S1	Weakness of ankle plantar flexion (gastrocnemius and soleus)
	Patient finds walking on, or repeatedly rising onto, tiptoe difficult*
	Sensory deficit over sole of foot
	Reduced ankle reflex

* Maneuvers may be affected by pain, making interpretation difficult.

- Osteonecrosis of an os trigonum or posterior talar process or tarsal navicular may be identified by radiographs. It is invariably located by bone scan and can be characterized further, usually with soft tissue swelling, by MR.
- A plantar spur does not denote current plantar fasciitis.
- Plantar heel pain may be due to a fracture in a spur. Erosions just above the spur may be seen. The thickness of heel fat pad can be gauged from its X-ray attenuation (thin = risk for plantar fasciitis). A fat pad >23 mm thick in men and >21.5 mm thick in women is associated with acromegaly.
- Calcaneal fractures or an osteoid osteoma can be seen in some cases with radiographs alone. Bone scans/CT are more sensitive.
- Patterns of joint, enthesis, and tendon inflammation can be documented using MR or bone scan. This is useful information when characterizing an arthropathy.
- Bony abnormalities in the mid and forefoot are generally revealed by radiographs alone, though metatarsal stress fractures may be missed. MR can discriminate a plantar neuroma from interdigital bursitis and MTP joint synovitis. The former are probably best initially demonstrated by US.

Other Diagnostic procedures
- Neurophysiology is a useful adjunct to clinical examination in diagnosis of lower limb neuropathies, and can help discriminate between peripheral (common peroneal or sciatic) or nerve root causes of foot drop, and also S1 root or tibial nerve entrapment causes of paresthesias of the sole of the foot.

- Joint/bursa fluid aspiration is mandatory in suspected cases of sepsis and should be sent for culture (remember to consider gonococcus in young adults and TB in patients from endemic or inner-city areas). Fluid should be sent for polarized microscopy if a crystal-induced disease is suspected.
- Laboratory tests requested should reflect suspicion of specific infective, inflammatory, metabolic, or malignant pathology.

Treatment

Lower leg disorders

- Anterior shin pain should be treated according to cause. If there is also a problem of foot alignment then orthoses that support both the hind foot and mid arch may be very useful. Patients may volunteer that good walking shoes or sneakers help (as is the case with plantar fasciitis).
- Exercise-induced lower leg pain has a number of causes and includes shin splints and compartment syndrome. The latter may require further investigation with pressure readings or exercise scintigraphy (^{99m}Tc-MIBI). In cases resistant to rest, analgesia, and modification of triggering factors, decompressive surgery may be required.
- Patients with Paget's disease of the tibia may require treatment with high-dose bisphosphonates and will need a biomechanical assessment.

Ankle and hindfoot disorders

- Tendonitis around the ankle should respond to treatment of its underlying cause. Chronic posterior tibial tendonitis left untreated will eventually accelerate the development of hindfoot valgus. Consider heel and arch support orthotics early.
- Plantar fasciitis may respond to a number of conservative measures:
  - heel pads and/or supportive shoes
  - modification of weight-bearing activity
  - Achilles tendon stretching
  - hindfoot strapping
  - resting night splint (preventing ankle plantar flexion)
  - steroid injection around medial calcaneal tubercle
  - surgery

Forefoot disorders

- Localized forefoot pain, e.g., metatarsalgia, may respond to support pads and a change to a wider, more supportive, low-heel shoe. The opinion of a podiatrist or orthopedic surgeon should be sought as required.
- Forefoot stress fractures and metatarsal head osteochondritis require rest, supportive footwear and time to heal.
- Patients with chronic forefoot pain may benefit from a podiatric assessment. "Stress offloading" foot orthoses for metatarsalgia and other biomechanical abnormalities (e.g., hallux rigidus) can be individually molded using thermoplastic materials.

Steroid injections (see also Corticosteroid Injection Therapy)

Steroid injections may be of value in the following:
- Ankle joint inflammation (e.g., RA, OA, gout)

- Subtalar joint inflammation
- Tarsal tunnel syndrome
- Achilles peritendinitis (local steroid injections for Achilles' nodules should be avoided if possible as the risk of rupture is high. The same concern, though probably lesser risk, applies to Achilles' peritendinitis)
- Calcaneal apophysitis (Sever's disease—Achilles' tendon insertion)
- Retrocalcaneal bursitis
- Plantar fasciitis
- Gout/OA/enthesitis at first MTP joint

Surgery
- Minor surgical techniques can be curative in tarsal tunnel syndrome and in excising an interdigital (Morton's) neuroma. Consider excision of painful exostoses and troublesome rheumatoid nodules and amputation of deformed or overriding toes.
- Major surgical procedures with good outcomes in appropriate patients include fusion of hindfoot joints and forefoot arthroplasty in chronic inflammatory arthritides. Osteotomy realignment of a hallux valgus deformity can be successful in the long term.

Child and adolescent foot disorders

For a review of classification criteria of autoimmune juvenile arthritides see Chapter 7.

Background

Lower limb and foot deformities of babies may be noticed first by parents. Diagnostic evaluation needs to focus on ruling out major congenital disease and exploring biomechanical factors.

- Neonatal deformities of the leg are uncommon.
- Talipes equinovarus (club foot) is an important deformity, which presents at birth. It is most commonly idiopathic and it is associated with wasting of the lower leg muscles. Causes to consider and rule out are spina bifida, spinal dysraphism, cerebral palsy, and arthrogryposis.
- With babies, persistence of certain sleeping postures is associated with patterns of angular and torsion deformity involving the whole leg. Postures include prone sleeping with knees tucked up under the chest, hips extended, or in a "frog's-legs" position.
- In children able to walk, the most common conditions that present to pediatric orthopedic clinics are in-toeing and flat feet, though serious causes of flat feet usually affect only older children. Important points in evaluating an in-toeing deformity and flat feet are shown in Table 2.23. Some deformities in this group have been associated with persistence of sitting postures, e.g., cross-legged or "reverse tailor" (floor sitting, knees bent and legs splayed out/back) positions.
- Achiness in the feet is the typical symptom in young children with torsional leg deformities of significance. If the biomechanical problem is sufficiently severe, shoes can wear out quickly.
- Regional musculoskeletal lesions in children <3 years of age are rare but most inflammatory arthritides can affect foot joints. Pain from an inflamed joint results in a miserable child and a refusal to walk.
- Periosteal pain (hyperostosis) in the tibia and other long bones occurs in Caffey's disease. There is usually symmetric limb enlargement in this rare condition, which usually occurs before the baby is 6 months old.

Taking a history

Ask about the site and quality of the pain

- Lower leg pain may be due to one of the causes of "shin splints", a bone lesion, or complex regional pain syndrome.
- Localized anterior lower leg pain occurs in lesions of the anterior tibia e.g., stress fractures, periostitis, tibial tubercle osteochondritis, but deeper more diffuse anterior pain (often also medial) occurs in "shin splints" (see below).
- Minimal or nontraumatic tibial fracture associated with fracture or bony deformity elsewhere raises the possibility of osteogenesis imperfecta.
- Localized or diffuse burning pain suggests a neurogenic cause. In children, disc prolapse is rare. Superficial burning pain may be due to peripheral neuropathy or complex regional pain syndrome.

Table 2.23 Common patterns of foot deformity in babies and infants

Deformity	Most common causes	Features
In-toeing	Metatarsus varus	Presents age 0–3 months or when starts to walk. Examination: forefoot varus only (heel is in neutral or valgus). Over 80% correct without surgery though predicting which will is difficult: "wait and see until age 3" is appropriate
	Torsional lower limb deformity—medial tibial torsion and/or excessive femoral anteversion	Often related to regular prone knee–chest (fetal) sleeping position in babies and toddlers, and persistently sitting on the floor with legs forward internally rotated and knees bent out/backwards in children (see Fig. 2.21)
	Cerebral palsy	Most often caused by excessive femoral anteversion
	Spinal dysraphism	Rare
Flat feet (pes planus)	Idiopathic or familial, hereditary connective tissue diseases, hindfoot disease: tarsal coalitions, arthritis, osteochondritis, infection etc.	Very common—often asymptomatic. Children often develop medial arch with time (passive big toe extension or standing on toes often reveals it). It is associated with conditions of general tissue laxity. If it occurs with pain and/or stiff flat feet look for peroneal muscle spasm and hindfoot pathology as the cause
Talipes equinovarus (club-foot)	Idiopathic, spina bifida, spinal dysraphism, tibial dysplasia, cerebral palsy, arthrogryposis	Incidence 1–2:1000 overall. Presents at birth. Idiopathic (etiology unknown) is most common. Often a family history. Examination: calf wasting, hindfoot and forefoot in equinus (plantaris) and varus
Pes cavus	Idiopathic, peroneal muscular atrophy	High arch (medial and lateral sides), toe clawing. Associated with neurologic disease rarely e.g., Friedrich's ataxia

- Complex regional pain syndrome (see Chapter 18) typically gives burning pain, although it can occur with dull, aching pain or paroxysms. Pain often disturbs sleep. In children it is more common in the lower leg and foot than in the upper limb. Diffuse swelling and skin changes may be present. In many cases trauma is a triggering event but anything from simple sprains to arthroscopic knee surgery can trigger it; 25% are idiopathic.
- In children, complex regional pain syndrome may occur in the limb distal to an arthritic joint.

- Unremitting, sleep-disturbing pain that is worse on weight bearing suggests bone or bone marrow pathology e.g., bone tumors, osteomyelitis, or periostitis (hypertrophic pulmonary osteoarthropathy, Gaucher's disease).

Ask about pain onset during sports

There are typical sports injuries of the lower leg that occur relatively often in active children and adolescents. Ask about pain onset during sports or recurrence during or after specific activities:

- Adolescents may refer to "shin splints." Possible conditions include: tibial stress fracture, Osgood–Schlatter's disease, tibialis posterior fasciitis, compartment syndrome, popliteal artery stenosis, and malalignment of the hind- and midfoot.
- Tibial fascial inflammation and pain typically occurs as running begins. Patients can run through it, but it often returns severely after exercise and takes days to wear off. It is associated with hyperpronation of the foot (which increases stretch forces on the tendon).
- Compartment syndrome can be acute (due to muscle necrosis) or chronic. The chronic form occurs almost exclusively in endurance sports. Pain is absent at rest but builds as exercise progresses. It diminishes gradually—usually within a few hours. The pattern of pain and findings from perfusion scintigraphy suggest the cause of pain is ischemic. Increased compartment pressures can be demonstrated by invasive monitoring.
- Pain from major vessel ischemia (i.e., claudication) typically occurs with exercise. Muscle or a fibrous band in the popliteal fossa can compress the popliteal artery.
- Stress fractures occur in young athletes. In girls there may be an association with amenorrhea and generalized osteopenia.

Are there regional traumatic lesions?

In the foot, regional traumatic lesions are quite common, particularly in active children and athletes. Chronic arthritides should be considered:

- Apophysitides (osteochondritides) are quite common (see Table 2.24). Most present with localized pain during exercise. There is tenderness and often swelling and pain on resisted movement of the appropriate tendon.
- Proximal midfoot pain may be caused by an accessory navicular, navicular osteochondritis (Köhler's disease), and tarsal coalitions (abnormal joins between bones leading to joint hypomobility, bilateral in 50% of cases). All lesions may be associated with a rigid flat foot (peroneal spastic flat foot) and will be more painful on weight bearing.
- Joint synovitis (pain with immobility-related stiffness) is often difficult to detect clinically. Ankle synovitis is the easiest to be confident about. Soft or springy swelling with tenderness over the dorsal skin crease often suggests an effusion. Synovial thickening can be felt in florid cases circumferentially or just around the lower margins of the malleoli. In oligoarticular JIA the ankle joint is sometimes painlessly swollen.
- Juvenile SpA/ERA is rare in children aged <8, and up until that age oligo/polyarticular JIA is a more likely cause of joint synovitis in the

Table 2.24 Localized painful foot disorders specific to school-age children and adolescents. Tumors are rare but osteoid osteoma should be considered

Site of pain	Disorder	Characteristics of disorder
Posterior heel	Calcaneal apophysitis (Sever's disease)	Traction osteochondritis. Both sexes age 8–10 years
Dorsal midfoot	Accessory navicular	Common finding in all children (50%). In 75% it fuses with main navicular. Majority not painful. Rarely it is associated with exercise-related pain
	Navicular osteochondritis (Köhler's disease).	Boys > girls. Presents with pain, limp and weight bearing on the outside of the foot
	Tarsal coalitions	Asymptomatic or with peroneal spastic (rigid) flat foot (8–16 years)
Medial side of foot (may be diffuse)	Hypermobile flat foot	Children 1–5 years. May have generalized tissue laxity
Lateral side of foot	5th metatarsal base osteochondritis (Iselin's disease)	Children 10–12 years. Possibly due to tendon ossification and related to tight shoes
Dorsal and plantar distal midfoot	Stress fracture (rare)	Adolescents—2nd/3rd metatarsal
	Metatarsal head osteochondritis (Freiberg's disease)	Commonly 2nd metatarsal head. Affects active adolescent girls most frequently

foot. Juvenile SpA/ERA may present with synovitis in a single lower limb joint, enthesitis at the Achilles tendon insertion or plantar fasciitis.

- Dactylitis ("sausage toe") raises the possibility of psoriatic arthritis or sarcoid. History usually discriminates the pattern of arthritis that helps in the differential diagnosis.
- The most common other arthritides to involve foot joints are viral and poststreptococcal arthritis and Lyme disease.
- Diffuse foot swelling occasionally occurs with synovitis in oligo/polyarticular JIA. The major differential is complex regional pain syndrome. Both pains are worse at night. Sensory symptoms are prominent and skin changes common in established complex regional pain syndrome.
- Forefoot pain in adolescents may be due to an interdigital neuroma (Morton's metatarsalgia) or osteochondritis of a metatarsal head (Freiberg's osteochondritis). Neuroma pain is often associated with dysesthesia and numbness between the toes.
- Big toe pain from hallux rigidus (<50° passive dorsiflexion) is rare but can occur after injury and prevent running.
- Unlike in adults, gout occurs rarely in children and usually only in the context of renal failure, glucose 6-phosphatase deficiency (von

Gierke's), malignancy, or X chromosome-linked disorders of uric acid metabolism.

Examination

Observe the lower legs from front and back while the patient is standing:

- Lower leg muscle wasting occurs in hereditary sensorimotor neuropathy (bilateral) and typically accompanies spinal dysraphism. Diffuse muscle hypertrophy might suggest muscular dystrophy.
- Extremity swelling occurs in some forms of JIA (see Chapter 7), vasculitis (e.g., Henoch–Schönlein purpura (HSP)—see Chapter 14) and sepsis (see Chapter 17).
- Note the appearance and distribution of any rashes. Skin conditions from venous abnormalities are common. Other skin lesions that may be relevant include purpura (HSP) and panniculitis over the shins (erythema nodosum/sarcoid—see Chapter 18).

Observe the feet from front and back while the patient is standing

- Look for swelling and patterns of deformity. Patterns of deformity may require detailed orthopedic assessment. Check the gait.
- Look for localized edema—an occasional sign of underlying JIA but also present in nephrotic syndrome and in systemic vasculitides.
- Some torsional leg deformities are clinically significant. The most common pattern is with the hip internally rotated (usually excessive femoral anteversion), the tibia compensating in external rotation, and associated hindfoot valgus and forefoot varus.
- Flat feet are often asymptomatic and familial, and regress as the child grows (the medial arch becomes evident standing on tiptoe and with passive big toe dorsiflexion). Hindfoot pathology may be a cause.

Examine the sitting patient

With the patient sitting on the edge of the couch, check for tibial torsion:

- Tibial torsion is measured as the angle between an imaginary line through the tibial tubercle in the sagittal plane and the perpendicular of an imaginary line through the malleoli (see Figure 2.22).

Examine the supine patient

With the patient supine on the couch, examine the lower leg:

- Check for bruising, swelling, and tenderness around the fibular head in patients with foot drop (peroneal nerve palsy).
- Localized anterior tibial tenderness is often found in patients with stress fractures.

Examine for swellings in the foot

- Bony lumps (exostoses) that may have formed at sites of pressure (e.g., a "pump bump" at the posterior heel).
- Swelling, skin erythema and localized tenderness suggests infection, although synovitis, skin vasculitis and panniculitis (e.g., erythema nodosum) should also be considered.

Examine the hindfoot

In the hindfoot, examine for joint and tendon synovitis, palpate specific structures, and test passive hindfoot joint mobility:

- Synovitis of hindfoot joints is not always easily detected. With ankle joint synovitis thickened tissue may be felt anteriorly in the ankle crease (where there may be a "springy fullness", like foam rubber) or laterally around the malleoli.
- The pain of plantar fasciitis may be elicited by firm palpation of the medial underside of the calcaneum. ERA should be ruled out.
- Posterior tibial and peroneal tendonitis are associated with soft tissue swelling of the medial and lateral hindfoot, respectively. Synovial thickening from ankle and talocalcaneal joints may also be felt there and synovitis of structures may coexist in JIA or ERA. Resisting a tendon's movement to elicit specific tendon pain may not be a specific test.
- Painful posterior heel structures are usually easily palpated, though pain may be due to a number of causes including Achilles' enthesitis, mechanical damage to the tendon, retrocalcaneal bursitis, and apophysitis.
- The loss of passive hindfoot movements is not specific. Often due to ankle synovitis, stiffness may also occur in other causes of joint pain (e.g., osteochondritis dissecans) and cases of peroneal spastic flat foot. The hindfeet of children are more mobile than those of adults.
- Peroneal spastic (rigid) flat foot syndrome should be distinguished from flexible flat foot (when the medial longitudinal arch reappears when standing on the toes or with passive big toe dorsiflexion). Pain is centered on the dorsomedial side of the foot. The medial longitudinal arch is deficient. Associated peroneal muscle spasm may be painful. The age of presentation depends on the etiology, the most common cause being tarsal coalition. It is always important to consider cerebral palsy and spinal dysraphism as well as local lesions: tumors (e.g., osteoid osteoma of calcaneum); navicular osteochondritis (Köhler's); local osteomyelitis or pyogenic arthritis; ankle or talocalcaneal joint synovitis (e.g., JIA). AP, lateral, oblique, and axial talocalcaneal radiographs, a three-phase bone scan, and hindfoot CT may all be useful in defining associated hindfoot lesions.

Examine the midfoot

In the midfoot determine any sites of tenderness and stiffness:

- Twisting the midfoot may elicit pain from lesions, although this can be nonspecific.
- The major condition to rule out in teenagers is tarsal coalitions. These are fibrous, cartilaginous, or osseous joins between bones resulting in no or little mobility. The most commonly involved joints are the calcaneonavicular and the talocalcaneal. They may be tender. Passive movement with inversion is usually painful and increases spasm in peroneal muscles.
- A tender navicular may also be due to osteochondritis.
- Synovitis associated with some forms of JIA can occur at any joint. The precise location is often difficult to identify clinically.

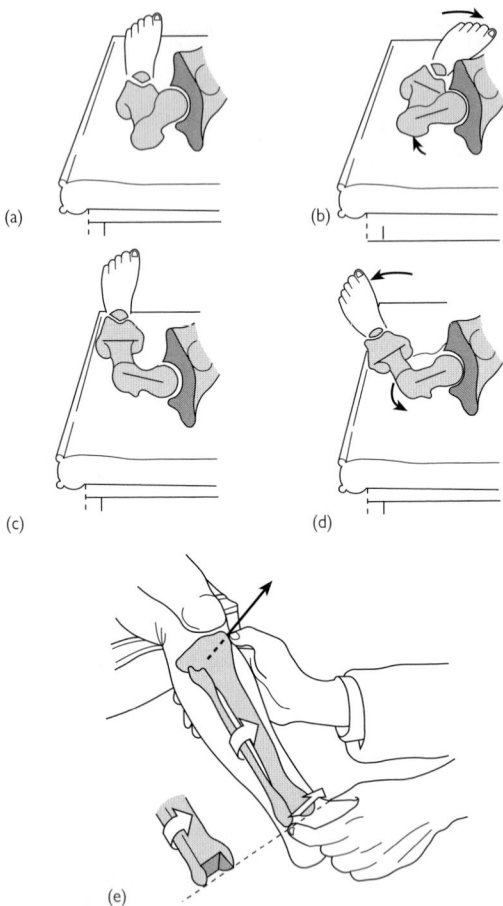

Fig. 2.22 Femoral anteversion, retroversion, and tibial torsion. (a) Where the femoral neck angulates excessively forward relative to an imaginary axis through the femoral condyles, the hip is anteverted. (b) Femoral neck anteversion can lead to a greater-than-usual range of hip internal rotation and a toe-in gait. (c) and (d) Retroversion, where the femoral neck angulates posteriorly relative to a femoral condyle axis, can cause a toe-out gait. (e) Toeing can also be caused by excessive medial tibial torsion. Normally the ankle mortise faces 15° externally relative to a sagittal plane axis through the tibial tubercle (arrow) but in medial torsion it faces forward or internally.

Examine the forefoot

Check for bony or other swelling, look for digit separation, examine the digits and the sole of the forefoot. Squeezing the whole forefoot at the line of MTPs is a useful but nonspecific screening test for painful forefoot lesions:

- Dactylitis (psoriatic arthritis or sarcoid) swelling is soft, not bony.
- Forefoot splaying and interdigital separation suggests MTP synovitis. MTPs may be tender when palpated (simultaneously with thumb below and finger above).
- Tenderness between two metatarsal heads is typical in Morton's neuroma. The differential (in adolescents) may be osteochondritis of the second or third metatarsal head.
- Extending the big toe passively can reveal an ability to form a medial longitudinal arch in patients with flat feet (Jack's test).
- Discrete bony tenderness without swelling may occur with stress fractures.
- Loss of sensation under the forefoot is rare. Full back and neurologic leg examination may be necessary.

Diagnostic procedures

Imaging of the lower leg

- Radiographs of the lower leg have characteristic patterns of abnormality in osteogenesis imperfecta, rickets, and some periosteal conditions, e.g., from stress fracture or periostitis, etc.
- Bone scan is a sensitive investigation for radiograph-negative cases of suspected bone disease. It is also a useful initial investigation in adolescents with shin splints as it will rule out stress fractures and can show tibialis fasciitis.
- Treadmill or cycle ergometer exercise scintigraphy using ^{99m}Tc-MIBI can be useful in revealing compartment perfusion defects in athletes with ischemic-type pain during exercise (another cause of shin splints).

Imaging of the foot

Local lesions require investigation with radiographs, but in patients with inflammatory or bony lesions, further imaging may be necessary:

- Routine AP and lateral hindfoot radiographs will reveal most cases of Sever's disease and osteochondritis dissecans of the ankle. Some cases of talocalcaneal coalition will require extra views and CT for diagnosis.
- In patients with a rigid flat foot, additional oblique and axial view radiographs of the hindfoot help show osteoarticular abnormalities if routine AP and lateral views do not. The gold-standard investigation is CT which is used to plan for surgery.
- Forefoot radiographs are a good screening test in those with forefoot pain. Radiographs are insensitive for detecting early synovitis, but are useful for identifying osteochondritides, hallux abnormalities, and the pattern of established arthritis.
- It is important to check a radiograph for first MTP osteochondritis dissecans in those with hallux rigidus.
- Isolated soft tissue swelling may be due to complex regional pain syndrome, underlying synovitis, or infection. Radiographs are

mandatory. Bone scan may be nonspecific in this setting, but can be useful to diagnose complex regional pain syndrome.
- MR of the whole foot or swollen area is the quickest way to an advanced differential diagnosis.
- Where swelling, pain, and tenderness coexist, infection must be ruled out using imaging. If it cannot and suspicion remains, tissue or fluid sampling should be undertaken. In most cases it is appropriate to do this under general anesthesia. Complex regional pain syndrome should be excluded before any intervention.

Laboratory tests

Any possibility of joint synovitis (most likely at the ankle), enthesitis, tendonitis, or infection requires investigation with laboratory tests:
- ESR and CRP are likely to be raised in cases of inflammatory arthritis and infection, and are more likely to be normal or only slightly increased in oligoarticular JIA and juvenile ERA compared with polyarticular and systemic JIA or infection.
- Normochromic anemia (± mild microcytosis) is a nonspecific sign of a systemic condition. CBC may be normal in oligoarticular JIA. Leukocytosis is typical with infection, with steroids and in systemic JIA.
- Thrombocytosis can be seen in all forms of JIA. If the ESR and CRP are elevated, but the platelet count is low, malignancy should be considered.
- Moderately elevated titers of ANA may be present in 40–75% of patients with oligoarticular JIA; a positive ANA is a risk factor for associated uveitis. Even minimally symptomatic uveitis can threaten vision if not treated.
- Check for circulating rheumatoid factor (RF) and anti-citrullinated protein antibodies (ACPA) in cases of synovitis. High titers are expected in (RF+) polyarticular JIA.

Treatment

Lower leg disorders
- Anterior shin pain should be treated according to cause.
- Treat foot alignment problems with appropriate orthotics.
- Review diagnosis if conservative treatment fails, e.g., is there an underlying stress fracture or periostitis? Consider obtaining a bone scan.

Ankle and foot disorders
- The management of bony anomalies/deformities should be discussed with an orthopedic surgeon and physical therapist early, to avoid missing an opportunity to prevent growth abnormalities.
- Be aware that soft-tissue steroid injection of a presumed local lesion may impair healing/growth at apophyses and may aggravate the symptoms of (missed) complex regional pain syndrome.
- Consider intra-articular steroid injection of specific joints in oligoarticular JIA if joints can be clearly identified by bone scan or MR. Use of sedation (adolescents) or light general anesthesia (toddlers/children) may be appropriate.

Corticosteroid injection therapy

Background

- Local anesthetic and steroid injection into joints or soft tissues is a very effective treatment for localized pain.
- Injection offers a local maximal anti-inflammatory effect with minimal systemic absorption.
- The indications for local steroid injection include: to reduce inflammation in joints, entheses, tendon sheaths and bursa; to relieve pain from inflammatory ligament lesions; to relieve inflammation at sites of nerve compression; to attempt to reduce the size of nodules and ganglia; to relieve pain at trigger points; and as part of epidurals.
- The contraindications are:
  - Absolute:
    — septic arthritis/septicemia
    — febrile patient, cause unknown
    — serious allergy to previous injection
    — sickle cell disease
  - Relative:
    — neutropenia, thrombocytopenia
    — anticoagulation or bleeding disorder.
- Hydrocortisone acetate is a short-acting, weak anti-inflammatory, useful for superficial lesions such as tendons and bursae. A dose of 25 mg is typical.
- Methylprednisolone acetate (40 mg/ml), prednisolone acetate (25 mg/ml), and triamcinolone acetonide (10 and 40 mg/ml) are long-acting synthetic agents suitable for joint injections.
- Small joints accept only a small volume; thus, for IPs, MCPs, MTPs, ACs, and TMs, 0.5 ml of triamcinolone acetate (10 mg) is appropriate. All other joints should accept at least 1ml. Choice of strength of steroid remains empiric. There may be merit in diluting the steroid in sterile saline, to increase volume for better distribution in larger joints.
- The patient should be warned of potential, though uncommon, side-effects:
  - exacerbation of pain for 24–48 h
  - septic arthritis and reactivation of TB
  - tissue atrophy (less likely with hydrocortisone than others)
  - depigmentation
  - anaphylaxis
  - nerve damage
  - tendon rupture
  - avascular necrosis
  - cartilage damage
  - soft-tissue calcification
  - temporary exacerbation of hyperglycemia in diabetes.
- As a general rule it is recommended that any one joint should not be injected more than four times in 12 months and there are at least 6 weeks between injections.
- Children and some adolescents usually require a light general anesthetic for most joint injections given the procedure can be quite

traumatic. An alternative for older children or those who have had many injections done before is to use local anesthetic gel pads (e.g., EMLA® patch) to numb skin adequately before the injection.

Principles of injection techniques

The procedure need not necessarily be done in a sterile environment. Some steps below illustrate the need to maintain relatively aseptic conditions:

- Mark the exact spot of needle insertion.
- Wash hands. Use sterile gloves for procedure.
- Clean the skin with povidone-iodine and allow to dry.
- Anesthetize the skin (either with local anesthetic or refrigerant alcohol spray).
- Insert clean needle with empty syringe and aspirate back.
- Leave needle in place, detach syringe, and place syringe containing drug onto end of needle.
- Pull back syringe plunger again before injecting to confirm placement.
- Introduction of steroid should be effortless. Resistance implies that the needle is in the wrong space.
- On completion, remove syringe and needle and throw away "sharps".
- Cover the injection site with clean gauze or bandage.
- Re-emphasize possible side effects and benefits.

The glenohumeral joint

- The anterior route gives reliable access in patients with adhesive capsulitis. It is also better suited for aspiration of joint effusions.
- Palpate the coracoid process anteriorly and the acromion posteriorly. The injection is made just lateral to the coracoid with the needle pointing toward the acromion.
- The posterior route requires the clinician to palpate the spine of the scapula with the thumb to its lateral end where it bends forward as the acromion. With the forefinger then palpate the coracoid anteriorly. The line between finger and thumb then marks the position of the joint line. The needle is advanced from behind, 1 cm below the acromion, and toward the coracoid. There should be no resistance.
- Withdrawing the needle slightly, and redirecting 30° upward will allow you to reach the rotator cuff with the same procedure!

Subacromial articulation and acromioclavicular joint

- The subacromial bursa is approached from the lateral side. To inject this space, the arm is placed in a neutral position, hanging to the side, and the gap between the acromion and the humeral head is palpated. The needle is directed medially and slightly posterior and not too deep (see Plate 13).
- The AC joint is located by following the clavicle laterally. The joint is often tender to palpate. The patient lies supine and a small gauge needle with 0.5 ml of steroid is directed into the joint at about 45° anteriorly.

The elbow joint and periarticular elbow structures

- Lateral humeral epicondylitis is injected with the elbow resting on the examination table and flexed at 90°. This superficial injection is

directed at 45° to the end of the common extensor tendon origin. A fair amount of pressure is required for this injection. It is often painful (see Plate 14).
- The medial humeral epicondylitis is managed similarly. The needle is directed to the flexor tendon origin. However, care should be taken to avoid the groove just behind the medial epicondyle—the site of the ulnar nerve.
- An olecranon bursa can be aspirated and injected superficially with minimal effort. Needle position is confirmed by the aspiration of fluid.
- The elbow joint is most easily reached by a posterior approach. Place the thumb on the lateral epicondyle and the third finger on the olecranon. The groove between the two fingers identifies the joint line. Inject at 90° to the skin, just above and lateral to the olecranon. Alternatively the radial head can be palpated (with forearm pronation/supination) and the needle sited tangentially just under the capsule (anterolateral approach).

Lesions of the wrist
- The radiocarpal joint is best felt with the patient's hand held palm down and the wrist in slight flexion. A triangular gap is felt between the radius and the carpal bones. The needle is pointed proximally and at 60°.
- The carpal tunnel is injected on the palmar surface of the wrist in the first crease. If the palmaris tendon is present the injection should be sited just medial (i.e., closer to the "little finger") to the midline, by about 1 cm, and toward the palm at 45°. There should be no resistance on injection or nerve pain (see Plate 15).
- De Quervain's tenosynovitis should be injected at the point of maximal tenderness, tangentially along the line of the tendon sheath.

The hand
- The small joints of the hand will normally only accept 0.5–1 ml of injected fluid.
- It is important to remember that the joint line of an MCP is about 1 cm distal to the crest of the knuckle. The approach to a PIP is from the lateral side.
- PIPs and DIPs are often difficult to inject. Accuracy of needle placement within a joint space might be improved by using US guidance.
- Efficacy may be greater using US-guided injection though as yet this is unproved.

Hip joint and periarticular hip lesions
- Hip injection is not a routine outpatient procedure and aspiration and injection under US or fluoroscopic guidance is recommended.
- Meralgia paresthetica occurs as a consequence of lateral cutaneous nerve entrapment as it traverses the fascia 10cm below and medial to the anterior superior iliac spine. If this spot can be clearly demarcated because of localized tenderness, steroid injection has a greater chance of success.
- The ischial tuberosities are located deep in the medial side of the buttocks. The overlying bursae can become inflamed, causing pain on

sitting. These tender points can be injected. The differential diagnosis is enthesitis or possibly coccydynia.
- The coccyx can be palpated centrally (with the patient prone or lying on their side). This site is also amenable to local anesthetic and steroid injections.
- Adductor apophysitis occurring from a sports injury can be injected simply although it can be difficult to access. An inflamed symphysis pubis is best injected under US guidance.
- Trochanteric bursitis or enthesitis at the greater trochanter can be injected with the patient lying on their good side. The injection site can be very deep and to reduce the risk of fat atrophy from a "blind approach", it is reasonable to try using hydrocortisone first. The site of injection should be chosen based on the point of maximal tenderness. Injection failure should raise the possibility of poor needle position or a different diagnosis, e.g., gluteus medius muscle tear at its insertion or pain referred from a lumbosacral disorder.

The knee joint and periarticular lesions
- The most common technique for injection of the knee joint is either the lateral or medial retropatellar approach.
- From the lateral side, the joint line is marked between the upper and middle third of the patella. Access to the joint space may be improved by depressing the medial aspect of the patella, tipping it up laterally. The needle is advanced tangentially between the patella and the femoral condyle.
- The entry site for the medial approach is below the midline of the patella, with the needle advanced tangentially toward the suprapatellar pouch.
- In both techniques, aspiration as the needle is inserted will reveal fluid as soon as the capsule is entered, so reducing the risk of forcing the needle too far forward causing cartilage damage.
- Prepatellar bursitis, painful ligaments, and trigger points around the knee may all respond to local steroid and anesthetic.
- Popliteal cysts can be directly aspirated and injected but due to the risk of damaging superficial neurovascular structures, should be done under US guidance.

Ankle and foot disorders
- The ankle joint is located most easily with the patient supine on a couch. The joint line can be palpated just lateral to the extensor digitorum tendon as it crosses the ankle crease. The needle is initially advanced downwards over the talus.
- Tendon sheaths and the tarsal tunnel can all be injected; the latter is injected under the flexor retinaculum between the calcaneum and the medial malleolus.
- Painful points under the heel should be injected from the medial side after carefully localizing the position of maximal pain. Never inject through the sole of the foot. Some clinicians will numb the area by local anesthetic to the posterior tibial nerve, in the tarsal tunnel.
- The MTPs are injected from the lateral side. Care should be taken as these joints have a greater than normal risk of infection after the procedure.

Principles of rehabilitation

Adults

- It is beyond the scope of this book to address the many techniques employed in rehabilitation. The reader is encouraged to discuss and observe the management of patients with arthritis with the rehabilitation team.
- In the last decade, the development of a multidisciplinary approach to rehabilitation has transformed the way most rheumatologists think about disability.
- Two main types of measurement exist for assessing outcome in rehabilitation (beyond the various scoring systems for particular diseases).
- Generic measures take a global view of disability and afford later comparison. Generic measures also help in assessing different programs, populations, and practices. Specific measures deal with the individual patient and their function in their own environment.
- No one instrument will suffice and there are now many well-validated disability scores:
  - Ritchie index—impairment
  - Health Assessment Questionnaire—disability
  - SF36
  - Beck depression score—depression
  - Spielberg score—anxiety
  - Sickness Impact Profile (SIP)
  - Multidimensional pain inventory—psychological response to pain and disability.
- Important components of rehabilitation for patients with arthritis include:
  - a coordinated team
  - problem-solving approach
  - functionally relevant program
  - education
  - community orientated
  - cognitive and psychological behavioral therapy
  - addressing social factors e.g., work, housing etc.
  - access to support services
  - commitment to long-term follow-up and reassessment.
- Ideally, the team will consist of doctors, specialist nurses, physical therapists, occupational therapists, counselors, psychologists, dieticians, physiatrists, and social workers.

Childhood

There are important additional issues to consider in the management of children:

- A child's rheumatic disease always has an impact on their family. Many normal activities are impossible or time-consuming, and financial hardship is common.
- Siblings may feel neglected and parents are often overburdened with tasks and worries to focus completely on the family. The "team" aims to share that burden and assist the whole family.

- The child should be integrated in school ("mainstream" preferably) and social life as much as possible. It is important to achieve the highest level of integration, hopefully ceasing a child's perception of sickness and difference, acquiring a sense of belonging and purpose.
- The therapist will spend as much time preventing deformity in early disease as dealing with chronic disability, the aim being to maintain or restore function.
- For a child with chronic progressive disease, a regular, often daily, therapy program is necessary. The best way to guarantee this is to involve the parents or care provider. With education on the role of splints/exercise and the impact of rehabilitation on disease progression, most parents are eager and capable participants in the therapy.
- Joint protection training is important—proper positioning, use of several joints in a task, safe transfer of loads, avoidance of prolonged position, planning of rest breaks, and adapted aids and devices should all be addressed.
- Chronic diseases may elicit different emotions in different children—often frustration with lack of mobility in the young, and peer group issues and psychosexual anxieties in the adolescent. Positive adjustment, focusing on strengths not weakness, is important, as is the constant awareness of such issues in those that make up the support structure. Competence comes in many forms, not simply physical ability, and should be praised at every level, building a child's self-esteem.
- Many children who have learned to cope with their disease develop a more mature personality earlier than others in their age group. As such, the adolescent may be earlier and better qualified to bid for an independent life despite physical limitations. It is important to ensure they are not held back.

Adolescents

At some point in a patient's development from childhood to adulthood, the pediatric physician must start to relinquish care to the adult physician. This phase of patient management, the transition, should be handled carefully. Some important principles to consider are stated below.
- Transfer should only occur when a young person feels ready to function in an adult clinic.
- From an early stage, adolescents should be encouraged to take responsibility for medications.
- The whole concept of independence should be introduced well ahead of an anticipated transfer time. This could be introduced at about the age of 11 years and encouraged by trying to see the adolescent by themselves for part of their consultation by the time they are 13–14 years of age.
- A schedule of events leading to "transition" and finally to transfer of care should be drawn up.
- Adolescents should be given information on health care rights and taught how to recognize changes in their disease (good or bad) and how to seek help from health professionals.

Patterns of disease presentation: making a working diagnosis

Monoarticular pains in adults

- When evaluating a patient with joint pain, it helps to know the number of joints involved, i.e., monoarticular (one joint), oligoarticular (2–5 joints), or polyarticular (> 5 joints). Each of these patterns is associated with its own differential diagnosis.

- The assessment of specific joints is discussed in detail in chapter 2. However, the evaluation of a single, hot swollen joint—particularly the knee—comes up so frequently, a few points bear repeating.

- When evaluating an acute monoarthritis, it is helpful to remember that the most common causes include infection, crystals, and fracture.

- Diagnosis of fracture may be obvious from the clinical history, but may require a high index of suspicion. Stress fractures occur as the result of repetitive loading of bone, and can be found with occupational, recreational, or athletic activities. Stress fractures may be small, and, therefore, can be missed on plain radiographs; MRI may be more sensitive and should be considered if the patient is at risk.

- The most common cause of an acute monoarthritis in a young adult is gonococcal arthritis. This most frequently affects the knee, although other joints may be affected as well. Gonococcal arthritis responds rapidly to antibiotic therapy; the speed of the response often helps confirm the diagnosis.

- Crystalline arthropathies such as gout or pseudogout should be considered in older adults. Gout in particular can lead to a highly inflammatory arthritis; it can be accompanied by a gouty tenosynovitis that can mimic a cellulitis. In addition to causing a monoarticular arthritis, pseudogout may also mimic rheumatoid arthritis and osteoarthritis.

- Nongonococcal septic arthritis is particularly important to consider in the elderly, who may not present with the signs and symptoms expected with infection. Nongonococcal septic arthritis is a rheumatologic emergency, and should be treated with intravenous antibiotics and joint aspiration. Although *S. aureus* is the most common culprit, in the elderly, it is prudent to consider less common infections (e.g., Gram negative). Also remember that the presence of crystals does not completely exclude the possibility of a co-existing infection.

- Finally, remember that rheumatic disease that is destined to evolve into an oligoarticular or polyarticular disorder may initially present as a problem with a single joint. Because long-term outcomes of rheumatoid arthritis in particular are improved by early treatment, it is always appropriate to consider at least a serologic screening for this disorder (e.g., RF, ACPA) in a patient with a monoarthritis for whom the underlying etiology is unclear.

Oligoarticular pains in adults

Background

The assessment of an inflamed joint

- The clinical features of inflammation and pain at any given synovial joint and the differential diagnosis in the context of other possible regional musculoskeletal diagnoses are discussed in Chapter 2.
- Synovitis is the term given to inflammation of the synovial lining. This inflammation may be a consequence of a range of cellular processes, and is not specific for any one diagnosis. Joint effusions often accompany synovitis.
- Inflammation of periarticular tissues may accompany synovitis. Enthesitis (i.e., inflammation where tendon inserts into bone) or tenosynovitis may be the most prominent feature.
- The differential diagnosis of synovitis includes hemarthrosis, which can be due to a number of causes, including trauma, bleeding disorder, vitamin C deficiency, synovial hemangioma, and pigmented villonodular synovitis (PVNS).

Table 3.1 lists the most common causes of oligoarticular joint pain.

History: general points

- Pain and stiffness are typical features of synovitis and enthesitis; both are often worse in the morning, or after other periods of immobility. The presence or absence of stiffness does not discriminate between different causes of synovitis.
- Pain is often severe in acute joint inflammation. In chronic situations, pain may be less severe (due to mechanisms that increase physical and psychological tolerance). There are no specific descriptors that discriminate pain from synovitis or enthesitis.
- Swelling, either due to synovial thickening or effusion, often accompanies synovitis. Enthesitis may be associated with periarticular soft tissue swelling.
- A patient's report of swelling is not always reliable. Patients with carpal tunnel syndrome, for example, will frequently report that their hands are swollen, even when no swelling is visible.
- Reduced mobility in a joint affected by enthesitis/synovitis is almost universal regardless of its cause.

Examination: general points

- Swelling may be observed or detected by palpation. Its absence does not rule out synovitis or enthesitis. Synovial swelling needs to be discriminated from bony swelling, fat, and other connective tissue swellings (e.g., ganglia, nodules, etc.). Without imaging or attempting to aspirate joint fluid, it may be difficult to discriminate synovial thickening from effusion.
- Skin erythema (implying periarticular inflammation) and warmth do not always accompany joint inflammation, but they are common with crystalline and septic arthritis. Erythema can also occur in reactive arthritis, rheumatic fever, and with nascent Heberden's/Bouchard's nodes in OA.

Table 3.1 The most common causes of monoarticular and oligoarticular joint pain and typical patterns of presentation

Disease	Typical pattern
Gout (Chapter 7)	Age >40 years. Initially presents as an acute monoarthritis. Strong association with hyperuricemia, renal impairment, and diuretics. Possible general symptoms mimicking sepsis. Possible family history. Acute phase reactants and serum WBC often high. Joint fluid urate crystals seen by PLM. Joint erosions (radiographically typical) and tophi occur in chronic disease
Spondyloarthritis (Chapter 8)	Age <40 years, men more than women. Mostly oligoarticular lower limb joint enthesitis/synovitis. May occur with sacroiliitis, urethritis or cervicitis, uveitis, gut inflammation, psoriasis (scaly or pustular). Possible family history. ESR/CRP may be normal. More severe course if HLA B27-positive.
CPPD arthritis (Chapter 7)	Mean age 72 years. Oligoarticular, acute monoarticular (25%) and occasionally polyarticular patterns of synovitis
Hemarthrosis	Obvious trauma does not always occur. Swelling usually considerable. Causes include trauma (e.g., cruciate rupture or intra-articular fracture), pigmented villonodular synovitis, bleeding diatheses, and chondrocalcinosis
Osteoarthritis (Chapter 6)	Soft tissue swelling is usually not as obvious as bony hypertrophy (i.e., osteophytes). Typical distribution (e.g., first carpometacarpal and knee joints)
Rheumatoid arthritis (Chapter 5)	Can initially present with an oligoarthritis that evolves into a symmetric polyarthritis. Can rarely present as an acute monoarthritis.
Septic arthritis (excluding N. gonorrhea) (Chapter 17)	Most common cause = Staphylococcus aureus. Associated with chronic arthritis, joint prostheses, and reduced host immunity. Peak incidence in elderly. Systemic symptoms common and sometimes overt, but may not occur. Synovial fluid is Gram stain positive in 50% of cases and culture positive in 90% of cases
Gonococcal arthritis (Chapter 17)	Age 15–30 in urban populations and with inherited deficiency of complements C5 to C9. One form presents as an acute septic monoarthritis. Organism detected by Gram stain of joint fluid in 25% and by culture in 50% in the second group

- Tenderness of thickened synovium is common but is not always present. Severely tender swelling suggests joint infection, hemarthrosis or an acute inflammatory reaction to crystals. Inflammation of entheses results in 'bony' tenderness at joint margins and sites of tendon or ligament insertion.
- Decreased range of motion is almost always demonstrable in a joint affected by synovitis or enthesitis. The degree to which passive and active range of motion is reduced depends on a number of often interdependent factors (e.g., pain, size of effusion, periarticular muscle weakness or pain).
- Movement of a joint affected by synovitis or enthesitis will induce pain. Affected joints will demonstrate reduced range on active or passive range of motion exercises.

Taking a history

Age, sex, and occupation

The age, sex, and occupation of the patient give nonspecific but important clues in many cases:

- Oligoarthritis is uncommon in young adults. SpA, especially reactive arthritis, is likely to be the main cause. 75% of patients who develop reactive arthritis are less than 40 years old.
- Gout typically occurs in those more than 40 years old, and is the most common cause of inflammatory arthritis in men (self-reported in 1 in 74 men and 1 in 156 women).
- The mean age of patients with calcium pyrophosphate dihydrate (CPPD) arthritis is about 72 years (range 63–93 years).
- Patients in areas endemic for tick infection with *Borrelia* are at risk of Lyme arthritis. In 2003–2005, 93% of Lyme cases in the United States occurred in 10 endemic states: Connecticut, Delaware, Maryland, Massachusetts, Minnesota, New Jersey, New York, Pennsylvania, Rhode Island, and Wisconsin.

Which joints are affected?

Some processes are more common in certain joints than others:

- Shoulder synovitis is typical in hydroxyapatite arthritis (Milwaukee shoulder/knee syndrome) and AL amyloidosis.
- Involvement of a shoulder or hip is extremely unusual in gout.
- CPPD arthritis (as pseudogout) occurs rarely in the small finger joints.
- The knee is the commonly involved in acute crystalline arthropathy and septic arthritis (both gonococcal and nongonococcal).
- Large knee effusions are common with Lyme arthritis, but this is a nonspecific finding. Large effusions can also be seen with septic and psoriatic arthritis.
- In theory, there are many causes of synovitis in a single first MTP joint but the majority of cases are due to gout; 50–70% of first attacks occur in this joint.

Preceding factors

Factors preceding swelling of a single joint or oligoarthritis may be highly relevant. These include infection and trauma:

- Acute nontraumatic monoarticular synovitis is most commonly due to crystal-induced synovitis or synovitis associated with SpA.
- A preceding history of trauma typically suggests intra-articular fracture (which may cause hemarthrosis), a meniscus tear (knee), or an intrarticular loose body such as an osteochondral fragment (which may cause the patient to complain about a "locking" knee).
- Twinges of joint pain often precede an acute attack of gout. Acute arthritis occurs in 25% of patients with CPPD arthritis.
- In hydroxyapatite arthritis, synovitis is usually mild-to-moderate, gradual in onset and typically worse at night.
- An acute monoarthritis with fever in familial Mediterranean fever (FMF) is a mimic of septic arthritis. Such joint manifestations are present in up to 75% of cases.
- Septic arthritis should always be considered (and promptly ruled out) as a cause of acute joint swelling (see Chapter 22).

Crystal arthritides

Crystal arthritides are associated with nonmusculoskeletal conditions:

- Hyperuricemia, causes of which include obesity, renal insufficiency, tumor lysis syndrome, myeloproliferative diseases, and hemolytic anemia, is associated with gout.
- Saturnine gout, which is associated with lead exposure (e.g., moonshine, welders), is more likely to lead to polyarticular attacks.
- Hypertension and hypertriglyceridemia are associated with gout.
- A history of renal stones (urate) may be a clue to hyperuricemia and associated gout.
- Attacks of gout and CPPD arthritis can be precipitated by any nonspecific illness, trauma, or surgery. The most common associated metabolic disorder is hyperparathyroidism (10% of cases).
- Though uncommon, hypomagnesemia, hypophosphatasia (low alkaline phosphatase activity), hemochromatosis, Wilson's disease, and ochronosis are all associated with CPPD arthritis. Calcium oxalate crystal arthritis can be seen as a rare complication of hemodialysis.

Link with infection

Many types of infection are linked to oligoarticular arthritis. Often a high index of suspicion is needed to make a link:

- Specific infections are directly or indirectly associated with arthritis.
- Viruses, bacteria, protozoa, helminthes, and fungi can all directly invade joints. The range of systemic features is wide and pathogens can cause both polyarticular and oligoarticular patterns of joint involvement.
- The infections recognized to trigger reactive arthritis are *Salmonella, Yersinia, Shigella, Campylobacter* and *Chlamydia*. The development of reactive arthritis in those who acquire chlamydial (nongonococcal) urethritis is relatively uncommon (about 1 in 30).
- Acute HIV infection is associated with a subacute oligoarthritis commonly involving knees and ankles.
- Chronic arthritis, diabetes, immunodeficiency, and joint prostheses are all risk factors for septic arthritis.

- Lyme disease should be considered a cause of oligoarthritis in patients with a remote history of erythema chronicum migrans (i.e., macule/papule initially, expanding 0.5–1 cm/day to a mean diameter of 15 cm (range 3–68 cm), often fading without treatment in 3–4 weeks).
- Migratory arthritis is typical in untreated rheumatic fever; however, persistent monoarthritis is a common finding in treated patients.
- A history of circumcorneal eye redness with pain, photophobia, and blurred vision may be due to anterior uveitis most commonly associated with SpA but also seen with sarcoid, Behçet's, and Whipple's disease.

Family and social history

There may be important clues from the family and social history:

- Both gout and SpA have a familial component. Between 6 and 18% of patients with gout also have a family history of gout. There may be a family history of SpA or uveitis in patients who have reactive, psoriatic, or enteropathic arthritis or AS.
- Gout in young adults suggests an inherited abnormality (usually increased urate production from 5-phosphoribosyl-1-pyrophosphate synthetase activity, since the other enzyme deficiencies present in childhood).
- Excessive alcohol consumption is associated with gout. Alcohol can also contribute to lactic acidosis that inhibits urate breakdown.
- Consider Lyme disease if patients live, work, or visit endemic areas. Outside of the United States, this includes Europe, Russia, China, and Japan. Peak incidence occurs during the summer.
- Brucellar arthritis is generally monoarticular and occurs primarily in areas where domesticated animals are infected and poor methods of animal husbandry, feeding habits, and hygiene standards coexist.

Ask about other associated features

Associated extra-articular features include previous eye, gastrointestinal, cardiac, and genitourinary symptoms:

- Low-grade fever, malaise, and anorexia occur commonly in both septic arthritis and gout. Marked fever can occur in gout and only occurs in about a third of patients with septic arthritis.
- Ask about any current or previous features which might suggest SpA: back or buttock pain (enthesitis or sacroiliitis); swelling of a digit (dactylitis); plantar heel pain (plantar fasciitis); red eye with irritation (anterior uveitis); urethritis, balanitis, cervicitis or acute diarrhea (reactive arthritis); psoriasis; symptoms of inflammatory bowel disease.
- Behçet's disease (see Chapter 18) can cause an oligoarthritis. Other features include painful oral and genital ulcers and uveitis.
- The involvement of more than one joint does not rule out septic arthritis. In up to 20% of cases, multiple joints can become infected.

Examination

General

- Always compare sides, to establish if the changes are symmetric or asymmetric.

- It is important to establish from the examination whether there is true synovial swelling. A history of swelling is not always reliable and other, nonsynovial, pathology can present with single or oligoarticular joint pain.

Examine the affected joints

Examine the affected joints for tenderness. Check passive range of motion for evidence of locking or instability:

- Acute processes such as crystal arthritis, infection and post-traumatic effusion often lead to painful swelling, marked tenderness of swollen soft-tissues, and painfully restricted active and passive movement of the joint. These features are usually less overt with chronic arthritis.
- Instability of an acutely inflamed joint or tests for cartilage damage in the knee may be difficult to demonstrate. Further examination will be necessary after drainage of joint fluid.
- Detection of enthesis tenderness around the affected joints or at other sites is a useful clue to the diagnosis of SpA.

Examine other musculoskeletal structures

- Examine the low back and typical sites of bony tenderness—sacroiliitis and enthesitis are common features of SpA.
- Tendonitis is not specific and can occur in gout, CPPD arthritis, SpA, and gonococcal infection.

Look for skin rashes and any inflammation

Oligoarthritis may be part of a systemic inflammatory or infectious condition.

- Fever and tachycardia can occur with some noninfectious causes of acute arthritis (e.g., crystal arthritis), but their presence in the context of oligoarticular joint swelling requires exclusion of joint infection.
- Gouty tophi may be seen in the pinnae and in other peripheral locations. They can be difficult to discriminate clinically from rheumatoid nodules. Polarized light microscopy of material obtained by needle aspiration will be diagnostic for tophi.
- The hallmark of relapsing polychondritis is lobe-sparing, full thickness inflammation of the pinna.
- Mouth ulcers are common; however, crops or large painful tongue and buccal lesions associated with oligoarticular arthritis suggest Behçet's disease.
- A typical site for the osteitis (tender swelling of bone) of SAPHO syndrome is around the sternum and clavicles.
- Skin erythema over a joint suggests crystal arthritis or infection.
- Associated skin rashes may include erythema nodosum (associated with ankle/knee synovitis in acute sarcoid), purpuric pustular rashes (Behçet's, gonococcal infection, and SAPHO syndrome), erythema marginatum (rheumatic fever), or keratoderma blennorrhagica (aggressive-looking rash of the sole of the foot in Reiter's disease).
- Psoriasis may be associated with both synovitis and enthesitis.

Diagnostic procedures

The presence of synovitis can be confirmed by obtaining US or MR of the joints in question. At larger joints, both are sensitive for the detection of effusion and synovial thickening. Inflammation at periarticular or capsular entheses can also be seen.

Joint aspiration

The most important investigation of a patient with monoarticular synovitis is joint aspiration and prompt examination of fluid. Fluid should be sent in sterile bottles for microscopy and culture:

- The appearance of synovial fluid is not specific; however, blood or bloodstaining suggests hemarthrosis from trauma (including the aspiration attempt), a hemorrhagic diathesis, hemangioma, PVNS, and synovioma.
- Turbidity (i.e., decreased clarity) of fluid relates to cellular, crystal, lipid, and fibrinous content. Synovial fluid in septic arthritis and acute crystal arthritis is frequently turbid due to the high number of neutrophils.
- Cell counts give some diagnostic guidance but are nonspecific (see Table 3.2). There is a high probability of infection or gout if the PMN differential is >90%.
- Joint fluid eosinophilia is not specific.
- Polarized light microscopy of fluid can discriminate urate (3–20μm in length, needle-shaped and negatively birefringent—initially blue, and then yellow as the red plate compensator is rotated through 90°) and calcium-containing crystals such as calcium pyrophosphate (positively birefringent crystals, typically small and rectangular or rhomboid in shape).
- Lipid and cholesterol crystals are not uncommon in joint fluid samples, but their significance is unknown.
- Crystals appearing in synovium less commonly but in typical settings include hydroxyapatite associated with Milwaukee shoulder (and knee) syndrome (which can be visualized by staining with alizarin red S), calcium oxalate in end-stage renal failure on dialysis (may need scanning electron microscopy to confirm), cystine in cystinosis, and xanthine in xanthosis.
- The presence of crystals in joint fluid does not exclude infection.
- The most common causes of nongonococcal septic arthritis in Europe and North America are *Staphylococcus aureus* (40–50%), *Staphylococcus epidermidis* (10–15%), *Streptococcal* species (20%), and Gram-negative bacteria (15%).

Radiographs

Radiographs can confirm an effusion, show characteristic patterns of chondral and bone destruction (e.g., in infection or erosive gout) and can reveal intra-articular calcification associated with CPPD or hydroxyapatite arthritis:

- Septic arthritis causes patchy osteopenia and loss of bone cortex.
- "Punched-out" erosions (within joints or around metaphyses), soft tissue swellings (tophi), and patchy calcification are hallmarks of chronic gout.

- Intra-articular calcification may be associated with either chondrocalcinosis (fine linear or punctate fibrocartilage calcification) or larger loose bodies (often with prolific osteophytes)—both are associated with CPPD arthritis.
- Numerous regularly shaped calcific masses in a joint may be due to synovial chondromatosis (most common in middle-aged men; 50% of cases affect the knee).
- The presence of erosions does not implicate RA. The arthritis may be due to an enthesitis associated with SpA.

Further imaging

Further imaging should be discussed with your radiologists:
- MR confirmation of traumatized structures such as meniscus damage in the knee and labral damage in the shoulder should be sought if suspected.
- MR can confirm synovitis, although appearances are usually nonspecific. MR can also identify enthesitis and PVNS.

Laboratory tests to consider

- CBC, acute phase response (ESR, CRP). Neutrophilia is not specific for infection and can occur in crystal arthritis.
- Blood urea, electrolytes, creatinine, and urate (e.g., hyperuricemia and renal impairment associated with gout).
- Blood calcium, phosphate, albumin, alkaline phosphatase (±iPTH), thyroid function tests and ferritin to screen for hyperparathyroidism, thyroid disease, and hemochromatosis, all of which can be associated with CPPD arthritis.
- Autoantibodies: rheumatoid factor and ACPA, such as cyclic citrullinated peptide (CCP) may help identify early rheumatoid arthritis.
- IgM *Borellia burgdorferi* serology may help diagnose Lyme disease in patients at risk (e.g., acute arthropathy or migratory arthritis).

Table 3.2 Characteristics of joint fluid

Characteristic	Normal	Group I (noninflammatory)	Group II (inflammatory)	Group III (septic)
Viscosity	Very high	High	Low	Variable
Color	None	Straw	Straw or opalescent	Variable with organisms
Clarity	Clear	Clear	Translucent or opaque	Opaque
Leukocytes (cells/mm$_3$)	200	200–2000	2000–50000	>50000
PMNs (%)	<25	25	Often >50	>75

- Antibodies to the streptococcal antigens streptolysin O (ASOT) DNAse B, hyaluronidase, and streptozyme may be useful in patients who have had sore throat, migratory arthritis, or features of rheumatic fever.

Synovial biopsy
- If there is a hemarthrosis or suspicion of PNS, MR of the joint is wise before undertaking a biopsy to characterize the vascularity of a lesion.
- Consider a biopsy to evaluate a monoarthritis of unclear etiology. Biopsy may be helpful to diagnose sarcoid arthropathy, infectious arthritis, or crystalline arthropathy when the usual diagnostic procedures are negative.
- Formalin fixation of samples is sufficient in most cases. Samples for polarized light microscopy are best fixed in alcohol (urate is dissolved by formalin). Snap freezing in nitrogen is essential if immunohistochemistry is required.
- Arthroscopic biopsy will yield more tissue than needle biopsy, and will allow joint irrigation.
- Congo red staining of synovium, ideally with polarized light microscopy, should be requested if AA, AL, or β_2-microglobulin amyloid is a possibility. This should be considered in patients with myeloma (AL) and long-term dialysis patients (β_2-microglobulin). AA amyloid is an uncommon but recognized complication of rheumatoid arthritis, ankylosing spondylitis, familial Mediterranean fever, and Crohn's disease.

Oligoarticular pains in children and adolescents

Background

Disease classification

In 2001, a working group under the auspices of the International League of Associations for Rheumatology (ILAR) met to establish a consensus regarding classification criteria for pediatric and adolescent arthritides (see below). For a review of these new and old autoimmune arthritis classifications, see below and Table 3.4, and under the relevant diagnostic headings in Chapter 9.

Important issues pertinent to children and adolescents

- Compared to adults, it may be quite difficult to establish whether there is synovitis in a child's joint (see Table 3.3).
- An awareness of injuries and mechanical conditions that affect specific joints, notably at epiphyseal or apophyseal growth plates, is essential.
- In very young children, a history from both the child and the main care provider is important.
- It is important to note that monoarticular or oligoarticular synovitis:
  - may present with limb pain
  - may not necessarily present with joint pain and stiffness
  - may result in nonuse, altered use, or irritability, any of which may be the main or only complaint.
- Systemic juvenile idiopathic arthritis (JIA) (previously systemic onset juvenile rheumatoid arthritis (JRA)) is defined as arthritis preceded by (or occurring with) daily recurring fever of more than 2 weeks' duration (documented for greater than 3 days) plus one or more of the following: an evanescent, nonfixed, erythematous rash; generalized lymphadenopathy; enlarged liver or spleen; or serositis.
- Persistent oligoarthritis is defined by the involvement of no more than four joints throughout the disease course. Extended oligoarthritis affects a cumulative total of five joints or more after the first 6 months of disease. Excluded from each group are those with: a family history of psoriasis (first- or second degree relative); a positive RF; HLA B27 (males >8 years old); or systemic arthritis.
- Under the new system, enthesitis has a key-classifying role in the group of conditions previously classified as spondyloarthropathy (SpA), now called enthesitis-related arthritis (ERA).
- The definition of psoriatic arthritis has been broadened under the new ILAR classification (see Table 3.4). The classification criteria require arthritis beginning before 16 years of age and either typical psoriasis or at least three of the following: dactylitis, nail pitting, psoriasis-like rash, family history of psoriasis (first- and second-degree relatives). Enthesitis, iritis, and HLA B27 are absent from this classification.

Table 3.3 The major causes of monoarticular/oligoarticular joint synovitis or swelling in children

Condition	Distinguishing features
Septic arthritis	Systemically unwell child. With TB—pulmonary disease, lower limb, insidious onset, and rapid joint destruction
Trauma	Direct blow/forced hyperextension, hemorrhage into joint
Foreign body synovitis	History of injury
PVNS	Recurrent joint hemarthrosis
Thalassemia	Episodic and migratory arthritis
Malignancy	Acute monoarticular joint swelling, associated with leukemia and neuroblastoma
Viral arthritis	Associated with rash or immunization
Lyme disease	Exposure in endemic area, rash, positive serology
Post-streptococcal	Sore throat, migratory arthritis, signs of rheumatic fever
FMF	Ethnic grouping and familial aggregation, acute febrile episode with chest/abdominal pain
Behçet's disease	Rare. Orogenital ulceration and skin rashes
Oligoarticular JIA	Monoarticular in 60% of cases and involves two joints in 31% of cases. Diagnosis of exclusion, associated with asymptomatic uveitis
Enthesitis-related arthritis	Usually age 8 or over, boys > girls, iritis, most have enthesitis, HLA B27. Sacroiliac joint involvement, low back stiffness
Psoriatic arthritis*	Rash, nail pitting, or other changes
Sarcoid	Usually associated with rash and ocular symptoms
Vasculitis	Rash, high ESR/CRP
SLE	UV-sensitive skin rash, ANA

* In the ILAR classifications, psoriatic arthritis is distinguished from enthesitis-related arthritis (see below).

Taking a history

Epidemiology

Recall epidemiological features associated with different groups and ages:
- The peak incidence of oligoarticular JIA (or pauciarticular JRA) is between the ages of 1 and 3. It is relatively very rare after 12 years of age.
- Enthesitis-related arthritis (ERA or SpA) is more common in boys (ratio up to 10:1) and typically occurs after the age of 8.

Table 3.4 ILAR classification of arthritis in childhood (juvenile idiopathic arthritis)

ILAR classification of juvenile idiopathic arthritis (JIA)	Previous classification
Systemic arthritis*	Systemic onset JRA
Oligoarthritis* which is either: persistent (always 4 joints or less) extended (after 6 months >4 four joints affected)	Oligoarticular JRA Pauciarticular JRA
Polyarthritis (RF+)* 5 or more joints affected	Polyarticular JRA Polyarticular JRA (RF+)
Polyarthritis (RF–)	Polyarticular JRA (RF–)
Psoriatic arthritis*	Psoriatic arthritis
Enthesitis-related arthritis (ERA)*	SpA

JCA = juvenile chronic arthritis; JRA = juvenile rheumatoid arthritis; RF = rheumatoid factor.
* See text for notes.

Trauma

Monoarticular synovitis may be associated with trauma:
- Time to onset of joint swelling after trauma (<2 h) and intensity of pain (severe) may help discriminate whether a hemarthrosis is present. Intra-articular fracture should then be suspected.
- An absence of a history of trauma does not rule out the possibility of osteochondritis dissecans (only 10% are associated with trauma).
- Be aware that nonaccidental trauma can present with traumatic joint swelling.

Infection/malignancy

Infection and malignancy must be ruled out in all cases of atraumatic monoarthritis:
- An insidious onset does not rule out infection. This pattern is well recognized in TB. Joint destruction, however, may not be insidious.
- The most common neoplastic causes of monoarticular joint swelling in children are leukemia and neuroblastoma.

Rare causes of symptoms

The rarer causes of monoarticular synovitis, joint swelling, or pain, and joint-specific causes of pain in a single joint should not be forgotten:
- Intra-articular hemangiomas, osteoid osteomas, synovial chondromatosis, and lipomatosis arborescens can occur in most joints.
- Anterior knee pain (common in growing adolescents, especially girls).
- Isolated hip pain conditions such as Perthes' disease.
- Oligoarticular JIA (Pauci-JRA) of the hip is very rare.
- Osteochondritides/avulsion fractures, e.g., Osgood–Schlatter's.
- Osteonecrosis at typical sites, e.g., tarsal navicular, carpal lunate.

Preceding symptoms

Ask about preceding symptoms of infection and rashes. Consider viral, streptococcal, and enteric infections, and Lyme disease:

- Oligoarthritis (or monoarthritis) may be a reaction to an infection and may be short-lived usually lasting 3–6 weeks, but occasionally up to 8 weeks.
- A streptococcal sore throat can lead on to a migratory arthritis. The differential diagnosis would include rheumatic fever and Lyme disease.
- The most distinctive features of acute rheumatic fever should be sought in patients with oligoarthritis, especially if it has been partially treated with aspirin or NSAIDs, which can mask its migratory nature; these include: carditis with prolonged PR interval, chorea, skin nodules, erythema marginatum.
- *Salmonella, Shigella, Yersinia*, and *Campylobacter* enteric infections are associated with reactive arthritis.
- *Escherichia coli* and *Clostridium difficile* infections have the potential for triggering reactive arthritis.
- A facial rash occurs in rubella—coalescing erythema that clears as the limbs become affected; in most patients, however, a facial rash should make you think about parvovirus B19 infection (erythema infectiosum—'slapped cheek' syndrome).
- Pink or faintly red erythema on the trunk or limbs but not the face is typical of the erythema marginatum of rheumatic fever. The outer rash margin is often distinct and continuous. Firm, nontender skin nodules, which may have regressed, may also suggest rheumatic fever.
- Lyme disease causes erythema chronicum migrans, a spreading erythema from a tick bite. Because of heightened awareness, patients may present early, before the classic targetoid rash has a chance to evolve.
- Live attenuated rubella vaccines are associated, in up to 15% people, with subsequent arthralgias and myalgias. Arthritis may occur 2 weeks after the injection and clears in a week, but symptoms can remain for a year or so.

Family history

Ask about a history of illness in the family or a family history of enthesitis-related (SpA) features:

- In children suspected of having septic arthritis due to TB, establishing a history of contact with sources may be important.
- Due to a link with HLA B27, there may be a history of similar musculoskeletal features in family members.

Examination

General principles of pediatric musculoskeletal examination

- Ensure that the child is comfortable in the environment and with the people present at the time of examination.
- Reassure the child that the examination will not persist if it is painful.
- Observe small children playing at first.
- Try to leave the painful area until last.

Confirmation of synovitis/enthesitis in a joint

Review the features that help to confirm synovitis/enthesitis in a joint:

- It is important to establish from the examination whether there is true synovial swelling. Remember, a history of swelling is not always reliable and other, nonsynovial, pathology can present with single or oligoarticular joint pain (e.g., enthesitis).
- Always compare both sides. Even subtle differences in range of motion may be important and denote synovial thickening.
- Doubt about synovial swelling can be addressed by obtaining US.

Additional musculoskeletal examination

Additional musculoskeletal examination must include a search for muscle atrophy, tenosynovitis, enthesitis, and spinal limitation:

- Adjacent muscle wasting may be a clue to the severity or chronicity of joint inflammation.
- Tenosynovitis is unusual in oligoarticular JIA, but can occur in sarcoid, occasionally in ERA/SpA, and in the polyarticular conditions.
- Enthesitis should discriminate between oligoarticular JIA and ERA/SpA. Commonly involved sites include Achilles, patellar tendon, and plantar fascia insertions.
- Clinical detection of spinal disease in patients who develop AS or ERA/SpA is not always possible at the time of presentation of the first musculoskeletal manifestations of the disease, i.e., enthesitis, although spinal examination assessing localized pain and impaired mobility should be done.

Look for skin rashes and any inflammation

Oligoarthritis may be part of a systemic inflammatory/infective condition. Look closely for skin rashes:

- Skin erythema overlying a joint suggests infection.
- Associated skin rashes may include erythema nodosum, the purpuric pustular rashes of Henoch–Schönlein purpura (HSP) (extensive lower limb) or Behçet's (less florid than HSP), gonococcal infection (single pustules), SAPHO syndrome, erythema marginatum (rheumatic fever) and psoriasis.

Diagnostic procedures

Although synovitis may be obvious clinically, its presence in any joint needs to be confirmed if there is doubt:

- The soft tissue appearances of joint radiographs are sufficient in confirming effusion and synovial thickening in many instances.
- US and MR can identify effusion and synovial thickening.

Joint aspiration

The most important investigation of a child with monoarticular synovitis is joint aspiration and prompt examination of fluid. Fluid should be sent in sterile bottles for microscopy and culture. This procedure may be psychologically traumatic. Consider using sedation (at least) in older children and a light general anesthetic in younger ones.

- Synovial fluid appearances are not specific. However, the following guidelines may be helpful:
- Blood or bloodstaining suggests hemarthrosis from: trauma (including the aspiration), hemorrhagic diathesis, PVNS, synovioma, or hemangioma.
- Turbidity (decreased clarity) of fluid relates to cellular, crystal, lipid, and fibrinous content; the joint fluid of septic arthritis and acute crystal arthritis is turbid due to the high number of neutrophils present.
- Crystals in synovial fluid in children are rare.
- The most common causes of nongonococcal septic arthritis in Europe and North America are *Staphylococcus aureus* (40–50%), *Staphylococcus epidermidis* (10–15%), streptococcal species (20%), and Gram-negative bacteria (15%). Gonococcal infection should be considered a possibility in teenagers.

Radiographs

Radiographs can confirm an effusion and show characteristic patterns of chondral epiphyseal and bone destruction (e.g., in infection or malignancy):

- In septic arthritis, osteopenia and loss of bone cortex are classic signs (although their absence does not rule out septic arthritis). The main differential diagnosis is malignancy.
- If calcified, loose bodies due to osteochondritis dissecans may be visible.
- Erosions can occur in oligoarticular JIA or in ERA/SpA (entheseal).
- Discriminating erosions from ossifying cartilaginous epiphyses in normal joints (which can appear irregular) is sometimes difficult. Bilateral views are sometimes helpful in this respect.
- Joint space narrowing is difficult to confirm from radiographs because of normal changes in epiphyseal cartilage thickness, operator error, and difficulty in weight bearing on painful joints.
- Joint destruction is a characteristic of polyarticular JIA.

Further imaging

Further imaging should be discussed with your radiologist. US and scintigraphy can confirm synovitis and its pattern of joint involvement. CT and MR are useful in discriminating against the causes of synovitis:

- US is a very sensitive investigation for detection of synovitis and is particularly useful in evaluating the hip.
- US and MR can detect erosions earlier than radiographs.
- When malignancy and infection are suspected, bone scan may help identify or rule out additional lesions.
- Because of its high sensitivity, bone scan can be useful in establishing whether significant bone/joint pathology is present in children with joint symptoms but few clinical findings.
- In a normal joint, MR differentiates all the major joint structures including epiphyses. Sedation may be needed in young children.
- MR is an accurate and sensitive tool for identifying joint and epiphyseal damage at an early stage of a disease process. This may be invaluable for example if there is any doubt about the status of oligoarticular JIA

or peripheral joint involvement in ERA/SpA, since early treatment can prevent permanent deformities and disability.

Laboratory tests

Laboratory tests should provide or exclude evidence of infection, give dis-criminatory diagnostic information, and exclude nonrheumatic diseases:

- A predominance of bands on CBC implies infection. Neutrophil predominance may be seen with a variety of inflammatory states, and is less specific for infection. Interestingly, monoarticular JIA can be associated with normal indices.
- A low platelet or white cell count but elevated acute phase indices may be suggestive of an underlying malignancy.
- Antibodies to streptolysin O (ASOT) may be helpful in patients who have had sore throat, migratory arthritis, or features of rheumatic fever. If there is persistent clinical suspicion despite a normal ASOT, antibodies to streptococcal DNAase B, hyaluronidase, and streptozyme may be of value.
- Autoantibodies: a single positive test for RF has little value. Repeatedly positive tests might suggest (RF+) JIA. ANAs are present in 40–75% of children with oligoarticular JIA (JCA). They are not disease-specific, but identify a subset within it at particular risk of (often asymptomatic) uveitis.
- Lyme serology may be helpful in a patient with an acute arthropathy or migratory arthritis.

Synovial biopsy

- If there is a hemarthrosis or suspicion of PVNS, MR of the joint is wise before undertaking biopsy to characterize the vascularity of a lesion.
- Biopsy may be helpful to evaluate a persistent monoarthritis of unclear etiology; biopsy may help diagnose sarcoid arthropathy, malignancy, and chronic infectious arthritis due to atypical pathogens.
- Arthroscopic biopsy will yield more tissue than a needle biopsy. Direct viewing may add diagnostic information and allow joint irrigation.

Widespread pain in adults

Widespread (musculoskeletal) pain is a common reason for adults to seek medical advice (see Table 3.5). Although some of these patients will have a polyarticular arthritis, many conditions are characterized by musculoskeletal symptoms, some of which may be diffuse or multicentric. In addition, the interpretation and reporting of symptoms varies considerably and can be a source of confusion.

Such patients are often referred to rheumatologists for evaluation. A referral may (or may not) be made with a working diagnosis in place.

In the following section, we have aimed to review important aspects of the history, examination, and initial investigations in the initial evaluation of patients who present with nonlocalized, multicentric pains.

Initial impressions
- Think broadly about the possible diagnoses.
- Use what you know about the epidemiology of likely conditions. For example, a 25-year-old man with joint pains is more likely to have SpA than systemic lupus erythematosus (which occurs mostly in women age 14–50) or PMR (which is a condition of the elderly), although joint pains are characteristic of all of these diagnoses.

Age, sex, and racial background
What clues can be drawn from the age, sex, and racial background?

The degree to which these factors influence the likelihood of disease varies according to the prevalence of the disease in the local population.
- Review what you know about the epidemiology of the major diseases. For example:
  - there is a very low incidence of ankylosing spondylitis (AS) in patients over 65 years old with back and joint pains.
  - generalized OA is rare in young men.
  - polymyositis is 100 times less common than polymyalgia rheumatica
  - SLE is up to five times more common in Hispanics and African Americans than in Caucasians.

Previous diagnoses
Presenting features may be put in context early if you have knowledge of musculoskeletal associations of diagnoses that have already been made. For example:
- Synovitis in patients with (radiological) chondrocalcinosis.
- Arthropathy in patients with hyperparathyroidism and hypercalcemia (see Chapter 16).
- Enthesitis/synovitis in patients with Crohn's disease or ulcerative colitis (see Chapter 8).
- Polyarticular synovitis and myalgia in patients with lymphoma.
- Crystal-induced or β_2-microglobulin deposition arthritis and osteodystrophy in chronic renal disease.

Taking a history

First, establish whether pains arise from joints or tendons/entheses, muscles, bone, or are neurologic (see Table 3.5).

Table 3.5 Broad categories of conditions that may present with widespread musculoskeletal pain

Common	Inflammatory polyarthritis (e.g., RA—see Chapter 5, SpA—see Chapter 8)
	Generalized (nodal) OA (see Chapter 6)
	Fibromyalgia/chronic pain syndromes (see Chapter 18)
	Nonspecific myalgias and arthralgias* associated with infection (e.g., viruses)
Less common	Myalgias and arthralgias* due to autoimmune connective tissue disease
	Myalgias, increased muscle inflammation (e.g., polymyositis) (see Chapter 14)
	Myalgias and arthralgias* associated with neoplasia (e.g., lymphoma)
	Skeletal metastases
	Polyostotic Paget's disease (see Chapter 16)
Rare	Metabolic bone diseases (e.g., osteomalacia, renal osteodystrophy) (see Chapter 16)
	Metabolic myopathies (e.g., hypokalemia)
	Neurological disease (Parkinson's disease)

* In certain situations/conditions patients may complain of both muscle and joint pains. This is easily appreciated if you've ever had influenza!

- Although the patient (or referral letter) may report "joint pains," take time to establish whether the pains are truly articular.
- Listen carefully to the description of the pains; try to determine if the patient has a single condition or a number of overlapping causes of pain.

Obtain a detailed history of the pain at different sites

- A good history should help narrow the differential diagnosis considerably. For example, a 70-year-old man referred with "widespread joint pains mostly in his legs", could have multiple weight-bearing joint OA or lumbosacral nerve root claudication symptoms. A middle-aged woman with "hand and neck pain" could have an arthropathy or radicular pain associated with cervical spondylosis.
- Widespread pain due to bone pathology could be due to skeletal metastasis. Bony pain is often unremitting, and changes little with changes in posture and movement.
- One pitfall is to assume that all pains arise from a single pathological process. For example, in an older patient, shoulder pain could be caused by PMR, OA, shoulder impingement syndrome, radicular pain, or a combination of all of these.

Joint pain at rest, after rest, or with joint use?

How do you establish whether pains arise from joints or tendons/entheses, and are likely to reflect a single process?

- Pain occurring with inflammation is conventionally regarded as being associated with morning stiffness or stiffness after periods of rest. It tends to be prominent in conditions such as RA, SpA, PMR, and myositis. Inflammatory joint pain often improves during the day.
- Mild degrees of immobility-associated pain and stiffness occur in some other conditions such as OA and fibromyalgia, although such forms of stiffness generally last for less than 1 hour. Stiffness may also be a feature of muscle spasm and soft-tissue edema.
- Mechanical joint damage such as OA is also painful. Unlike inflammatory joint pain, mechanical joint pain is worsened by use, and improves with rest.

Ask, and document in detail, which joints are affected

- A symmetric polyarthritis affecting the small joints is typical for RA. RA can also present with carpal tunnel syndrome, tenosynovitis, tennis elbow, or an asymmetric pattern of joint involvement, and can be preceded by a palindromic pattern of joint pain (see below).
- Arthritis from parvovirus B19 infection may also be polyarticular and symmetric.
- Small joint pain in the hands occurs in nodal generalized OA. DIPs, PIPs, and thumb joints are usually affected. OA is also associated with pain in the spine, hips, and knees.
- The combination of sacroiliac (low back and buttock), pelvic, and lower limb joint/enthesis pain, typically in an asymmetric oligoarticular pattern, is suggestive of SpA. Typical sites of involvement include the anterior knee, posterior heel and inferior foot (plantar fascia).
- Enthesitis (as the hallmark of SpA) can affect the wrists and small joints of the hand and feet (e.g., plantar fascia origin and insertion at metatarsal heads) and may be difficult to distinguish from RA on clinical grounds alone.
- CPPD typically favors the large and medium-sized joints, but a picture of multiple joint involvement similar to that in RA is possible (including tenosynovitis).
- Widespread arthralgias/arthritis occurs in patients with leukemia, lymphoma, myeloma, and certain infections.

Ask about the pattern of joint symptoms over time

- A short, striking history of marked, acute polyarticular symptoms often occurs with systemic infection (see Table 3.6). Prominent malaise and fever should raise suspicion of infection.
- There may be a longer history than is first volunteered. Autoimmune rheumatic and connective tissue diseases may evolve over a period of time and often naturally relapse and remit; the first symptoms of disease may be dismissed by the patient as irrelevant.
- RA may initially present as a monoarticular or oligoarticular disease, and should be considered for any inflammatory arthritis when an underlying disorder is not readily identified.

- Migratory arthralgias occur in 10% of RA patients initially: a single joint becomes inflamed for a few days then improves and a different joint becomes affected for a few days and so on. A similar pattern can occur in poststreptococcal arthritis, granulomatosis with polyangiitis (Wegener's), sarcoidosis, Lyme disease, and Whipple's disease.
- The onset of enthesopathy may be insidious or acute.
- Recurrent pains from various musculoskeletal lesions, which have occurred from injury or have developed insidiously, are typical in patients with underlying hypermobility (benign joint hyper-mobility syndrome or other heritable diseases of connective tissue such as Ehlers–Danlos, see Chapter 16).

Is there widespread muscle pain?

If you think there is widespread muscle pain, remember to consider that:
- The myalgias may be fibromyalgia or enthesitis.
- Pain locating to muscle group areas may be ischemic or neurologic in origin, and not necessarily due to intrinsic muscle disease.
- The differential diagnosis of PM and dermatomyositis (DM) is broad, but many of these conditions are rare (see Table 3.7 and Chapter 14).

Ask about the distribution and description of myalgias and weakness

- True weakness may denote either myopathy or a neurological condition. However, patients may report a feeling of weakness if muscles are painful, therefore, rely more on your examination before deciding muscles are weak.
- PMR (rare in patients less than 50 years old), myositis, and endocrine/metabolic myopathies typically present with proximal weakness.
- PMR does not lead to objective weakness; instead, patients experience proximal muscle pain and stiffness that is worse in the morning, and is frequently described by the patient as "weakness."
- Though rare, truncal muscle pain and stiffness can be a presenting feature of Parkinson's disease.
- Cramp-like pains may be a presenting feature of any myopathy (e.g., hypokalemic) or even motor neuron disease. However, some patients may interpret radicular (nerve root) pains as muscle cramps.
- Inflammatory and endocrine/metabolic myopathies are often not painful.
- Occasionally some genetic muscle diseases (e.g., myophosphorylase, acid maltase deficiency), can present atypically late (in adults) with progressive weakness that may be mistaken for PM.

Ask about the pattern of muscle pains over time

- Severe, acute muscle pain occurs in a variety of conditions. The most common causes are viral, neoplastic, and drugs. Some toxic causes may result in rhabdomyolysis, myoglobinuria, and renal failure.
- Usually PM/DM is characterized by slowly evolving but progressive proximal muscle weakness (e.g., weeks to months); pain is an uncommon feature.
- Low-grade episodic muscle pains may denote a previously undisclosed hereditary metabolic myopathy.

Are the pains ischemic?
- Lay persons may have little concept of ischemia and might describe their symptoms in the context of muscles and in a muscular distribution.
- Ischemic muscle pain often occurs predictably in association with repeated activity and eases or resolves on rest ("claudication"). Consider this especially if pains are confined to a single limb or both legs.
- The distribution of pains may give clues as to sites of underlying pathology, e.g., upper extremities are affected by subclavian artery stenosis and thoracic outlet syndrome; lower extremities are affected by atherosclerotic vascular disease or lumbar nerve root stenosis.
- Ischemic pains in the context of a highly inflammatory state may suggest systemic vasculitis, such as polyarteritis nodosa.

Widespread pain may be due to bone pathology
- Bone pains are unremitting and disturb sleep. They could denote serious pathology—radiographic and laboratory investigations will be important.
- The major diagnoses to consider include disseminated malignancy, multiple myeloma, metabolic bone disease (e.g., renal osteodystrophy, hyperparathyroidism, osteomalacia) and polyostotic Paget's disease.

Past medical history
Specific questions are often required because previous problems may not be regarded as relevant by the patient. For example:
- For those with joint pains a history of the following may be of help: other autoimmune diseases (increased risk of RA, SLE, etc.); Raynaud's phenomenon (association with scleroderma, RA, and SLE); dry eyes (possible Sjögren's syndrome); uveitis or acute 'red eye' (association with SpA); recurrent injuries/joint dislocations (association with hypermobility); genital, urine, or severe gut infection (associated with SpA); psoriasis (association with SpA); diabetes (cheiroarthropathy).
- For those in whom myalgias/myositis seems likely: preceding viral illness (possible viral myositis); foreign travel (tropical myositis); other autoimmune disease (associated with PM/DM); previous erythema nodosum (sarcoid); drugs and substance abuse (see below).
- For all patients: weight loss or anorexia (association with malignancy); fevers or night sweats (association with infection); sore throat (possible poststreptococcal condition); persistent spinal pain (association with fibromyalgia); rashes (association with Lyme disease, SLE, DM, vasculitis).
- For those with widespread bony pain: history of rickets (association with osteomalacia); chronic renal disease (will precede renal osteodystrophy and may predispose to crystalline arthritis and osteoarticular deposition of β_2-microglobulin).

Psychosocial and sexual history
- Preceding sexual activity and genital infection is important primarily because of an association of *Chlamydia trachomatis* infection with reactive arthritis and enthesitis/SpA (see Chapter 8).
- Reactive arthritis has an association with HIV. HIV is also associated with polymyositis, and is a risk factor for pyomyositis.
- There is an association of anxiety and depression with fibromyalgia (see Chapter 18).

Table 3.6 Common infections that can present with acute polyarthritis and a raised acute phase response

Infection	Common extra-articular clinical features	Key laboratory diagnostic procedures in acute infection
Rheumatic fever (group A β -hemolytic streptococci)	Acute infection 1–2 weeks earlier, fever, rash, carditis	Positive throat swab culture. High ASOT (in 80%). Anti-DNAseB IgM
Post-streptococcal (?rheumatic fever)	Acute infection 3–4 weeks earlier, tenosynovitis	As above
Parvovirus B19 (adults†)	Severe flulike illness at onset, various rashes	Anti-B19 IgM
Rubella (also post-vaccine)	Fever, coryza, malaise, brief rash	Culture. Anti-rubella IgM
Hepatitis B	Fever, myalgia, malaise, urticaria, abnormal liver function	Bilirubin+, ALT+, AST+, anti-HBsAg, anti-HBcAg
Lyme disease (Borrelia burgdorferi)	Tick bites, fever, headache, myalgias, fatigue, nerve palsies	Anti-Bb IgM (ELISA + immunofluorescence)
Toxoplasma gondii	Myositis, paresthesias	Anti-Toxo IgM

Even if serological tests have high sensitivity and specificity, the positive predictive value of the test is low if the clinical likelihood of the infection is low. Therefore, do not use serological tests indiscriminately.

ASOT = antistreptolysin O titer.

†The presentation of parvovirus B19 illness may be quite different in children.

Ask about travel
- Residence in, or travel to, rural areas populated by deer might be important in indicating a risk of exposure to *Borrelia burgdorferi* and contracting Lyme disease (the spirochete is carried by ticks which colonize deer, boar, and other animals and bite other mammals).
- *Plasmodium falciparum* (intertropical areas), trypanosoma (mainly South America), trichinella, and cystercercicae infections are associated with myalgias/myositis.

Family history
Ask about family with arthritis or autoimmune diseases:
- There is a hereditary component to large joint and generalized nodal OA and hyperuricemia/gout.
- The risk of developing any autoimmune condition is higher in families of patients with autoimmune diseases than generally.

Table 3.7 The major causes of myopathies and conditions associated with diffuse myalgia (see also Chapter 14.)

Infectious myositis	Viruses (e.g., influenza, hepatitis B or C, coxsackie, HIV, HTLV-I)
	Bacteria (e.g., Borrelia burgdorferi (Lyme))
	Other (e.g., malaria toxoplasmosis)
Endocrine and metabolic	Hypo/hyperthyroidism, hypercortisolism, Hyperparathyroidism
	Hypocalcemic, hypokalemic
Autoimmune diseases	Polymyositis, dermatomyositis, SLE,
	scleroderma, Sjögren's, RA, PMR
	Vasculitis (e.g., PAN, Wegener's granulomatosis, rheumatoid)
	Myasthenia gravis
	Eosinophilic fasciitis
Carcinomatous myopathy	
Idiopathic	Fibromyalgia (muscles should not be weak)
	Inclusion body myositis
	Sarcoid myositis
Drugs	Lipid-lowering drugs (e.g., lovastatin, clofibrate, gemfibrozil, niacin)
	Immunosuppressants (e.g., colchicine, cyclosporine, D-penicillamine*)
	Rhabdomyolysis (e.g., alcohol, opiates)
	Others (e.g., AZT chloroquine*)
Muscular dystrophies	Limb girdle, facioscapulohumeral
Congenital myopathies†	Mitochondrial myopathy
	Myophosphorylase deficiency Lipid storage diseases

*Drugs most likely to cause painful myopathy.

†Because of variable severity, some conditions may not present until adulthood.

Note: Guillain–Barré and motor neuron disease may be considered in the differential diagnosis of nonpainful muscle weakness.

Drug history
- The following drugs have been reported to cause a myopathy (those marked * are more likely to be painful): lithium, clofibrate, statins, penicillin, colchicine, D-penicillamine*, sulfonamides, hydralazine, cyclosporine, phenytoin, cimetidine* (muscle cramps), zidovudine, carbimazole, and tamoxifen.

- The myositis that occurs with D-penicillamine is not dose- or cumulative dose-dependent. It can be life threatening.
- Drug-induced SLE, which is characterized commonly by arthralgias, aching, and malaise, and less commonly by polyarthritis, can occur with a number of drugs including hydralazine, procainamide, isoniazid, and minocycline. Quinidine, labetalol, captopril, phenytoin, methyldopa, and sulfasalazine may also cause similar symptoms.
- Mild myalgias and arthralgias may be caused by a number of commonly used drugs, e.g., proton pump inhibitors, bisphosphonates and quinolone antibiotics.
- Alcohol in excess and some illegal drugs are associated with severe toxic myopathy occasionally resulting in rhabdomyolysis (see Table 3.7).

Ask about chest pain, dyspnea, palpitations, cough, and hemoptysis

- Cardiac abnormalities are features of autoimmune rheumatic and connective tissue diseases, but are infrequent at initial presentation. Cardiac infection is associated with widespread aches and pains (e.g., rheumatic fever/post-streptococcal myalgias/arthralgias, infective endocarditis).
- Chronic effort-related dyspnea due to interstitial lung disease occurs in many patients with autoimmune connective tissue and rheumatic diseases. Up to 40% of RA patients may have CT evidence of lung disease. In many sedentary patients, however, symptoms are not prominent. Dyspnea may be present at presentation.
- Respiratory failure and aspiration pneumonia can occur as a result of a combination of truncal striated, diaphragmatic, and smooth muscle weakness in PM.
- There is an association between bronchiectasis and RA.
- The most common neoplasm in patients diagnosed with malignancy-associated myositis is of the lung.

Ask specifically about dysphagia, abdominal pain, and diarrhea

- Patients may not mention gastrointestinal symptoms if they have resolved. There are many links between bowel disease and polyarthralgias or polyarthritis.
- Ask specifically about previous severe diarrheal or dysenteric illnesses; *Campylobacter, Yersinia, Shigella,* or *Salmonella*, may be relevant to diagnosing reactive arthritis/SpA.
- Gut smooth muscle may be affected in polymyositis and give rise to dysphagia and abdominal pain.

Examination

In patients with widespread pain a full medical examination is always necessary.

Skin and nails (see Chapter 4)

In all patients, look carefully at the skin and nails:

- Nails may show prominent ridges or pits in psoriatic arthropathy, splinter hemorrhages in infective endocarditis, systemic vasculitis or antiphospholipid syndrome (APS), or periungual erythema in scleroderma and the inflammatory myopathies.

- Look for skin rashes in conditions characterized by widespread pain. For example:
  - erythema migrans in Lyme disease
  - erythema marginatum in rheumatic fever
  - UV sensitive rash on face/arms in SLE
  - violaceous rash on knuckles/around eyes/base of neck in DM
  - livedo reticularis in SLE and APS
  - purpuric rash in vasculitis (e.g., HSP)
  - erythema nodosum in sarcoidosis.
- Lymphadenopathy may be present with either infection or inflammation and is nonspecific. However, if prominent it may denote lymphoma.
- Signs of anemia are a nonspecific finding in many chronic systemic autoimmune diseases.
- Clubbing of the digits may be present in Crohn's disease and ulcerative colitis (associated with SpA) and bronchiectasis (associated with RA).
- Edema can occur in both upper and lower extremities in a subset of patients presenting with inflammatory polyarthritis/tenosynovitis. The condition has been termed RS_3PE (remitting seronegative symmetric synovitis with pitting edema). This condition is striking in that it occurs suddenly, often in patients between 60–80 years old and is very disabling. It may be associated with other conditions e.g., hematologic or gynecologic malignancy.

Examination of the joints

Important points to note when examining joints (detailed examination techniques that help discriminate synovitis from other pathology at specific joints are included in sections in Chapter 2):

- Each joint should be compared to the joint on the opposite extremity, first by observation, then palpation, then by its active and passive range of motion exercises.
- Useful examination tools include a tape measure to record swelling (circumferential) and a goniometer (protractor with arms) to measure the range of joint movement.

Patterns of abnormality

Note the specific cause of joint swelling and site of tenderness, distribution of affected sites, and hypermobility

- In nodal generalized OA, osteophytes (bony swelling—may be tender) can be noted at DIPs (Heberden's nodes) and PIPs (Bouchard's nodes). Periosteal new bone at sites of chronic enthesitis may be palpable and tender.
- Nodules may occur in nodal OA, RA, polyarticular gout, ANCA-associated vasculitis (Churg-Strauss nodules), multicentric reticulohistiocytosis (see Plate 16), or hyperlipidemia (xanthomata).
- Soft tissue swelling with tenderness and painful restriction of the joint on movement suggests an inflammatory arthritis. There is often adjacent muscle wasting. This is most easily appreciated in the interosseous muscles in patients with hand arthritis, or the quadriceps in patients with knee arthritis.

- The "painful joints" may be inflamed tendons or entheses. Tender tendon insertions and periarticular bone tenderness, often without any joint swelling, may denote enthesis inflammation associated with SpA.
- Tendonitis may be part of many autoimmune rheumatic or connective tissue diseases. Look specifically for thickening of the digital flexors and swelling of the dorsal extensor tendon sheath in the hand, and tenderness/swelling of both peroneal and posterior tibial tendons in the foot.
- Gross swelling with painful restriction of small joints is unusual in SLE. Often there is little to find on examination of joints.
- General joint hypermobility may lead to joint and other soft tissue lesions. An examination screen for hypermobility (see Chapter 16) may be helpful (see Table 3.8). Check also for associated features.

Examination of patients with widespread myalgias
- Check for muscle tenderness and weakness. Document the distribution. Is there evidence of neurologic or vascular disease?
- In the past, fibromyalgia was diagnosed based on tenderness at characteristic sites (see Figure. 3.1). However, a diagnosis of fibromyalgia should be considered in any patient with chronic, widespread pain. Despite discomfort, the muscles should be strong.
- Examine the strength of both truncal and limb muscle groups (see Figure 3.2). In the presence of pain it may be difficult to demonstrate subtle degrees of muscle weakness.
- Patterns of muscle weakness are not disease specific; however, there are some characteristic patterns: symmetric proximal extremities in polymyositis and dermatomyositis; quadriceps and forearm/finger flexors in inclusion body myositis; limb muscles in mitochondrial myopathy. (Note: using specific apparatus physical therapists can help document isometric muscle strength in certain muscle groups.)
- Muscles in PMR are not intrinsically weak.
- Muscle wasting is not specific. If wasting is profound and rapid, consider neoplasia. Wasting will occur in most long-standing myopathies.
- Check for increased limb tone and rigidity—most evident by passive movement at a joint—consistent with extrapyramidal disease. There may be resting tremor in the hand, facial impassivity, and "stiff" gait. Muscular tone in the limbs may also be increased in motor neuron disease (MND); however, if presenting with muscle pains, the patient with MND is more likely to have a lower motor neuron pattern of neuronal loss (progressive muscular atrophy) with muscular weakness/wasting, flaccidity, and fasciculations.
- The fatigability of myasthenia gravis can be identified by determining the length of time the patient can keep his arms extended in front of him, or maintain an upward gaze.
- Muscle pains or cramps due to large-vessel ischemia are likely to be associated with muscles that are nontender at rest and strong. Look for diminished pulses or bruits on your examination, and confirm your findings by imaging (e.g., ultrasound, CT angiogram, or MR).
- In suspected cases of polymyositis and dermatomyositis, carefully examine for cardiopulmonary abnormalities. Other associated signs

Table 3.8 Features of the benign joint hypermobility syndrome (BJHS). See also p. 486, for new "Brighton" criteria.

Examination screen (scored out of 9)	Ability to extend fifth finger >90° at MCPJ (score 1 + 1 for R + L)
	Ability to abduct thumb (with wrist flexion) to touch forearm (score 1 + 1)
	Extension of elbows >10°(1 + 1)
	Extension of knees >10°(1 + 1)
	Ability to place hands flat on floor when standing with knees extended (1)
Associated features	Prolonged arthralgias
	Skin striae, hyperextensibility, and abnormal scarring
	Recurrent joint dislocations
	Varicose veins
	Uterine/rectal prolapse
	Recurrent soft-tissue lesions
	Marfanoid habitus (arm span > height)
	Eye signs: drooping eyelids, myopia, down-slanting eyes

- Tenderness of skin overlaying trapezius
- Low cervical spine
- Midpoint of trapezius
- Supraspinatus
- Pectoralis, maximal lateral to the second costochondral junction
- Lateral epicondyle of the elbow
- Upper gluteal area
- Low lumbar spine
- Medial fat pad of the knee

Fig. 3.1 Typical sites of tenderness in fibromyalgia.

in dermatomyositis include periungual erythema/telangiectasias, erythematous violaceous rash and skin calcinosis; include dysphonia and swallowing abnormalities in both polymyositis and dermatomyositis.

- Because of its associations (see Table 3.7), patients with myositis should be carefully examined for the following signs: dry eyes/ mouth (Sjögren's—see Chapter 12), skin thickening/tenderness or discoloration (scleroderma—see Chapter 13), skin rashes (SLE—see Chapter 10), thyroid tenderness or enlargement (endocrine myopathy).

Diagnostic procedures

General points

- ESR and CRP may be higher than normal in the setting of infection, malignancy, or active rheumatic disease. A slightly elevated ESR is a common finding in healthy elderly people.
- A positive ANA may occur in association with many autoimmune conditions, in other diseases (see Table 3.9) and in some healthy people. It is, therefore, not diagnostic for SLE or any single condition; however, high-titer ANA may be significant and conversely, ANA-negative SLE is rare.
- ACPA (such as CCP) are more specific for RA than is RF, which can be positive in a number of inflammatory conditions.
- Controversy exists about the diagnosis of fibromyalgia. It is prudent only to make a diagnosis of fibromyalgia only when inflammatory disorders can be confidently excluded.

Basic tests in patients with polyarthropathy

- Urinalysis (dipstick) may show proteinuria or hematuria. Both glomerular and tubular damage are possible. Glomerulonephritis (in SLE, vasculitis, or endocarditis, for example) is usually associated with significant proteinuria and hematuria simultaneously. These patients will need urgent evaluation by a nephrologist.
- ESR and CRP are nonspecific and may be normal in the early stages of these conditions. If very high (e.g., ESR >100), consider infection or malignancy. There is often no evidence of an acute phase response in patients with enthesitis (even though pain and bony tenderness may be widespread). A mild anemia and thrombocytosis may accompany inflammation.
- Throat swab, anti-Streptolysin O titer (ASOT), and anti-DNAseB antibodies may be useful to identify a post-streptococcal condition.
- Other simple blood tests that should be considered in the appropriate setting: random blood sugar (diabetes); TFTs/thyroid antibodies (hyper/hypothyroidism); prostatic specific antigen (malignancy).
- Joint fluid aspiration and culture is mandatory for patients in whom sepsis is a possibility. Fluid should be examined by polarized light microscopy in suspected cases of crystal-induced synovitis.
- In patients who are ANA-positive, testing serum for extractable nuclear antigens (ENAs) may be useful for characterizing the type of autoimmune process. Ro, La, Sm, and RNP positivity are each found in a slightly different spectrum of disorders.
- In many patients presenting with a short history of widespread joint pains, radiographs will be normal. An early sign of joint inflammation is periarticular osteopenia, but this is not specific for any particular disorder. Recognized types of erosions and their distribution can be noted by experienced radiologists in specific conditions (e.g., RA, psoriatic arthritis, gout).

(a) Functional

Stand from low chair.
Arms folded

Sit from lying. Arms folded

(b) Specific resisted

(i) Patient resists downward force on abducted arms

(ii) Patient lifts head and neck against a resistance on the forehead

(iii) Patient resists force downwards on thigh

Fig. 3.2 Screening examination for proximal myopathy. (a) Functional movements requiring truncal and proximal lower limb muscle strength. (b) Resisted movement testing of deltoid (i), longitudinal flexors of the neck (ii), and iliopsoas/quadriceps (iii) strength.

- Referral to a sexual health clinic for further detailed investigations if there is a suggestion of recent or recurrent genital infection may help to strengthen the evidence for a diagnosis of reactive arthritis.

Basic laboratory tests in patients with widespread muscle pain/weakness

- Dipstick urinalysis: to screen for hematuria or myoglobinuria.
- CBC and measures of acute-phase response.
- An endocrine and metabolic screen: urea/electrolytes, creatinine, free thyroxine and TSH, blood calcium, phosphate and 25-hydroxyvitamin D, LFTs.
- Elevated CK or aldolase occurs in most cases of PM. ALT, AST, and LDH are nonspecific markers of muscle damage. Note that specific muscle isoenzymes of CK and LDH exist and the normal range of all enzymes may vary in different populations. Muscle enzymes may be elevated after noninflammatory causes of muscle damage, e.g., exercise/trauma.
- Check for ANA and, if positive, screen for ENAs. Antibodies to certain (cytoplasmic) tRNA synthetases (e.g., Jo-1) are myositis-specific.
- All of the procedures just mentioned may reasonably be done in cases where you think muscle pains are due to fibromyalgia but want to rule out other pathology.
- Think of checking for urinary myoglobin in cases where acute widespread muscle pain may be associated with excessive alcohol or ingestion of certain drugs (cocaine, amphetamines, ecstasy, heroin), exercise, or trauma. Such patients may be at risk of renal failure.
- Polymyositis can be a presenting feature of HIV. In HIV-positive patients, infections causing muscle disease include TB and microsporidia.
- Viral myositis may be clinically indistinguishable from PM. Serology may yield diagnostic clues.

Electrophysiology and imaging in patients with muscle conditions

- Electromyographic abnormalities occur in two-thirds of patients with muscle inflammation. More information is likely if studied in the acute rather than the chronic phase of the illness. In the acute phase, denervation and muscle degeneration give rise to fibrillation potentials in 74% of polymyositis and 33% of dermatomyositis patients. Other features include: low-amplitude short-duration motor unit and polyphasic potentials.
- Electromyography is poor at discriminating on-going muscle inflammation in myositis from steroid-induced myopathy.
- There are characteristic MR patterns of abnormality in polymyositis and dermatomyositis. MR can be used to identify potential muscle biopsy sites to avoid false-negative results associated with patchy muscle inflammation.

Muscle biopsy

- Muscle biopsy should be considered in all patients evaluated for polymyositis or dermatomyositis.
- In polymyositis, inflammatory infiltrates predominate in the endomysial area around muscle fibers without perifascicular atrophy. In

Table 3.9 Examples of the prevalence of antinuclear antibodies (ANA) in some diseases using Hep2 cells as substrate

Population group		Prevalence of ANA
Normal population		8%
SLE		95%
Other autoimmune rheumatic diseases	Systemic sclerosis	90%
	Sjögren's syndrome	80%
	Rheumatoid arthritis	60%
	Polymyositis	40%
	Polyarteritis nodosa	18%
Other diseases	Chronic active hepatitis	100%
	Drug-induced lupus	100%
	Myasthenia gravis	50%
	Waldenstrom's macroglobulinemia	20%
	Diabetes	25%

dermatomyositis, inflammation is more prominent in the perimysial area and around small blood vessels and there is typically perifascicular atrophy.
- Routine tests do not reliably distinguish polymyositis from cases of viral myositis. Some of the glycogen storage diseases will become apparent from light microscopy of biopsy material.

Investigations for malignancy
Investigations in adults with widespread bony pain should aim to rule out malignancy, particularly myeloma and malignancies from breast, renal and prostate cancers:
- Investigations may include: mammography, urine cytology, PSA, renal US, serum and urinary protein electrophoresis.
- Hypercalcemia may accompany these conditions; check blood calcium, phosphate and albumin (also PTH).
- Intact PTH should also be checked in suspected cases of osteomalacia (raised due to calcium/vitamin D deficiency) together with 25-hydroxyvitamin D levels (low or low/normal), alkaline phosphatase (high/normal), and 24h urinary calcium (low).
- Radiographs of affected sites are important. Include a CXR.
- Bone scintigraphy can identify sites of neoplasia, Paget's disease, polyostotic osteoporosis, or osteomalacia (see Plate 17). Although characteristic patterns exist, it is generally not specific for any condition.

- Bone biopsy (maintained undecalcified by placing sample in 70% alcohol) of affected sites will be diagnostic in some, but not all, cases of osteomalacia, osteoporosis, renal osteodystrophy, malignancy, and Paget's disease as good samples are hard to obtain. The best samples are obtained from a transiliac biopsy. Bone marrow can be aspirated for examination at the same time.

Widespread pain in children and adolescents

Background

Disease classification

A working party, under the auspices of the International League of Associations for Rheumatology (ILAR) met in 2001 to establish a consensus about a unifying classification of arthritis in childhood termed juvenile idiopathic arthritis (JIA). A comparison of old and new classification is shown in Table 3.4. For details of each condition, see the relevant diagnostic headings in Chapter 9.

- Systemic JIA (previously systemic onset JRA) is proposed to be classified as arthritis preceded by or occurring with daily recurring fever of more than 2 days (documented for greater than 3 days) plus one or more of the following: an evanescent, nonfixed, erythematous rash; generalized lymphadenopathy; enlarged liver or spleen; serositis.
- Persistent oligoarthritis is defined by the involvement of no more than four joints throughout the disease course. Extended oligoarthritis affects a cumulative total of five joints or more after the first 6 months of disease. Excluded from these groups are patients with a family history of psoriasis (first- or second-degree relative); a positive RF; HLA B27 (male >8 years of age); systemic arthritis.
- The definition of psoriatic arthritis has been broadened under the new ILAR classification.
- Enthesitis has a key-classifying role in the group of conditions previously classified as SpA.

Assess the distribution of the pain

Are the pains in a joint distribution? What is their pattern?

- Arthralgias may accompany any infection, although they are generally short lived. Persistent (>6 weeks) joint pains raise the possibility of many other diseases (see Table 3.10).
- Poststreptococcal arthralgias are often migratory. Skin overlying joints often appears red in acute rheumatic fever but not in systemic JIA (systemic onset JCA).
- The presentation of polyarticular JIA (RF/ACPA+ or RF/ACPA−) is often profound, with several weeks' history of worsening joint stiffness and swelling.
- Stiffness is a prominent associated feature of the joint pain in both (RF/ ACPA+) and (RF/ACPA−) polyarticular JIA.

Taking a history

Are the pains due to myalgias or myositis?

The differential diagnosis is wide (see Table 3.11):

- Acute viral myositis is distinguished from chronic myositis by its localization to calf muscles, severe pain, and its resolution within 4 weeks.

Table 3.10 The differential diagnosis of (RF−) JIA

Infection (multiple sites in immunodeficiency)	Staphylococcus septic arthritis
	Haemophilus influenzae septic arthritis
Reactive to an infectious agent	Parvovirus B19, hepatitis, rubella, rubella vaccination
	Post-streptococcal, rheumatic fever
Autoimmune connective tissue disorders	SLE
	MCTD, overlap syndromes
	Poly/dermatomyositis
Systemic vasculitis syndromes	Kawasaki disease (young child, high fever, desquamating extremity rash)
	Polyarteritis nodosa
	Granulomatosis with polyangiitis (Wegener's)
	HSP, Behçet's disease
Sarcoid arthritis (polyarthritis, rash, uveitis)	
Hematological disorders	Sickle cell disease
	Constitutional bleeding disorders
	Acute leukemia (bone and joint pain)
Other causes	Chronic recurrent multifocal osteomyelitis
	Diabetic cheiroarthropathy
	Familial Mediterranean fever

- Chronic muscle weakness suggests an autoimmune connective tissue disease such as juvenile dermatomyositis. Myalgias and muscle cramps occur in hypothyroidism, uremia, and electrolyte imbalance.
- Myalgias are common in pediatric SLE, but myopathy occurs rarely (10%).
- Episodic cramping or muscle pain related to exercise in early childhood might reflect muscular dystrophy, congenital myopathy, myotonic disorders, or genetic defects in glycogen or glucose metabolism.
- A pain syndrome (e.g., fibromyalgia) is a diagnosis of exclusion. Enthesitis (ERA) should be carefully excluded.

Is there bone pain?

Do the pains represent bone pain—persistent, deep-seated pains which change little with posture or movement?

- Night-time pain is typical of bony involvement in malignancy or osteomyelitis. Acute lymphoblastic leukemia, lymphoma, and neuroblastoma are the most common malignant lesions.
- Achy "bony" pain around joints may be due to enthesitis. Patients with ERA/SpA can present with enthesitis alone.
- Migratory bone pains are typical in multifocal osteomyelitis.

Is the child with arthritis systemically unwell?

- Malignancy should be ruled out and vasculitis and autoimmune connective tissue diseases considered in all children with persistent polyarthritis or widespread pains who have systemic symptoms.
- Fever is nonspecific but essential to making a diagnosis of systemic JIA (see Figure 3.3), which is associated with spiking fevers, chills, and sweats. Anorexia and weight loss are common. Vasculitis (see Chapter 15) and FMF (see Chapter 18) should be considered in appropriate patients.
- There may be several months between the onset of systemic features and the arthritis of systemic JIA.
- Serositis is typical in systemic JIA but also occurs in SLE.

Table 3.11 Classification of childhood disorders characterized by myalgias and muscle weakness

Muscular dystrophies	X-linked, e.g., Duchenne
	Autosomal dominant, e.g., fascioscapulohumeral
	Autosomal recessive: limb girdle
Congenital myopathies	e.g., myopathic arthrogryposis
Myotonic dystrophy	
Metabolic disorders	Glycogen storage disease, e.g., acid maltase/ phosphorylase/phosphofructokinase deficiency
	Familial periodic paralyses
	Due to endocrinopathies, e.g., Addison's disease, Cushing's disease
Inflammatory diseases	Postinfectious, e.g., viruses—influenza B, coxsackie B, echo, polio
	Autoimmune, e.g., juvenile RA, dermatomyositis, SLE
Genetic abnormalities	Osteogenesis imperfecta
	Ehlers–Danlos
	Mucopolysaccharidoses
Trauma	Physical, e.g., rhabdomyolysis
	Toxic, e.g., snakebite
	Drugs, e.g., steroids, hydroxychloroquine, diuretics
Neurogenic atrophies	Spinal muscular and anterior horn cell dysfunction
	Peripheral nerve, e.g., peroneal muscular atrophy
	Neuromuscular, e.g., congenital myasthenia

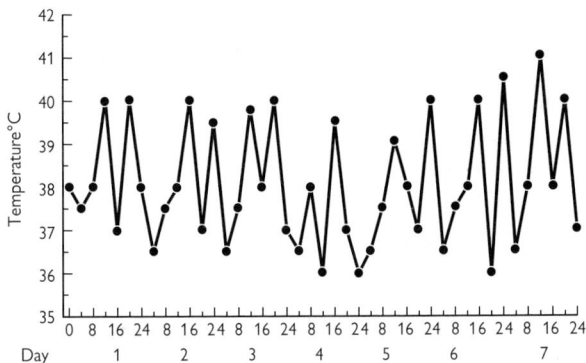

Fig. 3.3 Double-daily fever spikes with rapid return to below 37°C in systemic JIA (systemic-onset JRA)

- In children <1 year, fever and arthralgias raise the possibility of chronic infantile neurological cutaneous and articular (CINCA) syndrome (see Chapter 9) and hyperimmunoglobulin D syndrome.
- A catastrophic illness can occur in children with systemic JIA. It is termed macrophage-activation or hematophagocytic syndrome and is characterized by cytopenias, hepatic dysfunction, encephalopathy, and disseminated intravascular coagulation with bleeding.
- A history of recurrent infections and arthritis may suggest immunodeficiency. The most common is X-linked humoral deficiency.

Is there a rash?
Does the child have a rash or did one precede the onset of pains?
- Rashes raise the possibility of preceding infection: EBV, rubella, and adenovirus are common and are associated with myalgias, arthralgias, and fever.
- The rash of systemic JIA is a salmon-pink macular rash. Lesions may either persist or come and go and may exhibit Köebner phenomenon—the exaggeration of the rash at sites of trauma.
- UV skin sensitivity may indicate SLE or dermatomyositis.
- Check for a vasculitic rash (e.g., HSP, cutaneous PAN). Systemic vasculitis can be associated with recurrent fevers and joint pains.

Are there ophthalmic symptoms?
Eye symptoms are an important indicator of underlying autoimmunity in the context of persistent joint or muscle pains:
- Uveitis is associated with most forms of JIA (particularly in association with ANA), but also may indicate an ERA/SpA (uveitis = pain/ discomfort, blurring of vision, photophobia and a "red eye").

- Impairment of visual fields suggests a retinal abnormality—a typical manifestation in juvenile dermatomyositis (due to occlusive vasculopathy).
- The challenge is that most uveitis is generally asymptomatic in children with JIA. Screening is imperative to identify those with active disease.

Examination

Full medical examination

A full medical examination is essential:
- Pharyngeal erythema is nonspecific and swabs should be cultured for streptococci. Sterile pharyngitis is a known feature of systemic JIA.
- Lymphadenopathy is common but nonspecific.
- For skin examination in detail see the preceding sections under Widespread Pain in Children and Adolescents. UV sensitivity occurs in DM and SLE; healing psoriasis may mimic Gottron's lesions; calcinosis and pretibial hypopigmentation are signs of DM.
- The cardiovascular examination is important. Pericarditis is common in systemic and other forms of JIA but is infrequently detected clinically. Myocarditis and heart failure also occur (rarely) in systemic JIA. Persistent tachycardia without anemia/fever raises the possibility of myocarditis. Cardiac conduction defects are common in juvenile DM.
- A variety of cardiac conditions occur in (RF/ACPA+) JIA including aortic valve insufficiency. The latter also occurs in ERA/SpA (8–30%).
- Respiratory examination may be abnormal if the arthralgias/arthritis are associated with respiratory tract infection; however, fixed crackles may indicate fibrosis (e.g., (RF+) JIA, PM) and a simultaneous reduction in expansion, breath sounds, and vocal fremitus suggests pleural effusion (e.g., (RF+) JIA).
- Bedside eye examination may be unrevealing even in those with ophthalmic symptoms. Thrombosis of dilated blood vessels at the margin of the upper lid is characteristic of dermatomyositis and polymyositis. Dry eyes are a common complaint, and may be the result of medication side effects; dry eyes are also found in association with a number of rheumatic diseases.
- As with all chronic conditions of childhood, growth and maturation (skeletal, endocrine/pubertal, and psychological) assessments should be considered at regular intervals.

Musculoskeletal examination—general principles

- Synovitis of a joint is characterized by soft-tissue swelling, effusion, and a reduced range of joint movement.
- Enthesitis may not be accompanied by an effusion; it can appear alone at bony insertions of ligaments/tendons with joint stiffness but without swelling.
- Tendonitis can be difficult to distinguish from synovitis. Its diagnosis requires a precise knowledge of anatomy. The inflamed tendon may be more painful on active range of motion exercises.
- If the condition is chronic, an assessment of limb growth should be done, e.g., measuring leg length discrepancy (see Plate 18).

Musculoskeletal examination—patterns of joint, tendon, and enthesis involvement

A full examination should be undertaken:

- Ligament/tendon insertion tenderness, not necessarily associated with swelling, may denote enthesitis. Enthesitis, which is probably more common (or at least more commonly recognized in lower limbs) raises the possibility of ERA/SpA.
- Almost any joint can be involved, including those in the cervical spine. Hip joint involvement is almost always symmetric.
- There is no consistent pattern of joint or tendon involvement that distinguishes polyarticular (RF+) JIA from the majority of conditions associated with, or characterized by, polyarticular (RF−) JIA.
- Subsets of polyarticular (RF−) arthritis have been suggested on the basis of features such as "painful" or "dry" synovitis, stiffness, and other laboratory and genetic indices.
- Muscle tenderness is not specific. If confined to the calves, consider viral myositis. Weakness can accompany metabolic and endocrine myopathies and is not specific for inflammatory myopathy.
- Muscle weakness at rest may be present in children with severe forms of inherited metabolic muscle diseases. Often weakness only becomes apparent after exercise in these conditions (see Table 3.12).

Laboratory tests

- Laboratory abnormalities are nonspecific in polyarticular (RF−) JIA.
- Because RF may appear in association with infections, ILAR criteria propose that significant titers of RF should be demonstrated on two occasions at least 3 months apart to make a diagnosis of polyarticular (RF+) JIA.
- ACPA, on the other hand, are sensitive and specific for a diagnosis of polyarticular JIA.
- A range of laboratory investigations is suggested when considering a diagnosis of systemic JIA (see Table 3.13).
- Lymphopenia is a hallmark of DM and SLE, and is not a feature of inflammatory arthritis.
- Neutrophilia and thrombocytosis are invariably present and can be marked in systemic JIA whereas leukopenia and thrombocytopenia are uncommon.
- Urinalysis is important in all children with widespread pains and may detect blood or hemoglobinuria in some muscle diseases (actually is myoglobin). Protein and blood may be a sign of underlying kidney inflammation in connective tissue diseases.
- Conventional acute phase markers can be normal in PM/DM. A sensitive indicator (though nonspecific) of active disease is von Willebrand factor.
- A raised CK, ALT/AST, or aldolase is a sensitive but not specific sign of autoimmune myositis.
- A positive ANA is found in association with many autoimmune connective tissue diseases and some JIA subsets. ANA (speckled) is positive in 60–70% of children with polymyositis and dermatomyositis.
- Additional initial investigations in those suspected of having myopathic pains include bone biochemistry and TFTs.

Imaging tests: radiographs
- Employ specialist pediatric radiologists and technicians if possible.
- Proper X-ray beam coning, high-speed intensifying screens, gonadal shielding, and digital radiography all reduce radiation dose.
- Soft tissue swelling and joint-space widening are important, but nonspecific, signs of early arthritis in young children.
- The most easily recognized sign of early polyarthritis in an older child will be periarticular osteopenia.
- At joints also look for joint space narrowing, erosions, growth abnormalities, subluxation, and ankylosis. All occur at multiple joints in systemic JIA and polyarticular JIA.
- In children with abnormalities in stature/skeletal morphology look for diffuse but subtle changes in bone quality and epiphyses.
- Destruction of bone cortex at sites of pain in patients with myalgias, arthralgias, or polyarthritis may suggest malignancy.

Table 3.12 Characteristics of rare inherited causes of muscle pain and/or weakness

Condition	Musculoskeletal features	Other features
Malignant hyperthermia (muscle sensitivity to severe physical or metabolic stress)	Acute rigidity and subsequent rhabdomyolysis	Acute—fever. Hyperkalemia
McArdle's disease (myophosphorylase deficiency)	Painful (temporary) muscle contractures triggered by exercise	Autosomal recessive. Genotypic and phenotypic heterogeneity
Tauri's disease (phosphofructokinase deficiency)	Similar to McArdle's	Hemolytic anemia (reticulocytosis)
Von Gierke's disease (glucose 6 phosphatase deficiency)	Skeletal myopathy	Hepatomegaly. Growth retardation. Hypoglycemia. Lactic acidosis
Pompe's disease (acid maltase deficiency)	Severe skeletal muscle weakness and cardiomyopathy	Death in first year
Cori–Forbes disease (debrancher enzyme deficiency)	Variation from severe childhood myopathic to symptomless adult forms	
Mitochondrial myopathies	Severely limited exercise capacity	Dyspnea. Lactic acidosis

Table 3.13 Useful tests in investigating suspected systemic JIA

In all patients:	CBC, ESR, CRP
	Renal and liver biochemistry, serum albumin
	Serum immunoglobulins
	Clotting screen
	Blood cultures
	ECG, CXR, abdominal/pelvic US
	ANA
	Bone marrow aspiration and biopsy
	Ocular slit-lamp examination
	Joint aspirate (single joint)
	Radiographs of selected affected joints
In selected patients:	Muscle enzymes (CK, ALT/AST, and aldolase)
	RF/ACPA
	Isotope bone/gallium scan
	Upper GI series/small bowel follow-through
	Tissue biopsies
	Viral serology—parvovirus, adenovirus, others
	Echocardiogram
	ASO/antihyaluronidase antibodies
	Urinary homovanillic/vanillylmandelic acid
	Serum IgD

Imaging: US, skeletal MR, and bone scan
- The role of US is expanding. It is noninvasive, nonionizing, can be done at the bedside, and is generally accepted well by children.
- With US, cartilaginous forms of bones can be visualized. This is especially advantageous in the hip where femoral head position and abnormal movement can be seen in young children.
- US is very useful for identifying effusions, notably in the hip, and for discriminating effusion from synovial thickening.
- Bone scan provides critical information in musculoskeletal pain when radiographs are unrevealing. Though of less use when joints are involved, bone scan should be considered when pain originates in bone or infection is a possibility.
- CT is a reliable way of documenting sacroiliac disease in children suspected of having ERA (SpA).

- MR has become the imaging modality of choice, especially when the diagnosis of JIA is not straightforward. It is more sensitive than radiographs for detecting soft-tissue and most bone lesions.
- MR is more sensitive than radiographs for detecting changes in joints associated with chronic arthritis. MR should provide diagnostic information if there is doubt about the presence of arthritis in a joint after clinical examination and radiographs.
- The discrimination of synovitis and enthesitis by MR may have implications for the diagnosis of ERA (SpA) compared with JIA.

Investigations of muscle pains

- EMG patterns of abnormality occur in muscular dystrophy, myasthenia gravis, and autoimmune myositis but each is not specific.
- Evidence of an inflammatory myopathy on EMG is not specific to juvenile dermatomyositis and may be due to a myositis-component of another autoimmune connective tissue disease.
- MR can confirm myositis and reveal potential sites of biopsy in what can be a patchy process.

The spectrum of presentation of rheumatic disease

Skin disorders and rheumatic disease

The importance of examining the skin

- The skin is the most accessible organ to examine.
- Pattern recognition of skin symptoms and lesions is valuable in aiding diagnosis (e.g., acute or chronic sarcoid) and prognosis of rheumatic diseases (e.g., nodules and vasculitis in RA).
- Musculoskeletal abnormalities may be mirrored by skin abnormalities (e.g., joint hypermobility and skin laxity with bruising, scarring, and striae).
- Some antirheumatic drugs produce highly specific and potentially serious cutaneous reactions that require prompt diagnosis and management.

Regional abnormalities

The scalp

Scalp symptoms and lesions may be subtle:

- Scalp tenderness and the description of scalp "lumps" (due to temporal artery aneurysms) are recognized in giant cell arteritis.
- C2 root/occipital neuropathy (e.g., in RA) or shingles may be associated with dysesthesias over the scalp and occipital neuralgia.
- Alopecia may be localized (areata) or diffuse (e.g., in SLE or iron deficiency). Scarring alopecia is typical of discoid lupus.
- Scalp psoriasis may be evident along the hairline
- A "salt and pepper" pattern of hyperpigmentation and hypopigmentation may be seen in scleroderma.

Face and ears

Face and ears are in sun-exposed areas. Consider UV skin sensitivity:

- A variety of patterns of SLE-associated, UV-sensitive rashes may occur. The rash is often diffuse. Shaded areas (e.g., nasolabial folds) may not be affected (see Chapter 10).
- As in SLE, rosacea can present with an erythematosus facial rash, but does not spare the nasolabial folds. Distinction is sometimes difficult without biopsy.
- Periorbital edema occurs in dermatomyositis, angioedema (which may be a presenting feature of SLE), and in nephrotic syndrome.
- Heliotrope rash refers to violaceous edema/erythema of the eyelids in dermatomyositis (see Chapter 14).
- The cutaneous infiltration of chronic sarcoid (lupus pernio) (see Chapter 18) across the nose and cheeks may be overt (papular) but also may be quite subtle (see Plate 19).
- Saddle nose deformity/nasal cartilage destruction has a number of causes: granulomatosis with polyangiitis (Wegener's) (see Chapter 15), relapsing polychondritis (see Chapter 18), sarcoidosis, hereditary connective tissue disease (e.g., Stickler's syndrome see Chapter 16), and lethal midline granuloma. Nasal septal and palatal perforation can also occur in the setting of cocaine use.
- Ear deformities ("cauliflower ear") may be associated with relapsing polychondritis.

- Purpuric lesions on the ears (in the absent of overt auricular deformity) may be due to levamisole, which is a common adulterant in cocaine.
- The pinna is a common site for gouty tophi and discoid lupus.
- Oral aphthous ulcers are common. Oral ulceration may follow disease activity (e.g., in SLE or granulomatosis with polyangiitis (Wegener's granulomatosis)) Ulcers in reactive arthritis are typically painless. Oral aphthous ulcers are frequently idiopathic, and not associated with systemic disease.
- Large punched-out and numerous tongue and buccal ulcers that scar are a hallmark of Behçet's disease (see Chapter 18). They may remain for several weeks.
- Strawberry erythema of the tongue and lips should not be missed in children. It may denote self-limiting streptococcal infections but may also herald the desquamating palmar (and sole) rash of Kawasaki disease (see Chapter 15).
- Strawberry (i.e., erythematous/swollen) gums may be a sign of granulomatosis with polyangiitis (Wegener's granulomatosis).
- Lacy white streaks on the buccal mucosa suggest lichen planus.
- Lipid skin deposits around the eye occur in hyperlipidemia and multicentric reticulohistiocytosis

Hands and nails

Hands and nails should be examined closely:
- A photosensitive eruption spares the finger webs and palms.
- Erythema on the back of the fingers may help distinguish dermatomyositis from SLE.
- In patients with Raynaud's phenomenon (RP), finger ulceration, finger pulp atrophy (with smooth tapering of the finger tips), induration, and tethering of the skin indicates scleroderma (see Chapter 13). Unlike normal skin, the skin of scleroderma does not form fine wrinkles when pinched.
- Onycholysis, pitting, salmon patches, and subungual hyperkeratosis are typical of psoriasis (see Chapter 8).
- Subungual splinter hemorrhages may be associated with trauma, infective endocarditis, systemic vasculitis, or thromboangiitis obliterans.
- Nailfold capillaries can be examined with an ophthalmoscope at 40 diopters after applying a drop of oil (or surgical lubricant) to the cuticle. Enlarged (dilated) capillary loops and capillary "dropout" suggests an underlying autoimmune connective tissue disease, particularly scleroderma and dermatomyositis.

Types of eruption

Macular rashes

Macular rashes are flat (nonpalpable) areas of altered skin color. Papules are lumps <1 cm in diameter:
- Maculopapular rashes are typical of viral infections.
- A short-lived, pinkish ("salmon-colored"), maculopapular eruption occurs on the trunk and limbs in Still's disease. It is often prominent in

the late afternoon, and coincides with temperature spikes. If scratched, the rash may blanch ("Köebner phenomenon").
- Erythema that enlarges to form erythematosus patches with pale centers suggests rheumatic fever ("erythema marginatum").
- A "bulls-eye" erythematosus lesion around a tick bite may be the erythema migrans of Lyme disease.
- Maculopapular eruptions can occur from NSAIDs, gold, D-penicillamine, sulfasalazine, azathioprine hypersensitivity, and leflunomide (see Chapter 5).

Pustules and blisters
Blisters may be vesicles (<0.5 cm diameter) or bullae (>0.5 cm diameter):
- The most common pustular rash is due to folliculitis.
- Pustules confined to the hands and feet suggest reactive arthritis, although local forms of psoriasis may be indistinguishable. Psoriasis can also occur as "raindrop" erythematous lesions, also known as guttate lesions.
- Generalized pustular rashes can occur in vasculitis, the neutrophilic dermatoses, intestinal bypass syndromes, Behçet's disease, and gonococcal bacteremia.
- Bullous eruptions may be due to SLE, drug reactions, pemphigus and pemphigoid.

Plaques
Plaques are slightly raised, circumscribed areas of skin, often disc shaped:
- Plaques are the hallmark of psoriasis. Skin may be scaly and flake off easily. Lesions are often red.
- Psoriatic plaques can occur anywhere on the skin, but typical sites are over the extensor surfaces of the joints, in the intergluteal cleft, and the umbilicus.
- Scaling may be a feature of discoid lupus; scaling tends to occur at the periphery of the lesion.

Vascular lesions
Bleeding into the skin that does not blanch is called purpura. It may sometimes be palpable. Telangiectasias are dilated small vascular lesions that blanch on pressure:
- Nonpalpable purpura may be due to thrombocytopenia, platelet dysfunction, trauma (± capillary/skin fragility, e.g., chronic steroid use), hemophilia, anticoagulation, and hereditary connective tissue diseases (e.g., Ehlers-Danlos—see Chapter 16).
- Palpable purpura suggests vasculitis, including drug-induced (see Chapter 15).
- Widespread telangiectasias occur in limited cutaneous scleroderma (see Chapter 13), hereditary hemorrhagic telangiectasia, and dermatomyositis.

Ulcers and ulcerating rashes
Ulcers are defined as a loss or defect of dermis and epidermis produced by sloughing of necrotic tissue:

- Cutaneous polyarteritis nodosa may cause painful ulcerating lesions in the lower extremities, as can other forms of systemic vasculitis that affect the medium-sized vessels.
- Cutaneous ulceration may have more than one cause in autoimmune diseases. For example, vasculitis, venous stasis in an immobile patient, and ulceration over nodules or pressure points may all contribute to the same set of lesions. Trauma may be an important cause of cutaneous ulcers in a patient who is already predisposed towards forming these lesions.
- A painful, indurated, expanding, plum-colored plaque or acneiform pustule that then ulcerates suggests pyoderma gangrenosum. The ulcer has irregular, bluish margins.
- Neurotropic ulcers are a classic sequelae of diabetes, but they can also occur in association with mononeuritis multiplex (from vasculitis) and other rheumatic diseases.
- Severe widespread ulceration developing rapidly in a child may suggest dermatomyositis.
- Vasculitic ulcers in the context of livedo reticularis and antibodies to phospholipids (e.g., cardiolipin) may be indicative of the antiphospholipid antibody syndrome (APS) (see Chapter 11).

Textural abnormalities

Abnormalities of the texture of the skin may be difficult to discern. Atrophy and thinning, laxity, thickening, and induration may all be associated with disease.

- Generalized skin atrophy and thinning is an age-related process, but this can be accelerated by chronic steroid use; heritable diseases of connective tissue should also be considered.
- Skin laxity can best be demonstrated over elbow and knee extensor surfaces. Generalized laxity of connective tissue may result in varicose veins and internal organ prolapse.
- True acral and digital puffiness in a patient with Raynaud's is suggestive of scleroderma. Skin thickening has a variety of causes (see below). Scleroderma and scleroderma-like skin may be localized, limited, or diffuse—this distinction is important (see Table 4.1).

Diagnostic issues in patients with skin thickening

- Raynaud's phenomenon (RP) invariably precedes the onset of systemic sclerosis (scleroderma), but is not a characteristic of morphea, linear scleroderma, or scleroderma mimics.
- In patients with RP, abnormal nailfold capillaries on capillaroscopy may indicate the presence of scleroderma or "prescleroderma" (see Plate 4).
- The specificities of autoantibodies are often predictive of the scleroderma subtype. In patients with RP, the ANA has predictive value for identifying patients who may progress to scleroderma; anticentromere antibodies are associated with limited cutaneous scleroderma; anti-topoisomerase I (SCL-70) and anti-RNA polymerase III antibodies are linked with progression to diffuse cutaneous scleroderma.

- Patients with diffuse cutaneous scleroderma have a preponderance of visceral organ involvement in the first 5 years of disease; screening investigations should include pulmonary function tests, an echocardiogram, and a high-resolution CT of the chest to screen for pulmonary hypertension and pulmonary fibrosis.
- Eosinophilic fasciitis may occur as a paraneoplastic syndrome, and is associated with hematologic malignancies. Clinically, eosinophilic fasciitis is associated with skin that takes on the appearance of an orange peel (*peau d'orange*).
- Linear scleroderma in children can produce lifelong deformities because limbs to develop correct length and bulk.
- Scleroderma-like syndromes may occur secondarily to exposure to some industrial chemicals: vinyl chloride, chlorinated organic solvents, and silicon and epoxy resins.

Table 4.1 Pattern recognition in patients with skin thickening

Classification	Skin features
Morphea may be localized (guttate) or generalized	Early small skin areas affected (itchy). Progression to hidebound skin, typically on trunk (areola spared) and legs. Lesions become waxy and hypo/ hyperpigmented guttate (small <10 mm) papules usually on neck and anterior chest
Linear scleroderma	Linear bandlike pattern often in dermatomal distribution. Atrophy of muscles is common. Fixed joint deformities and growth abnormalities can occur
"Coup de sabre"	Linear scleroderma on the face/scalp can be depressed; ivory in appearance. Hemiatrophy can occur
Systemic sclerosis (early)	Early morning "puffiness" in hands and feet, facial "tightness." Nonpitting edema of intact dermal and epidermal appendages. High degree of suspicion needed
Systemic sclerosis (classic)	Firm, taut, hidebound skin proximal to MCP joints. Skin may be coarse, pigmented, and dry. Epidermal thinning, loss of hair, and sweating can occur. Telangiectasias and skin calcinosis become obvious. Skin creases disappear. Such change proximal to elbows or knees in the limbs or below the clavicles (in those with face and neck involvement) classifies disease as diffuse as opposed to limited systemic sclerosis
Systemic sclerosis (late)	2–15 years after onset of classical phase, skin softens but pigmentation changes remain. Skin becomes atrophic and can ulcerate
Eosinophilic fasciitis	Phases: early—pitting edema; progressive—peau d'orange; late—induration ("woody feel") with venous guttering when limb elevated. Arms and legs most commonly affected but fingers mainly spared. Synovitis and low-grade myositis may occur. Eosinophilia is usually striking but not always present
Lipodermatosclerosis	Fibrotic induration of lower legs associated with venous stasis ("champagne-bottle legs")
Diabetes	Waxy thickening of extremities. Insidious progression. Joints of the hands become stiff, the tendons can thicken. Skin changes proximal to wrist and on the face very unlikely but stiffening of elbow and shoulder joints not uncommon
Dependent lymphedema	Feet/ankles/lower legs. Often pitting. Chronic presence may give hyperkeratosis. Main causes: R- or L-sided heart failure, renal failure, nephrotic syndrome, and low-protein states

Skin vasculitis in adults

Background

There are a variety of ways in which systemic vasculitis may present, including fever of unknown origin, organ infarction, gastrointestinal bleeding, and high acute phase reactants in a generally unwell patient. However, a vasculitic skin rash is one of the most common presenting features of systemic vasculitis, and can be an important diagnostic clue.

When to consider a diagnosis of vasculitis (see also Chapters 15 and 22)

- Systemic vasculitis is rare. Overall, the annual incidence is about 40 per million.
- Cutaneous vasculitis, however, is not rare; it can follow viral or bacterial illness, can be triggered by drugs, and is associated with malignancy.
- Biopsy generally demonstrates degranulation of neutrophils ("leukocytoclasis") and evidence of vessel destruction.
- The list of causes is long (see Table 4.2); however, in about 50% of cases, no cause may be found.
- Cutaneous vasculitis may also occur in association with another autoimmune disease not normally characterized by vasculitis, including SLE, rheumatoid arthritis, and Sjögren's syndrome.

Important considerations (see Table 4.3)

The following important points of clinical assessment should be followed in patients with possible vasculitic rashes.

- Determine whether the patient has been taking a new drug. Many antibiotics, including penicillins, sulfonamindes, and cephalosporins, commonly cause cutaneous vasculitis.
- Evaluate the patient for evidence of chronic infection; Hepatitis B, Hepatitis C, and HIV all are worth considering. Endocarditis should also be considered in the right host (e.g., the elderly, or patients who use intravenous drugs).
- Look for evidence of a primary autoimmune disorder that may be associated with cutaneous vasculitis. Inflammatory bowel disease, for example, can occasionally cause a leukocytoclastic vasculitis in addition to oral ulcerations and pyoderma gangrenosum. Because SLE is common, it may be worthwhile to check ANA and serum complements as well.
- Look for evidence of cryoglobulinemic vasculitis. Serum cryoglobulins tests are often mishandled, leading to false-negative results. Rheumatoid factor is detected in 80% of patients with mixed essential cryoglobulinemia, and may be a better screening test.
- Age-appropriate screening for malignancy should be performed. Serum and urine electrophoresis with immunofixation may be of value.
- Urinalysis may demonstrate an "active sediment"; evidence of hematuria, proteinuria, or red blood cell casts may be the first clue that a patient has a systemic vasculitis.

Table 4.2 Precipitants and associations of hypersensitivity (allergic) small vessel vasculitis

Drugs	Sulfonamides and penicillins, for example—there are many
Infections	Hepatitis B, hepatitis C, HIV
	β-hemolytic streptococcus
Foreign protein	e.g., serum sickness
Autoimmune disease	Rheumatoid arthritis
	Sjögren's syndrome (antiRo positive)
	Systemic lupus erythematosus
Inflammatory diseases	Sarcoid
	Crohn's disease, ulcerative colitis
	Chronic active hepatitis
Malignancy	Myelo- and lymphoproliferative disorders
	Solid tumors
Cryoglobulinemia	

Table 4.3 Laboratory tests in patients with suspected vasculitis

Hematology	CBC, ESR
Chemistries	Electrolytes, BUN, creatinine
	Liver function enzymes, serum ACE
	CRP, urine toxicology (cocaine)
	Serum and urine protein electrophoresis
Microbiology	Blood cultures
	Hepatitis B and C serology. Consider HIV
	Streptococcal antibodies
Immunology	Immunoglobulins, cryoglobulins, complement
	ANA (ENAs), rheumatoid factor
	ANCA (when relevant)

Systemic vasculitis

- Untreated primary systemic vasculitis is generally characterized by inflammation; many patients will complain of B-type symptoms, including fevers, weight loss, and night sweats.
- Patients with idiopathic cutaneous vasculitis, on the other hand, often feel quite well
- The extracutaneous signs and symptoms may provide clues to the correct diagnosis:
  - Henoch-Schönlein purpura: colicky abdominal pain
  - Churg-Strauss syndrome: adult-onset asthma, eosinophilia
  - Wegener's granulomatosis: chronic sinusitis
  - Microscopic polyangiitis: hemoptysis, red blood cell casts
- Mononeuritis multiplex, which presents as a "wrist drop" or "foot drop", is pathognomic for systemic vasculitis in a nondiabetic patient.

Diagnostic procedures

Skin biopsy

- Try to discuss the case with the pathologist first.
- Punch biopsy is simple, and may be sufficient to yield a diagnosis. Elliptical biopsy provides more tissue, and may increase yield.
- Use a needle to lift the skin sample—this avoids forceps-induced damage.
- Biopsy should extend to the subcutaneous fat, which generally includes the arterioles and venules affected by primary systemic vasculitis. Idiopathic leukocytoclastic vasculitis affects the capillaries but generally spares the arterioles and venules.
- Biopsy should be sent for routine histology and for direct immunofluorescence, which may yield important clues regarding the underlying cause:
  - IgA: Henoch-Schönlein purpura
  - IgM, C3: Cryoglobulinemic vasculitis
  - IgG, IgM, IgA, C3: SLE
  - Minimal immunoreactant staining: ANCA-associated vasculitis
- Samples for immunofluorescence should be snap frozen in liquid N_2 or dry ice or transported immediately to the laboratory, ideally in PBS. Immunofluorescence cannot be performed on samples that have been treated with formalin.

Skin vasculitis in children and adolescents

Epidemiology

- Classification of childhood vasculitis is difficult. A system that has clinical utility is shown in Table 4.4.
- Statistically, the most common form of vasculitis is HSP, followed by hypersensitivity angiitis.
- Kawasaki disease (KD) affects primarily children under 5 years of age.

Clues from the history

- All of the systemic vasculitides may be associated with features such as fatigue, fever, gastrointestinal symptoms, lymphadenopathy, myalgias, and arthralgias.
- Drugs or infection are often identified as a precipitant of a cutaneous leukocytoclastic vasculitis.
- Granulomatosis with polyangiitis (Wegener's granulomatosis) is rare. As in adults, it may be characterized by a limited localized form involving the respiratory tract. Subglottic stenosis, nasal septum disease, and respiratory infections may all have occurred.
- Testicular pain is a rare though fairly specific feature for polyarteritis nodosa. This can also occur with Wegener's granulomatosis.
- Abdominal pain is not specific. Gut bleeding can occur in Henoch-Schönlein purpura (HSP) and juvenile dermatomyositis especially.
- Vasculitis can occur in association with familial Mediterranean fever.

Examination

Characteristic examination features of the rash

- Erythematous rash with swelling progressing to desquamation of palms and soles of the feet is typical of KD.
- Lower limb and buttock palpable purpura is typical of, but not specific for, HSP and hypersensitivity angiitis.
- Skin nodules are not specific but are common in cutaneous polyarteritis nodosa and frequently occur in hypersensitivity vasculitis. A nodular, painful rash on the medial sides of the ankles is frequent in cutaneous polyarteritis nodosa.
- Extensive necrotic and ulcerative rash with notable muscle pains suggests dermatomyositis. Periungual erythema and both eyelid and nail bed telangiectasias are typical.
- Livedo reticularis is a feature of cutaneous polyarteritis nodosa (often with painful skin nodules), but also occurs with SLE and the antiphospholipid syndrome (see Chapters 10 and 11 respectively).

Other typical or specific examination features

- Bilateral conjunctival injection, lip/oral/buccal inflammation, and acute nonpurulent cervical lymphadenopathy are typical features of KD.
- The incidence of cardiovascular manifestations is 35% in KD. Murmurs, gallop rhythm, and coronary artery aneurysms (30%) can occur.
- Pulselessness may suggest a large vessel vasculitis.

Table 4.4 A classification of childhood vasculitis

Polyarteritis	Macroscopic
	Microscopic
Kawasaki disease (mucocutaneous lymph node syndrome)	
Granulomatous vasculitis	Granulomatosis with polyangiitis (Wegener's granulomatosis)
	Eosinophilic granulomatosis with polyangiitis (Churg-Strauss)
Leukocytoclastic vasculitis	Henoch–Schönlein purpura
	Hypersensitivity angiitis
Cutaneous polyarteritis nodosa	
Vasculitis and autoimmune connective tissue disease	SLE
	JIA
	Mixed connective tissue disease
	Dermatomyositis
	Scleroderma
Large vessel vasculitis	Takayasu's disease
Miscellaneous vasculitides	

- Severe oral aphthous ulceration raises the possibility of Behçet's syndrome. It is rare, but does occur in children.

Investigations

- Leukocytosis, thrombocytosis, anemia, and an acute phase response are typical in all forms of systemic vasculitis and are not specific.
- ECG and echocardiography are essential in suspected KD.
- In patients suspected of having a small vessel vasculitis, glomerulonephritis should be ruled out (urinalysis, urine microscopy, spot urine protein/creatinine ratio).
- In patients with an active sediment, or other unexplained renal abnormalities (e.g., worsening proteinuria or serum creatinine) kidney biopsy can be valuable to confirm the diagnosis.
- ANCA is not specific for vasculitis, but C-ANCA with antibodies to proteinase-3 (PR3-ANCA) in appropriate patients is highly suspicious for granulomatosis with polyangiitis (Wegener's granulomatosis), while P-ANCA with antibodies to myeloperoxidase (MPO-ANCA) is suggestive of microscopic polyangiitis or eosinophilic granulomatosis with polyangiitis (the Churg-Strauss syndrome).
- Biopsy of the skin rash is a key investigation in all patients.
- In patients suspected of having a medium vessel vasculitis, the most valuable investigation is often angiography of the affected region (e.g., renal, mesenteric, or extremity). Conventional angiography and CT-angiography are both acceptable; MR-angiography may not have

adequate resolution to exclude the presence of a medium vessel vasculitis.
- In patients suspected of having a large vessel vasculitis, MR-angiography is preferred, since MR may demonstrate vessel wall characteristics (e.g., edema, thickening, enhancement) that may not be visualized with other modalities.

Cardiac manifestations

Subclinical cardiac involvement is found in many of the rheumatic diseases, and it is not uncommon for a cardiac abnormality to be discovered incidentally. As our ability to treat the underlying rheumatic diseases improves, our ability to identify and to treat the cardiac complications of these diseases becomes increasingly important.

Pericardium

- Pericardial effusions are not uncommon, and have been reported in association with a large number of rheumatic diseases, including scleroderma, Sjögren's, polymyositis, mixed connective tissue disease, the spondyloarthropathies, and the systemic vasculitides.
- In the majority of cases, these effusions are discovered incidentally. These effusions are often small, clinically asymptomatic, and require no specific therapy.
- Pericardial effusions can also occur in the setting of nonrheumatic illness. When a patient with a known rheumatic disease presents with a symptomatic effusion, it is important to consider other possible explanations, such as infection (e.g., tuberculosis, viral, Whipple's disease), malignancy, and other unrelated conditions (uremia, hypothyroidism, cardiac amyloid).
- Pericardial effusions are a common manifestation of systemic lupus erythematosus (SLE), largely due to immune complex deposition into the pericardium. These effusions can be serous, serosanguinous, or hemorrhagic. Analysis of the pericardial fluid generally demonstrates evidence of complement, immune complexes, and leukocytes, consistent with an active inflammatory state.
- Although pericardial effusions are common with SLE, they are generally trivial. Cardiac tamponade is found in less than 1% of patients with SLE. Since the effusion tends to reflect the overall disease state, generally treatment of the underlying disease is adequate to resolve the effusion. Rarely, therapeutic pericardiocentesis may be required.
- Pericardial effusions are found in up to 30% of patients with rheumatoid arthritis, although only a small number of these patients will present with pericarditis or evidence of tamponade. Pericardial effusions are more common in RF-positive patients with a history of rheumatoid nodules. Chronic pericardial effusions can become superinfected, and in rare cases lead to a constrictive pericarditis.
- For both groups of patients, the presence of a symptomatic pericardial effusion is associated with increased mortality. In one study of patients with SLE who presented with cardiac tamponade, the 5-year survival was only 46%.

Myocardium

- Myocarditis is a relatively uncommon manifestation of rheumatic disease. Myocarditis can be found among patients with active SLE and RA, although it generally does not lead to clinically significant dysfunction.

- Cardiomyopathy among patients with RA and SLE is more likely to be due to premature coronary artery disease, followed by the development of ischemic heart disease.
- Although uncommon, the possibility of hydroxychloroquine-induced cardiomyopathy should be considered in a patient who develops congestive heart failure in the absence of coronary artery disease. This diagnosis can be confirmed with myocardial biopsy, and often responds to drug cessation.
- Eosinophilic granulomatosis with polyangiitis (the Churg-Strauss syndrome) can lead to an acute eosinophilic myocarditis that can be life-threatening if not treated promptly.
- One-third of patients with granulomatosis with polyangiitis (Wegener's granulomatosis) may have cardiac dysfunction as a consequence of the underlying vasculitis. The majority of these patients will have wall motion abnormalities on echocardiography, but valvulitis and ventricular aneurysm have also been reported. The majority of these lesions will be asymptomatic, but the 5-year survival rate for patients with cardiac lesions attributable to Wegener's granulomatosis is 57%.

Valvular disease

- Aortic regurgitation is an important potential consequence of aortitis, which can occur with any of diseases associated with large-vessel vasculitis (including Takayasu's arteritis, giant cell arteritis, Cogan's syndrome, and Behçet's disease). In these cases, aortitis leads to aneurysm formation, which creates valvular incompetence.
- Aortic regurgitation can also occur as a consequence of ankylosing spondylitis. Unlike the vasculitides, ankylosing spondylitis causes inflammation at the aortic root, which leads to dense scarring of the aortic valves. Although the mechanism is unique to this disease, it should be monitored and treated like any form of aortic insufficiency.
- Mitral regurgitation and mitral prolapse are common manifestations of SLE, particularly among patients who have antiphospholipid antibodies.
- A more serious valvulitis can occur in association with SLE. In the process of healing, the valves become scarred and calcified, a process that can eventually lead to clinically significant valvular disease.
- Libman-Sacks endocarditis is a classic manifestation of SLE. In this disease, vegetations form from immune complexes, mononuclear cells, and fibrin, which attach to the valves. Although not infectious, these vegetations can embolize
- Hemodynamically insignificant valve lesions have also been reported in association with RA, MCTD, scleroderma, and Sjögren's.

Coronary artery disease

- Surprisingly, the primary vasculitides rarely lead to coronary artery inflammation, although coronary artery vasculitis has been reported in association with polyarteritis nodosa and the ANCA-associated vasculitides.
- The antiphospholipid syndrome is associated with a substantial increased risk of myocardial infarction, even in the absence of true coronary artery disease.

- Both RA and SLE are strongly associated with coronary artery disease. This may be the result of systemic inflammation or a response to chronic immunosuppression. Regardless, patients with these diagnoses should undergo early cardiac evaluation to address modifiable risk factors for coronary artery disease.
- Accelerated atherosclerosis may be an important consequence of glucocorticoid exposure. Even chronic low dose prednisone may place some patients at increased risk of cardiovascular disease.

Conduction abnormalities

- Clinically insignificant arrhythmias and conduction defects are common among patients with inflammatory myopathies (dermatomyositis, polymyositis) and scleroderma.
- Clinically significant arrhythmias (including heart block) can be seen in patients with spondyloarthropathies as a result of the same scaring process that leads to the valvular abnormalities noted in the preceding section, Coronary Artery Disease.

Pulmonary manifestations

Pleura

- Pleural effusion is found in up to 50% of patients with SLE. These effusions can be unilateral or bilateral, and frequently are found in association with a pericardial effusion.
- Pleural disease is also a common manifestation of rheumatoid arthritis, which is associated with both pleural effusions and pleural thickening. These effusions are generally asymptomatic, and are found in the setting of active disease.
- Asymptomatic pleural effusions can also be found in 10–30% of patients with ANCA-associated vasculitis.

Pulmonary nodules/masses

- Both granulomatosis with polyangiitis (Wegener's granulomatosis) and sarcoidosis are often diagnosed incidentally, after the discovery of lung masses. Sarcoidosis is associated with hilar lymphadenopathy, while granulomatosis with polyangiitis (Wegener's granulomatosis) generally presents with multiple peripheral pulmonary nodules that can be mistaken for lung cancer or fungal infection.
- In a patient with a known rheumatic disease who presents with a lung mass, it is always important to consider the possibility of malignancy. Lung cancer risk is increased among patients with rheumatoid arthritis and scleroderma, and many rheumatic diseases are associated with an increased risk of lymphoma
- Granulomatosis with polyangiitis (Wegener's granulomatosis) – and less commonly, ankylosing spondylitis and rheumatoid arthritis – can lead to cavitating apical lesions that can be mistaken for tuberculosis.

Interstitial lung disease

- Pulmonary fibrosis (with a predilection for the lung bases and periphery) is a common feature of both scleroderma and the inflammatory myopathies (also known as the antisynthetase syndromes).
- Pulmonary fibrosis is found in 20%–65% of patients with scleroderma. Radiographically, the lesions take on the appearance of ground glass infiltrates that gradually lead to honeycombing and fibrosis.
- Pulmonary fibrosis may be the initial manifestation of an inflammatory myopathy, and pulmonary symptoms may precede clinical evidence of muscle involvement.
- Rheumatoid arthritis is also associated with an interstitial lung disease, although this has become increasingly rare.
- Apical fibrosis can be found in 1% of patients with ankylosing spondylitis. Apical fibrosis is also an uncommon feature of rheumatoid lung.
- Pulmonary fibrosis can also occur as the long-term sequelae of pulmonary capillaritis, which may occur in patients with granulomatosis with polyangiitis (Wegener's granulomatosis) and microscopic polyangiitis.

Vasculature

- Hemoptysis can be the result of pulmonary capillaritis, which can be found in association with the so-called "pulmonary renal syndromes": SLE, ANCA-associated vasculitis (predominantly microscopic polyangiitis), and antiglomerular basement membrane (GBM) syndrome.
- Cryoglobulinemic vasculitis can also cause pulmonary capillaritis, although this is not one of its more common manifestations.
- Pulmonary artery hypertension (PAH) is most commonly associated with limited cutaneous scleroderma. Isolated PAH can also be seen with diffuse cutaneous scleroderma, although it generally appears as a consequence of pulmonary fibrosis.
- Scleroderma causes PAH by narrowing of the small arteries and arterioles that gradually leads to obliteration of the pulmonary vascular bed.
- RA, SLE, inflammatory myopathy, mixed connective tissue disease, and Sjögren's syndrome can also be associated with PAH, but it is considered an uncommon feature of these diseases.

Airways

- RA can lead to laryngeal obstruction when it affects the cricoarytenoid joints. Such patients will present with hoarseness or odynophagia.
- Hoarseness and non-productive cough may also be an uncommon manifestation of giant cell arteritis, due to inflammation of the recurrent laryngeal nerve by the aortitis.
- Subglottic stenosis is a common feature of granulomatosis with polyangiitis (Wegener's granulomatosis), which can lead to significant stridor.
- Uncontrolled relapsing polychondritis can cause tracheomalacia or tracheal stenosis, which is a significant cause of morbidity and mortality for this disease.

Renal manifestations

Evaluation of renal failure: overview
- The kidneys are a key component to the evaluation and management of the rheumatic diseases.
- Many conditions affect the kidneys directly, and a careful examination may yield important clues to the correct diagnosis.
- For other patients, the kidneys must be considered because many treatments have renal toxicity or are renally cleared.
- In terms of time course, renal failure is frequently divided into "acute kidney injury" and "chronic kidney disease." Acute kidney injury describes the rapid loss of renal function, which might be reversible if the underlying cause is addressed; chronic kidney disease is the result of an irreversible loss of nephrons.
- Acute kidney injury (AKI) is often divided by the source of the injury. Acute renal failure due to renal hypoperfusion is called "prerenal"; acute renal failure due to urinary tract obstruction is called "post-renal."
- Intrinsic renal failure (i.e., renal failure due to direct involvement of the renal parenchyma) should be evaluated with a careful examination of the urine. The presence of red blood cells and protein, or red blood cell casts (i.e., an "active sediment") implies glomerulonephritis, which can occur with vasculitis and SLE.

Prerenal azotemia
- Hypovolemia is an important cause of prerenal AKI. Dehydration and anemia can both lead to prerenal azotemia.
- Renal hypoperfusion can also be caused by diminished blood flow to the kidneys. Diseases involving the renal artery (such as renal artery stenosis, polyarteritis nodosa affecting the renal artery, or renal artery thrombosis) may cause prerenal azotemia. If long-standing, this leads to intrinsic renal failure.
- Conditions associated with low cardiac output (including shock, congestive heart failure, myocarditis, tamponade, and pulmonary arterial hypertension) may all predispose the patient to prerenal AKI.
- Hyperviscosity, which is seen with type I (monoclonal) cryoglobulinemia, is a rare cause of prerenal azotemia.
- All of these conditions may be exacerbated by drugs that decrease renal perfusion, including NSAIDs and ACE-inhibitors.
- With prerenal azotemia, the fractional excretion of sodium
- $(FENa = (UNa \times PCr)/(PNa \times UCr))$ is less than 1.0; this test is not reliable in patients treated with diuretics.

Postrenal azotemia
- Nephrolithiasis is not a common cause of postrenal azotemia, but should be considered in a patient with gout. 5–10% of renal calculi in the United States are caused by uric acid; this is particularly common among patients with gout who have been treated with uricosuric agents (e.g., probenecid).

- Sarcoidosis can cause hypercalcemia and hypercalcuria, which in turn can lead to nephrolithiasis and nephrocalcinosis, both of which can rarely cause postrenal azotemia.
- Methotrexate and trimethoprim/sulfamethoxazole can cause crystalluria and renal obstruction.
- Ultrasound is a useful modality to evaluate both for the presence of obstruction leading to hydronephrosis and renal calculi.

Intrinsic renal failure—"active sediment"

- The nephritic syndromes are an important cause of rapidly progressive renal failure among patients with rheumatic diseases, particularly small vessel vasculitis and SLE.
- The presence of hematuria, proteinuria, and red blood cell casts strongly suggests the presence of glomerulonephritis, but a renal biopsy is crucial to determining the underlying diagnosis and the severity/chronicity of the disease.
- Nephritic syndromes can be divided into "focal proliferative" and "diffuse proliferative" based on histology.
- Causes of focal proliferative glomerulonephritis include SLE, Henoch-Schönlein purpura, and other forms of small vessel vasculitis.
- Diffuse proliferative glomerulonephritis is caused by cryoglobulinemia, SLE, anti-glomerular basement membrane (GBM) disease (Goodpasture's syndrome), and ANCA-associated vasculitis.
- Direct immunofluorescence can also provide valuable information regarding the correct diagnosis. SLE is associated with multiple immunoreactants ("full house" staining pattern). IgA deposition implies Henoch-Schönlein purpura. Cryoglobulinemic vasculitis leads to IgG and C3 deposition. Sparse or absent immunoreactants on biopsy is sometimes called "pauci-immune," and implies an ANCA-associated vasculitis.

Intrinsic renal failure—"bland sediment"

- A bland sediment refers to a urine sample that is acellular; transparent hyaline casts may be seen. Remember that a bland sediment is also seen in prerenal and postrenal azotemia.
- Acute tubular necrosis (ATN) is used to describe causes of acute, intrinsic renal failure associated with a urine sediment that has muddy brown casts and tubular epithelial cells.
- Nephrotoxic tubular injury from drugs is a common cause of ATN in patients with rheumatic disease.
- Prolonged prerenal azotemia can lead to permanent kidney damage; therefore, diseases of the renal artery (including polyarteritis nodosa and renal artery thrombosis from antiphospholipid antibody syndrome) should be considered.
- Interstitial nephritis is most commonly seen as a drug reaction (e.g., NSAIDs, azathioprine, allopurinol)
- Interstitial nephritis can also be seen as a manifestation of several rheumatic diseases, including Sjögren's, SLE, sarcoidosis, and eosinophilic granulomatosis with polyangiitis (the Churg-Strauss syndrome).

- NSAIDs cause renal vasoconstriction and interstitial nephritis, both of which can eventually lead to a chronic analgesic nephropathy.
- Unlike the other forms of ANCA-associated vasculitis, the mechanism of renal failure among patients with eosinophilic granulomatosis with polyangiitis (Churg-Strauss syndrome) is an interstitial nephritis; glomerulonephritis is relatively rare with this diagnosis.
- The most common causes of secondary renal amyloidosis are rheumatoid arthritis and familial Mediterranean fever. Glomerular deposits of amyloid lead to proteinuria (which can be nephrotic range) and progressive renal failure.

Scleroderma renal crisis

- Scleroderma renal crisis is a rheumatologic emergency characterized by acute renal failure and malignant hypertension.
- Patients with diffuse cutaneous scleroderma are at greatest risk; scleroderma renal crisis generally occurs within the first 4 years after diagnosis, but it can occur at any time. Patients who are treated with corticosteroids may be at the highest risk.
- Urinalysis generally demonstrates a bland sediment. Kidney biopsy demonstrates evidence of a thrombotic microangiopathy that histologically cannot be distinguished from malignant hypertensive nephrosclerosis, hemolytic-uremic syndrome, SLE, or the antiphospholipid antibody syndrome.
- The cornerstone of therapy is gradually escalating doses of ACE-inhibitors, followed by angiotensin II receptor blockers (ARB) and calcium channel blockers if adequate blood pressure control is not achieved.

Renal tubular acidosis

- Renal tubular acidosis (RTA) causes a nonanion gap metabolic acidosis caused by a failure of the renal tubules to maintain acid-base status.
- Type I RTA, caused by an inability to excrete acid, is found with Sjögren's syndrome and SLE.
- Type IV RTA is most commonly caused by hyporeninemic hypoaldosteronism, can occur as a result of treatment with NSAIDs, ACE-inhibitors, and ARBs. This is commonly associated with hyperkalemia.

Endocrine manifestations

Well-characterized musculoskeletal conditions occur in many endocrine disorders. Some are specific for certain disorders; others are nonspecific, but occur with greater frequency among patients with endocrine disease. Musculoskeletal manifestations occur either as a result of metabolic disturbances or are influenced by a common link through their autoimmune pathophysiology.

Diabetes

- Dupuytren's contracture, trigger finger, carpal tunnel syndrome, diffuse idiopathic skeletal hyperostosis (DISH), and adhesive capsulitis all occur with greater frequency among patients with diabetes.
- Some form of tissue or joint hypomobility/stiffness is common among patients with diabetes (see Table 4.5); in some cases, this can appear similar to scleroderma. These scleroderma-like skin changes are more prevalent among patients with type I diabetes.

Table 4.5 Patterns of joint and tissue hypomobility or stiffness in diabetes by reported series. Tissue changes are thought to occur from excessive hydration (a consequence of an excessive local production of sugar alcohols)

Patient series	Major abnormalities	Associations
Diabetics overall	In about 30–40% mainly in long-standing disease: slow decrease in hand mobility; waxy skin thickening ('scleroderma-like')	Occasional lung fibrosis. Microvascular diabetic complications
Adults	55–76% prevalence of joint hypomobility in type 1/type 2 diabetes, respectively	Not associated with diabetic complications
Mature onset diabetes (mean 61 years)	Stiffening of connective tissue (assessed in hands)	Diabetic nephropathy
Children with type 1 diabetes	31% have limited joint mobility	None with glycemic control, retinopathy, or proteinuria
Juvenile and young adult onset (age 1–24 years) diabetes	34% had skin thickening. Changes rarely proximal to MCPs and never proximal to wrists. Joint contractures in >50%, often third or fourth fingers	No flexor tendon rubs (as seen in scleroderma)

- Hand weakness may be due to diabetic neuropathy and may be mistaken for carpal tunnel syndrome. Nerve conduction studies help discriminate between these two diagnoses.
- Calcification of soft tissues around the shoulder occurs in approximately 20% of diabetics, and is associated with variable symptoms and disability.
- Diabetic amyotrophy (diabetic lumbosacral plexopathy) is uncommon. It presents acutely with pain, weakness, and wasting of the proximal lower limb muscles. It may be unilateral. Differential diagnosis includes myositis (see Chapter 14) and polymyalgia rheumatica (PMR—see Chapter 15). It is associated with uncontrolled hyperglycemia. The etiology is unknown, but it is probably a neuromyopathy.
- Though rare (1:500 diabetics), neuropathic arthritis (Charcot joint) can occur in advanced disease. Most patients are aged 40–60 years and have poor glycemic control. Tarsal and metatarsal joints are most frequently affected (60%). The usual presentation is of swelling of the foot with no or little pain. Trauma may have occurred. Early radiographic changes can resemble OA (see Chapter 6).
- Asymptomatic osteolysis can occur at the distal metatarsals and proximal phalanges with relative joint sparing. The etiology is unknown.
- Osteomyelitis is not uncommon and needs to be discriminated from cellulitis and neuropathic arthritis (Charcot's joint). MRI or a triple-phase bone scan is helpful to establish the diagnosis. Osteomyelitis is usually disclosed by prominent blood flow in the dynamic (first) phase and increased uptake of tracer by soft tissue and bone in later stages. Cellulitis is associated with minimal uptake of tracer in bone in the delayed (third) phase. Neuropathic joints display minimal first-phase abnormalities but prominent tracer uptake in the third phase.
- Diabetic muscle infarction can present as a painful muscle mass and is a result of arterial narrowing. Often mistaken for thrombophlebitis, myositis or vasculitis, this is a late complication of diabetes. Biopsy may be needed to confirm this diagnosis.

Hypothyroidism

- Over 25% of patients with hypothyroidism have an arthropathy. Because this arthropathy can lead to an erosive arthritis, it can be mistaken for RA (see Chapter 5).
- This arthropathy commonly involves the knees and hands; in children, the hips are most likely to be affected. It is characterized by pain, stiffness, effusions, and synovial thickening due to glycosaminoglycan deposition. Calcium pyrophosphate deposition may contribute to this arthropathy.
- Radiographically defined chondrocalcinosis is only marginally increased compared with controls (17% vs. 10%). About 1/10 patients with pseudogout are hypothyroid.
- Carpal tunnel syndrome is frequent (7%). Up to 10% of patients with carpal tunnel syndrome may have hypothyroidism.
- Hyperuricemia is common among patients with hypothyroidism but gout attacks are rare. However, screening for hypothyroidism in

patients with gout is recommended. Treated hypothyroidism then requires review of the need for uric acid-lowering therapy.
- Musculoskeletal symptoms are common, and may improve with treatment of hypothyroidism.
- Consequences of hypothyroidism in children included retarded bone age, short stature, and epiphyseal dysgenesis with premature epiphyseal plate closure and increased probability of slipped femoral epiphyses.
- Myopathy is relatively common. About 1 in 20 cases of acquired myopathy are due to hypothyroidism. The presentation can mimic polymyositis with elevation of muscle enzymes, but muscle biopsy typically shows no inflammatory cell infiltrate. Improvement with thyroxine replacement is sometimes complicated by muscle cramps, but these should resolve in a few weeks.
- The combination of weakness, muscular stiffness, and an increase in muscle mass in an adult with myxedema is termed Hoffman's syndrome. Muscle mass increase is sometimes striking and can take many months to resolve on treatment. The same condition occurs in children (Kocher–Debre–Semelaigne syndrome).
- Lymphocytic thyroiditis (Hashimoto's) is an autoimmune condition characterized by hypothyroidism and autoantibodies to thyroglobulin and thyroid microsomes. These antibodies are found in 40% of patients with primary Sjögren's disease but only about 10% are or have been overtly hypothyroid.

Hyperparathyroidism (see also Chapter 16)

Unless stated, points refer to both primary and secondary disease:
- Musculoskeletal symptoms are the initial manifestation in up to 16% of patients with primary hyperparathyroidism.
- Hyperparathyroidism, chondrocalcinosis, and pseudogout frequently coexist. Pseudogout (CPPD) can be triggered by parathyroidectomy.
- A polyarthropathy can occur that can mimic RA. Unlike RA, synovial proliferation is absent. Radiographically, erosions have a predilection for the ulna side of distal upper limb joints, the joint space is preserved, pericapsular calcification is often present, and reactive bone formation may be observed..
- An erosive polyarthritis favoring the large joints can occur with renal osteodystrophy in patients with chronic renal failure on dialysis. It does not appear to be related to CPPD.
- Hyperparathyroidism is associated with a specific shoulder arthropathy characterized by intra/periarticular erosions of the humeral head. This may be subclincial.
- Subjective muscle weakness and fatigability are common complaints. Typically, muscle enzymes are normal and biopsy shows type II fiber atrophy; the features of an inflammatory myopathy are generally absent.
- The hallmark of radiographic changes is bone resorption: subperiosteal (typically on the radial side of second and third phalanges), intracortical, subchondral, trabecular, subligamentous, and localized (Brown's tumors) resorption patterns are seen. Bone sclerosis, periostitis, and chondrocalcinosis also occur.

- Fragility fracture is common and often precedes a diagnosis of primary hyperparathyroidism. Although significant and fast accretion of bone occurs after surgery, bone mass often remains low long term.

Thyrotoxicosis

- Hyperthyroidism can cause a proximal myopathy (70%), shoulder periarthritis (7%), acropachy (thickening of extremities), and osteoporosis.
- Acropachy is rare (<2% of patients with thyrotoxicosis) and most often occurs in treated patients who are hypo/euthyroid. It consists of clubbing, painful soft tissue swelling of hands and feet, and periosteal new bone on the radial aspect of the second and third metacarpals. Clinically, this occurs most frequently in patients who have the ophthalmopathy or dermopathy associated with autoimmune thyroid disease.
- Graves' disease is frequently associated with fatigability and muscular weakness. It is associated with autoimmune rheumatic and connective tissue diseases.

Acromegaly

- Overstimulation of bone and connective tissue cells from excessive growth hormone can result in several features: bursal and cartilage hyperplasia, synovial and bony proliferation, an OA-like picture, backache, and hypermobility.
- Joint complaints usually manifest about 10 years after the onset of clinical acromegaly. Knees are frequently affected.
- Joint symptoms are not typical of an inflammatory arthritis—morning stiffness is not prominent and joint swelling is present in <50% of patients.
- Carpal tunnel syndrome (see Chapter 2) affects >50% of patients and is frequently bilateral.
- Back and neck pain and radicular symptoms from nerve root compression or spinal stenosis are not uncommon and are related to axial bony proliferation.
- A painless proximal myopathy occurs infrequently.
- Radiographs characteristically show widened joint spaces (e.g., >2.5 mm in adult MCPs) and a thickened heel pad (>23 mm in men and >21.5 mm in women).
- Diagnosis relies on demonstration of a failure of growth hormone to be suppressed by a glucose tolerance test, but a lateral skull radiograph is a good screening test as 90% have enlargement of the pituitary fossa.

Gut and hepatobiliary manifestations

- Musculoskeletal features frequently occur in patients with gut or hepatobiliary disease (see Table 4.6)
- Data on the frequency of rheumatologic features are largely based on studies of hospital patients with clinically overt gut or biliary disease. This may lead to an underestimate of the frequency of association.
- The most frequent associations are: sacroiliitis, arthritis, and enthesitis in patients with inflammatory bowel disease; inflammatory arthritis in celiac disease and viral hepatitis; and degenerative arthritis in hemochromatosis and Wilson's disease.
- The frequency of enthesitis in patients with inflammatory bowel disease may be underestimated. Enthesitis may be detected at the medial/lateral humeral epicondyles, Achilles' tendon insertion, calcaneal plantar fascia origin and insertion, and the patellar tendon origin and its insertion at the tibial tubercle.
- Radiology studies in patients with inflammatory bowel disease suggest that sacroiliitis is under-recognized by clinicians.

Severity of rheumatologic manifestations
- Optimal surveillance strategies for the musculoskeletal manifestations of gut or biliary disease are not known in many instances.
- Life-threatening vasculitis may occur from chronic viral infection. Hepatitis B is associated with polyarteritis nodosa, and hepatitis C may lead to cryoglobulinemic vasculitis.
- In most patients who develop joint inflammation or enthesitis after bacterial dysentery, the condition is self-limiting. Chronicity and severity may be linked to HLA B27. Progressive spondylitis is rare.

Gut and hepatobiliary conditions in patients with rheumatic diseases (see Tables 4.7 and 4.8)

- The most common problem among patients with RA is dyspepsia associated with gastroduodenal erosions or ulcers due to NSAIDs. Peptic lesions may be clinically silent and may present with dropping hemoglobin levels or an acute bleed.
- Rheumatoid arthritis may be the most common cause of AA amyloidosis. Biopsies of the upper gastrointestinal tract will demonstrate amyloid deposits in 13% of patients. There are numerous gastrointestinal manifestations of amyloidosis, including gastrointestinal hemorrhage, malabsorption, obstruction, and hepatomegaly.
- Scleroderma has numerous gastrointestinal manifestations including refractory gastroesophageal reflux disease, gastric antral vascular ectasia ("watermelon stomach"), esophageal dysmotility, bacterial overgrowth syndrome, and fecal incontinence. The reflux associated with scleroderma often requires treatment with high dose proton pump inhibitors. "Watermelon stomach" can lead to significant acute and chronic hemorrhage. The bloating and abdominal distension caused by bacterial overgrowth may respond to cyclic courses of antibiotics.

Table 4.6 Rheumatological features in patients with gut or hepatic disease

Gastrointestinal disorder	Rheumatic manifestation	Association
Enteric infection	Reactive arthritis: self-limiting in most	Arthritis in 2% who get shigella, salmonella, yersinia, campylobacter or C. difficile overall but in 20% of infected who are HLA B27+
Crohn's disease	Arthritis 20%, as 10%. Sacroiliitis in 26%	60% of spondyloarthropathy patients have histological evidence of bowel inflammation. See also below
Ulcerative colitis	Arthritis 20%. AS 7%. Sacroiliitis 15%	See also above. Severity of gut and joint inflammation varies in its association but SI joint/pine inflammation does not
Whipple's disease	Migratory arthritis in >60%	T. whippelii identified in small bowel. Diarrhea occurs in >75% ultimately
Intestinal by-pass surgery/(blind loop syndrome)	Polyarticular symptoms 50%in scleroderma	Intestinal bacterial overgrowth in small bowel. ?Associated with joint symptoms
Celiac disease	Arthritis is rare	?Increased intestinal permeability
Viral enteritis	Rare (<0.5%)	Most common: coxsackie or echo
Hepatitis A	Arthralgia 15%. Vasculitis rare	Causal association
Hepatitis B	Arthralgia 10–25%. PAN	Etiological.
Hepatitis C	Sialadenitis in >50%. Vasculitis (cryoglobulinemic)	?Etiological in Sjögren's. Hepatitis C identified in 27–96% of patients with cryoglobulinemia

(Continued)

Table 4.6 (Contd.)

Gastrointestinal disorder	Rheumatic manifestation	Association
Primary biliary cirrhosis	Polyarthritis 19%. Scleroderma 18%. Sjögren's 50%	Autoimmune "overlap." Features may be subclinical
Chronic active hepatitis	Polyarthralgia or arthritis in 25–50%	Autoimmunity
Hemochromatosis	OA 50%	Iron storage disease
Wilson's disease	OA in 50% adults. Chondrocalcinosis	Copper storage disease

Table 4.7 Gut and hepatobiliary manifestations in rheumatological diseases (I: General)

Disease	Abnormalities	Presentation with
Rheumatoid arthritis (Chapter 5)	TMJ arthritis Esophageal dysmotility	Impaired mastication Dysphagia, reflux
	GI vasculitis (0.1%)	Ulcers, pain, infarction
	Portal hypertension	Splenomegaly (Felty's)
	Liver involvement (Felty's)	Enzyme abnormalities
	Hepatosplenomegaly	Palpable viscera
Systemic lupus erythematosus (Chapter 10)	Esophageal dysmotility	Dysphagia, reflux
	GI vasculitis	Ulcers, pain, perforation
	Protein-losing enteropathy	Hypoalbuminemia
	Peritonitis	Ascites (10%), serositis
	Hepatosplenomegaly (30%)	Palpable viscera
Scleroderma (Chapter 13)	Esophageal dysmotility	Heartburn/dysphagia
	Delayed gastric emptying	Aggravated reflux
	Intestinal dysmotility and fibrosis (80%)	Malabsorption, pseudo-obstruction (<1%)
	Pseudo and wide mouth diverticula	Hemorrhage, stasis, bacterial overgrowth
Polymyositis and dermatomyositis (Chapter 14)	Muscle weakness	Aspiration, dysphagia
	Disordered motility	Dysphagia, constipation
	Vasculitis (rare)	Ulcers, perforation
MCTD	Hypomotility	Dysphagia, reflux, pseudo-obstruction
Sjögren's syndrome (Chapter 12)	Membrane desiccation	Xerostomia, dysphagia
	Esophageal webs (10%)	Dysphagia (>60%)
	Gastric infiltrates/atrophy	Masses, dyspepsia
	Pancreatitis	Pain, amylasemia
	Hepatic dysfunction	Hepatomegaly (≅25%)
	Hepatic cirrhosis	Primary biliary cirrhosis
Spondyloarthritis (Chapter 8)	Ileocolonic inflammation	May be asymptomatic
Adult onset Still's	Hepatitis, peritonitis, hepatosplenomegaly	Pain or abnormal enzymes (≅75%)
Systemic JIA (Chapter 9)	Serositis	Abdominal pain
	Hepatomegaly	Abnormal enzymes
Marfan, Ehlers-Danlos (Chapter 16)	Defective collagen	Hypomotility, malabsorption, visceral rupture/laxity

Table 4.8 Gut and hepatobiliary manifestations in rheumatic diseases (II: Vasculitis [see also Chapter 15])

Disease	Frequency of GI vasculitis and features
Polyarteritis nodosa	80% (mesenteric). Buccal ulcers, cholecystitis (15%), bowel infarction, perforation, appendicitis, pancreatitis, strictures, chronic wasting syndrome
Henoch–Schönlein purpura	44–68%. Abdominal pain, melena, hematemesis, ulcers, intussusception, cholecystitis, infarction, perforation, appendicitis
Eosinophilic granulomatosis with polyangiitis	≅40%. Hemorrhage, ulceration, infarction, perforation
Behçet's syndrome	Buccal and intestinal ulcers, hemorrhage, perforation, pyloric stenosis, rectal ulcers
Systemic lupus erythematosus	2%. Buccal ulcers, ileocolitis, gastritis, ulceration, perforation, intussusception, volvulus (1%), pneumatosis
Kawasaki disease	Abdominal pain, intestinal obstruction, noninfective diarrhea
Granulomatosis with polyangiitis	<5%. Cholecystitis, appendicitis, ileocolitis, infarction
Juvenile dermatomyositis	Well recognized. Perforation, pneumatosis
MCTD	Rare. Ulceration, perforation, pancreatitis
RA (including RF₊ JIA)	0.1%. Buccal ulcers, abdominal pain, peptic ulcers, acalculous cholecystitis, gut infarction, and perforation
Polymyositis and dermatomyositis	Very rare. Mucosal ulcers, perforation and pneumatosis
Cryoglobulinemia	Rare. Ischemia and infarction

- In SLE, serious gut and hepatobiliary manifestations are relatively uncommon (5%), but nausea, anorexia, vomiting, and diarrhea are quite frequent.
- Mesenteric vasculitis is classically caused by polyarteritis nodosa, but can be seen with a variety of rheumatic illnesses, including Takayasu's arteritis, ANCA-associated vasculitis, and (rarely) with SLE. Although mesenteric angina is the symptom most strongly associated with mesenteric vasculitis, the earliest sign of intestinal ischemia is diarrhea.
- Henoch-Schönlein purpura is an IgA-mediated small vessel vasculitis that presents with colicky abdominal pain and purpura. Although generally mild and self-limited in children, it can occasionally cause intussusception and bowel necrosis.

Gut and hepatobiliary side effects from drugs used in treating rheumatic and bone diseases

- Such side effects are common:
- NSAIDs are a common cause of gastrointestinal distress. COX-2 inhibitors were developed to decrease the risk of peptic ulcer disease; most have been withdrawn from the market due to concerns regarding increased risk of cardiovascular events. Only celecoxib remains on the market in the United States, but it may be no more effective than taking a conventional NSAID with a proton pump inhibitor.
- Glucocorticoids are also associated with gastritis, peptic ulcer disease, and gastrointestinal hemorrhage. Although the absolute increase in events is small, the combination of steroids and NSAIDs results in a synergistic increase in the risk of gastrointestinal sequelae.
- Methotrexate may cause stomatitis, which may respond to supplemental folate. Nausea, emesis, and altered taste may also occur, which may respond to dose reduction. Methotrexate can cause a transaminitis; therefore, we generally recommend that patients treated with methotrexate abstain from alcohol.
- Sulfasalazine: Gut and hepatobiliary side-effects are common and may occur in up to 20% of patients. The most frequent are mostly mild: indigestion, nausea, vomiting, anorexia, and abdominal pain. Gut ulceration, bloody diarrhea, and serious liver problems are rare. In about 65% of side-effects occur in the first 3 months of treatment.
- Azathioprine can cause nausea (15%), vomiting (10%), and abdominal pain (8%). Diarrhea is rare (5%). Liver enzyme abnormalities are often mild and may remit on lowering the dose. The GI side effects can occur in patients with normal levels of thiopurine methyltransferase.
- D-penicillamine causes altered taste (25% within the first 3–6 months), nausea or vomiting (18%), and stomatitis/mouth ulcers (5%). Hepatotoxicity and hemorrhagic colitis are rare.
- Chloroquine and hydroxychloroquine, used in mild SLE particularly, can cause nonspecific GI intolerance (10%). The onset is often insidious.
- Cyclosporine causes gingival hyperplasia, nausea, diarrhea, and elevation in hepatic enzymes.
- Effects of cyclophosphamide on the gut are frequent and include nausea, vomiting, diarrhea, and stomatitis. Serious hepatotoxicity is rare.
- Chlorambucil has a low incidence of GI side effects.
- Leflunomide can cause nausea (8–13%), diarrhea (up to 25%), and abnormal liver enzymes. In studies to date, most rises in transaminases have been mild (< two-fold) and are reversible on drug withdrawal.
- Oral bisphosphonates (such as alendronate and risedronate) can cause nausea, dyspepsia, and diarrhea. Esophageal ulceration has occasionally been noted with alendronate though it is thought this occurs only in people who do not follow the instructions for taking them. Myalgias and arthralgias can also occur.
- Calcitonin either given as subcutaneous injection or as nasal spray can give abdominal pains and diarrhea.

Malignancy

Rheumatic features may be clues to the existence of cancer; these may be caused directly (through tissue invasion) or indirectly (as a paraneoplastic phenomenon).

Primary and secondary neoplastic diseases of bone and joints

- Synovial tumors are rare. Sarcoma (synovioma) is more common in men than women and unusual in those over 60. It usually occurs in the legs (70%) and can occur around tendon sheaths and bursa. At diagnosis, pulmonary metastases are common.
- Para-articular involvement by bone tumors may give a monoarticular effusion. Invasion of synovium may occur and malignant cells can be detected in joint fluid. Breast, bronchogenic carcinoma, GI tumors, and melanoma can all metastasize to joints.
- Lymphomas and leukemias may simulate various conditions and cause synovitis in a single or in multiple joints.
- Arthritis complicating the presentation of myeloma or an acute leukemia is most likely to be polyarticular and asymmetric.
- In adults, arthritis complicating leukemia is rare (5% of cases).
- Leukemia is the most common cause of neoplastic skeletal symptoms in childhood and adolescence (15% of leukemia cases).
- Neuroblastomas are the most frequent cause of a solid tumor metastasizing to the skeleton in children.

Clues that may lead to a suspicion of malignancy directly causing musculoskeletal symptoms

- Constitutional symptoms.
- The coexistence of bone pain (also consider metabolic bone diseases, sarcoid, and enthesitis-related conditions).
- Hemorrhagic joint fluid (also consider trauma, pigmented villonodular synovitis (PVNS), chondrocalcinosis).
- Radiographs that show adjacent bone destruction, perhaps with loss of cortex (also consider infection).
- Radiographic calcification in soft-tissue mass (consider synovioma).

Paraneoplastic myopathies

Paraneoplastic myopathies may occur before, during, or after the diagnosis of malignancy:

- Myopathy is usually due to carcinomatous neuromyopathy.
- Polymyositis, dermatomyositis, Eaton–Lambert myasthenic syndrome (ELMS) and hypophosphatemic (oncogenic) osteomalacia are all found in association with malignancy (see Table 4.9).
- Carcinomatous neuromyopathy is a condition characterized by symmetric muscle weakness and wasting. The myopathy can pre-date malignancy.

Table 4.9 Myopathy and links with malignancy

Condition	Typical pattern of weakness	Common cancer associations	Other features
Carcinomatous neuromyopathy	Pelvic girdle—symmetric	Lung: 15% men, 12% women. Ovary: 16%. Stomach: 7% men, 13% women	Wasting, EMG abnormality, and increase in muscle enzymes are notvariable
Dermatomyositis (+?PM)	Proximal limb. Truncal	Reflects underlying cancer frequency in local population	Response to steroids is usual
Myasthenia gravis (MG)	Frequently ocular and bulbar muscles involved	Thymus. Any	Muscle strength fluctuates (fatigability). Responds to anticholinesterases
Eaton–Lambert myasthenicsyndrome (ELMS)	Pelvic girdle muscles. Altered gait. Ocular muscles not affected	Small cell lung. Can occur up to 2–3 years after ELMS	Autonomic disturbances. EMG + poor response to anticholinesterasesdistinguish from MG
Oncogenic osteomalacia	Generalized. Develops insidiously	Small, discrete mesenchymal tumors in bone, soft tissues, and sinuses. Neurofibromatosis	Bone pain and bone demineralization. Hypophosphatemia and lowcirculating 1,25 OH vitamin D

Nonmyopathic paraneoplastic syndromes

The nonmyopathic paraneoplastic syndromes are rare:

- Hypertrophic pulmonary osteoarthropathy (HPOA) consists of clubbing, periostitis of tubular bones, and an arthropathy (may range from arthralgias to diffuse polyarthritis). Suspicion of this should prompt a request for an isotope bone scan, which typically shows abnormally increased bone turnover in the long bones. Radiographs often show periosteal elevation. HPOA complicates 20% of primary lung tumors, but it is associated with other malignancies.
- Polyarthritis may be the presenting feature of cancer. Most cases occur in those over 60 years old. Unlike RA, the arthritis associated with malignancy tends to be asymmetric, and does not cause erosions.
- Eosinophilic fasciitis, severe bilateral palmar fasciitis (often mistaken for scleroderma), and fasciitis associated with panniculitis have been associated with malignancy. Cases of "shoulder–hand" syndrome (a form of reflex sympathetic dystrophy) that have been reported in association with malignancy probably reflect similar pathological processes.

Rheumatic diseases associated with an increased incidence of malignancy

There are a number of rheumatic diseases that are associated with an increased incidence of malignancy compared with healthy populations. These are dealt with briefly here and in more detail in Part 2 of this book.

- Non-Hodgkin's lymphoma is most strongly associated with RA. Myeloma and paraproteinemias are also found in RA patients.
- The relative risk of colon cancer among RA patients is 0.77; this may be due to the use of chronic NSAIDs in this patient population, which may be protective.
- Use of cyclophosphamide is associated with an increased risk of lymphoma and bladder cancer. Methotrexate may also be associated with an increased risk of lymphoma.
- Chronic azathioprine use is associated with an increased risk of skin cancer; patients taking azathioprine long term should be counseled about sun protection and monitoring for skin cancer.
- Non-Hodgkin's lymphoma develops in a subset of patients with Sjögren's syndrome (4%). Its onset may be indicated by rapid enlargement of salivary glands, the appearance of a paraprotein, or decrease in circulating immunoglobulins or RF titer.
- Scleroderma has been associated with an increased risk of both lung cancer and non-Hodgkin's lymphoma.
- Dermatomyositis is probably associated with malignancy in adults, though convincing evidence for an association of polymyositis with malignancy is lacking. Neither is associated with malignancy in children.

Rheumatoid arthritis (RA)

Disease criteria and epidemiology

There is no perfect test for rheumatoid arthritis (RA). The diagnosis rests on a composite of clinical and laboratory observations. It is a common systemic inflammatory disease characterized by the presence of a destructive polyarthritis with a predisposition for affecting the small joints of the hands and feet and the wrists (although it can affect any synovial joint).

Disease criteria are often developed for epidemiological work and for classification in the context of clinical trials. Classification criteria for RA in particular are dominated by signs and symptoms from the musculoskeletal system. It is important to remember, however, that there are a number of "extra-articular" manifestations to the disease, with involvement of, for example, the eyes, lungs, skin, heart, and nervous system.

The criteria for the diagnosis of RA ranges from the original American Rheumatism Association (ARA) scheme of 1958, through the development of the simpler New York criteria, to the 1987 ARA criteria (see Table 5.1) which replaced the 1958 ARA criteria. These criteria were not designed to diagnose patients with RA; in particular, it is often difficult to apply these criteria to the diagnosis of "possible," "early," or atypical RA. It is most straightforward to apply these criteria in clinical trials aimed at patients with well-established disease.

Significant evidence, however, indicates that early treatment of rheumatoid arthritis greatly improves the long-term outcomes associated with this disease, highlighting the importance of early diagnosis and therapy.

For this reason, in 2010, the American College of Rheumatology (ACR) and the European League Against Rheumatism (EULAR) developed a revised set of classification criteria (see Table 5.2), designed to identify patients with early RA, at the time of initial presentation. Therefore, the new criteria are not interchangeable with the old criteria; using the new criteria, for example, a patient who presents with 6 weeks of bilateral knee swelling or tenderness, in the setting of a high-positive rheumatoid factor and abnormal ESR, would be classified as having rheumatoid arthritis by the 2010 criteria, but not the 1987 criteria.

Table 5.1 The 1987 American College of Rheumatology criteria for the diagnosis of rheumatoid arthritis

	Criterion	Comments
1	Morning stiffness	Duration >1 hour lasting >6 weeks
2	Arthritis of at least three joints*	Soft tissue swelling/exudation lasting >6 weeks
3	Arthritis of hand joints	Wrists, MCPs, or PIPs lasting >6 weeks
4	Symmetrical arthritis	At least one area, lasting >6 weeks
5	Rheumatoid nodules	
6	Positive rheumatoid factor	
7	Radiographic changes	Erosions, particularly wrists, hands,and feet

At least four criteria must be fulfilled and there are no exclusion criteria.

* Possible areas: metacarpophalangeal joints (MCP), proximal interphalangeal joints (PIP), wrist, elbow, knee, ankle, metatarsophalangeal joints (MTP).

Table 5.2 The 2010 American College of Rheumatology/European League Against Rheumatism criteria for rheumatoid arthritis

Criterion		Score
Joint Involvement*	2–10 large joints	1
	1–3 small joints	2
	4–10 small joints	3
	>10 joints	5
Serology†	Low-positive RF or ACPA	2
	High-positive RF or ACPA	3
Acute phase reactants	Abnormal CRP or ESR	1
Symptom duration	≥6 weeks	1

For a definite diagnosis of rheumatoid arthritis, a total score of ≥6 is required, including at least one point from each of the first three categories. In patients with long-standing or inactive disease, it is adequate if the patient would have fulfilled these criteria at some point in the past.

* Large joints include the shoulders, elbows, hips, knees, and ankles. Small joints includes the metacarpophalangeal joints, proximal interphalangeal joints, second to fifth metatarsophalangeal joints, thumb interphalangeal joints, and wrists. The distal interphalangeal joints, first carpometacarpal joints, and first metatarsophalangeal joints are excluded from this assessment.

† RF, rheumatoid factor; ACPA, anti-citrullinated protein antibody, including anti-cyclic citrullinated peptide antibody (CCP)

Incidence, prevalence, and morbidity

- The disease has a worldwide prevalence, and has been identified in all populations that have been examined. Figures for prevalence range from 0.2 to 5.3%, but the age distribution in developing countries may be a confounding factor and perhaps contributes to low figures in, for example, some parts of Africa.
- Population studies on the incidence of the disease suggest figures of 3.4/10 000 in women and 1.4/10 000 in men. The incidence in men declines with age from age 45. In women, it increases until age 45, then plateaus and falls after the age of 75.
- RA is extremely heterogeneous with regard to severity and progression. Permanent remission can occur but is rare once joint damage has started. A distinction is sometimes made between cyclical disease and relentless progression, but in practice it is perhaps more useful to consider widespread versus limited chronic joint involvement.
- Without adequate treatment, life expectancy is reduced by approximately 7 years in men and 3 years in women. This is mainly due to cardiovascular disease, infections, respiratory disease, and RA itself.

The clinical features of rheumatoid arthritis

- A typical onset of insidious pain, stiffness, and symmetrical swelling of small joints is only one of several presenting patterns. Up to one-third of patients may have a subacute onset with symptoms of fatigue, malaise, weight loss, myalgias, morning stiffness, and joint pain without overt signs of swelling or radiological evidence of joint erosions.
- Traditionally, rheumatoid arthritis is described as a symmetric synovitis of the small joints of the hands, wrists, and feet (sparing the distal interphalangeal joints. Symmetry, however, develops later in the disease course, and one should not wait for symmetry to develop prior to initiating therapy. A mono- or bilateral arthropathy of the shoulder or wrist, for example, may account for up to 30–40% of initial presentations; 5% of initial presentations involve the knee.
- Any synovial joint can become involved in RA. The hands, wrists, elbows, shoulders, and knees are involved most commonly, followed by the hip and temporomandibular joints. RA also affects the clavicular joints and the cricoarytenoid.
- Atlantoaxial (C1-C2) subluxation is a known complication of RA, and may present with pain radiating towards the occiput, spastic quadriparesis, or sensory findings. Such patients are at high risk of progression, and patients with evidence of cord compression require immediate surgical stabilization.
- Patients may also present with a tenosynovitis or bursitis. The diagnosis and management of these conditions is covered in Chapter 2 of this book.
- "Classic" features of RA, such as "swan neck" and "boutonniere" deformity of the digits appear late in disease and are features of chronic disease; they are not usually seen at initial presentation where signs of synovitis and joint damage may be subtle.
- Though often suspected, there is no absolute evidence that stress, whether physical or psychological, triggers the disease.
- Pregnancy has a beneficial effect on RA in some women, especially during the last trimester. Arthritic symptoms usually return within 1–2 months postpartum and may be more severe than prior disease. Lactation has no effect and there is no evidence that RA patients have more medical complications during pregnancy per se. Therapeutics and pregnancy are discussed later in this chapter.

Organ disease in rheumatoid arthritis (see Table 5.2)

Lymph nodes

Lymph nodes are often enlarged but rarely palpable. In a few cases RA may present with widespread nodes mimicking Hodgkin's disease.

Pulmonary disease

- Pleuritis (like pericarditis) is frequent but often mild. Like other pulmonary and cardiac manifestations, it is more common in older men. Pleural effusions may also occur.
- Rheumatoid pulmonary nodules are usually an asymptomatic finding in seropositive RA. Radiographically they are coin-shaped lesions that can be difficult to distinguish from malignancy. In patients in whom malignancy is clinically suspected, further imaging or tissue biopsy may be required.
- Diffuse interstitial fibrosis and fibrosing alveolitis are rare associations. Methotrexate may be associated with the development of fibrosis, although this is controversial.

Cardiovascular system

There is increasing evidence that patients with RA suffer from increased cardiovascular disease, independent of the traditional risk factors. Inflammation is thought to play an important part in the development of atherosclerosis and the systemic inflammatory response in RA may explain the link. Epidemiological studies show that cardiovascular mortality is increased in patients with early and established disease and is worse in women, a group traditionally at lower risk. Standardized mortality ratios for cardiovascular disease in men are approximately 1.3 and 1.9 in women.

Skin

- Rheumatoid nodules occur in up to 30% of patients, and are found principally on the extensor surface of the forearm, Achilles tendon, and over pressure areas throughout the skin. Nodules are not specific for RA but are useful in diagnosis and prognosis, correlating with seropositivity, disease activity, and progression. The differential diagnosis includes tophaceous gout.
- Leukocytoclastic vasculitis also occurs and is seen as palpable purpura; most often this resolves spontaneously.
- Rheumatoid vasculitis can lead to large ulcerations on the lower extremities, although this is an uncommon manifestation.

Ocular involvement

- Rheumatoid vasculitis gives rise to a severe form of painful scleritis, leading to scleromalacia.
- Episcleritis is typically benign and resolves spontaneously. Uveitis and conjunctivitis are not associated with RA.

Table 5.3 Some organ disease in rheumatoid arthritis

Organ	Manifestation	Frequency (%)
Lymph nodes	Enlargement	>50
Spleen	Enlargement	25
	Felty's syndrome	<1
Lungs	Pleuritis	>30
	Nodules	5
	Fibrosis	Rare
Heart	Pericarditis	>10
	Myocarditis	>5
	Nodules	5
	Cardiovascular disease(RA is an independent risk factor)	Standardized mortality ratio: ♂ ~ 1.3 ♀ ~ 1.9
Muscle	Atrophy	Common
	Myositis	Rare
Bone	Osteoporosis	Common
Skin	Nodules	>20
	Vasculitis	1
Eyes	Sicca syndrome	10
	Scleritis	1
	Nodules	<2
Nervous system	Nerve entrapment	Common
	Mononeuritis multiplex	<1
	Cord compression	Rare

Neurological involvement

- Entrapment neuropathy secondary to synovitis is common. Median nerve compression can occur early in the disease. Other rarer examples included the ulnar nerve at the elbow, and the posterior tibial nerve at the tarsal tunnel.
- Mononeuritis multiplex, a peripheral and occasionally bilateral neuropathy causing a "wrist drop" or "foot drop", can present acutely. A sudden onset of motor neuropathy can signal the presence of aggressive vasculitis and poor prognosis.
- Rheumatoid vasculitis classically occurs in patients with with high titer RF and a history of erosive arthritis.
- Cervical subluxation at the atlantoaxial level is present in one-third of RA patients but is usually asymptomatic. Subluxation at lower levels is rare, but is more likely to cause pain and neurological symptoms.

- Cervical myelopathy due to cervical instability can be fatal. Symptoms include paresthesias, weakness, paralysis, sensory loss, incontinence, and syncope.
- Patients with gait dysfunction or clumsiness of the hands should be evaluated promptly for cervical myelopathy; most patients will not present with neck pain.
- Patients at risk for cervical myelopathy should be instructed to avoid prolonged cervical extension. Hairdressers should be instructed to allow the patient to face the sink when having hair washed. Anesthesiologists should be informed regarding this concern as well.

Fractures

- Cytokines, generated in inflammation, encourage bone resorption by osteoclast induction leading to periarticular osteoporosis.
- Inactivity, nutritional deficiency, glucocorticoids, and pre-existing osteoporosis constitute additional risk factors for vertebral fractures.

Tendons and ligaments

Spontaneous rupture is common, most often at the wrist, hand, and rotator cuff. More often, tenosynovitis and weakening of ligaments leads to joint instability and subluxation. Acute inability to raise the fourth and fifth digits may be seen with rupture of the extensor tendons due to wrist disease, and may be surgically corrected.

Infection

There is anecdotal evidence that infections may trigger flares in RA. More importantly, RA patients are more susceptible to septic arthritis, often compounded by the use of immunosuppressive drugs, including steroids (see later in this chapter). In such a situation, the usual signs of sepsis may be absent, delaying the diagnosis.

Secondary amyloidosis

Renal involvement is the most common type of organ failure, though the skin, liver, and GI tract are often affected. Intensive antirheumatic therapy now gives a more favorable outlook, with 80% 5-year survival rates.

Felty's syndrome

This is the association of splenomegaly and neutropenia with seropositive RA. Systemic disease, hepatomegaly, and lymphadenopathy are also common. In uncomplicated cases, treatment should be conservative, splenectomy remaining controversial and often only transient in effect.

Large granular lymphocyte (LGL) syndrome

Like Felty's syndrome, LGL syndrome is associated with neutropenia and splenomegaly. LGL syndrome is differentiated from Felty's syndrome by the presence large granular lymphocytes and a clonal lymphocytosis. Clonality can be demonstrated through PCR of the T-cell receptor-gamma gene. The arthritis that accompanies LGL syndrome is typically less destructive than that seen with Felty's syndrome, although this is not always the case.

The evaluation and treatment of rheumatoid arthritis

- A clearly documented assessment is invaluable for the ongoing monitoring of the disease and treatment (see Table 5.3).
- The ESR and CRP are useful measures periodically in the assessment of disease activity, and hematological and biochemical parameters will not only expose underlying organ disease but are also important in the regular monitoring of a number of drug treatments. That said, it is important to note that many patients can have active synovitis without elevation in acute phase reactants.
- Early erosive changes on plain radiographs of the hands and feet can be of great value in the assessment of patients with minimal clinical signs. The presence of typical erosions confirms the diagnosis of RA, and merits aggressive treatment with DMARDs.
- IgM rheumatoid factor (RF) is of value in establishing the diagnosis, however, a low positive result can be misleading and a negative result should not alter a diagnosis made on clinical grounds. Only 70–80% of patients with RA will be RF positive.
- RF is also found in association with other diseases, including hepatitis, monoclonal gammopathy, malignancy, tuberculosis, and syphilis.
- Anti-citrullinated protein antibodies (ACPA), including anticyclic citrullinated peptide (anti-CCP) antibodies are important markers for diagnosis and prognosis in RA. In both early and established disease, ACPA are more sensitive and more specific than RF. ACPA antibodies may be detected in roughly 50–60% of patients with early RA, and have a specificity for RA >99%. They are also a marker of erosive disease and may predict the development of RA in patients with nonspecific inflammatory symptoms.
- RF and ACPA measurements are not re-tested routinely, although repeat testing may be useful in patients whose initial test results are negative, but whose examination is strongly suggestive of RA, since patients with seropositive RA require more aggressive treatment.
- The ultimate goal is complete remission of disease; the standard of care is to "treat to target" of remission (or low disease activity).
- Patient reported outcomes may be more responsive than other measures in detecting disease activity.
- The management of RA requires a multidisciplinary approach. Working with physical therapists, occupational therapists, podiatrists, social services, and surgeons is an important part of management (see Table 5.4).

Disease activity assessment

- The current approach to the management of RA advocates for "treatment to target". Patients should be evaluated (and medications adjusted) monthly until remission (i.e., the absence of synovitis) or low disease activity is achieved.

Table 5.4 Comparison of clinical composite indices of disease activity for rheumatoid arthritis.

	DAS	DAS28	SDAI	CDAI	RAPID3
High disease activity	>3.7	>5.1	>26	>22	>12
Moderate disease activity	2.4–3.7	3.2–5.1	11.1–26	10.1–22	6.1–12.0
Low disease activity	1.6–2.4	2.6–3.2	3.3–11	2.8–10	3.1–6.0
Remission	<1.6	<2.6	<3.3	<2.8	0–3.0

- Key to this goal is the routine use of a validated measure of disease activity, which allows the clinician to compare disease activity between visits and assess response to therapy objectively.
- Disease activity may be quantified using clinical composite indices (e.g., DAS, DAS-28, SDAI, CDAI), patient-reported outcome measures (e.g., Health Assessment Questionnaire (HAQ), Routine Assessment of Patient Index Data (RAPID)), or imaging (e.g., radiographs, ultrasound, MRI).
- The Disease Activity Score (DAS) is a composite score using the Ritchie Articular Index (0–78), a swollen joint count (0–44 joints), ESR, and patient global assessment of disease activity using a 100 mm visual analogue scale. The DAS has been used in clinical trials to assess response to treatment, but is cumbersome. It provides a score from 1–10:

  DAS = 0.: 4, (Ritchie Articular Index)
  + 5.06, (number of swollen joints) + 0.33 ln(ESR)
  + 0.007 Global assessment (in mm)

- The DAS28 is calculated by surveying 28 joints (knees + upper extremities). The DAS28 provides a score from 0.49–9.07:

  DAS28 = 0.: 6, (number tender joints)
  + 5.28, (number of swollen joints) + 0.70 ln(ESR)
  + 0.014 Global assessment (in mm)

- The DAS-28 CRP uses the CRP in place of the ESR:

  DAS28 = 0.: 6, (number tender joints)
  + 5.28, (number of swollen joints) + 0.36 ln(CRP+1)
  + 0.014 Global assessment (in mm) + 0.96

- The Simplified Disease Activity Index (SDAI) is calculated by surveying the same 28 joints used in the DAS28. The SDAI provides a score from 0.1 to 86.0:

  SDAI=(number of tender joints) + (number of swollen joints)
  + CRP (mg/dL) +(patient global health on 10 cm VAS)
  + (evaluator global health on 10 cm VAS)

- The Clinical Disease Activity Index (CDAI) is calculated by without the use of lab data. The CDAI provides a score from 0 to 76.0:

    CDAI = (number of tender joints) + (number of swollen joints)
    + (patient global health on 10 cm VAS)
    + (evaluator global health on 10 cm VAS)

- The RAPID3 is an example of a patient-reported outcome measure that correlates with disease activity. It is derived from the MDHAQ, which was designed to facilitate clinic visits. The RAPID3 uses only 3 parts of the MDHAQ: patient self-assessed physical function, patient pain assessment, and patient global assessment. Even in the absence of physician input or laboratory tests, the RAPID3 correlates with the DAS and CD28, and can be completed more quickly than any of the preceding indices.

Fig. 5.1. RAPID3 Questionnaire. Used with permission of Ted Pincus

Table 5.5 Documenting the initial evaluation of RA

1	The duration of morning stiffness
	The degree of pain
	Fatigue
	Function (utilizing a score system such as Health Assessment Questionnaire—HAQ)
	Patient global assessment of disease activity
2	The distribution and number of painful joints, and the distribution and number of swollen joints, including periodicity
	The distribution and nature of mechanical joint disease noting loss of function, instability, and modifying factors
	The presence or absence of extra-articular disease
3	Radiographs of affected joints looking for erosive disease and mechanical damage
4	Laboratory tests
	ESR and CRP
	CBC
	Renal and liver function tests
	Urinalysis
	Rheumatoid factor
	Anti-citrullinated peptide antibodies (ACPA)

Which drugs, when, and what to monitor? (see Table 5.5)

Nonsteroidal anti-inflammatory drugs (NSAIDs)

- Most patients will either periodically or continuously be taking NSAIDs. These agents offer reliable, even if sometimes limited, relief of pain, swelling, and stiffness, improving quality of life in the majority of cases. These drugs do not, however, alter the natural history of RA. Adverse effects are, however, common and sometimes life-threatening; careful monitoring and patient education are essential. Combinations of NSAIDs should be avoided.
- Selective COX-2 NSAIDs are of similar efficacy to diclofenac or naproxen, and may be of value in patients intolerant of NSAIDs. Many agents in this class, however, have been withdrawn from the market due to concerns regarding COX-2 inhibitors and increased risk of myocardial infarction.
- Of concern is a study showing that even standard NSAIDs such as ibuprofen and diclofenac are also associated with an increased risk of myocardial infarction. It is therefore vital that these drugs are used appropriately and avoided for long-term use in patients with adverse cardiovascular or GI risk profiles (see Table 5.6). Further research is needed in this area.

Table 5.6 The main components in the treatment of RA

Modality	Examples
Education and counseling	Specialist registered nurse or nurse practitioner
	Self-care groups
	National organizations
Physical therapy	Exercise
	Joint protection
Occupational therapy	Adaptation
	Aids
	Splints
Podiatry	Orthotics
	Surgical shoes
Medication	Pain control
	Disease control
Nonmedical pain management	Transcutaneous nerve stimulation
	Acupuncture
	Psychotherapy
	Surgery
Surgery	Joint replacement
	Arthrodesis
	Tendon release/repair

Glucocorticoids
- IM and oral steroids are very effective in active RA, reducing active disease in an acute crisis or while waiting for a DMARD to take effect. Many patients are often on a combination of NSAID and DMARD with intermittent doses of systemic steroid.
- Local steroid injections are of value in symptom control both early in the disease and in an acute flare. The effect on joint recovery may be dramatic but short lived, with little impact on the overall process of RA, and should not be repeated any more than once every 3 months. It is sometimes of value to combine injections with a joint "washout" in refractory cases. There is no evidence to suggest an increased risk of joint infection, as long as aseptic technique is used.
- High-dose systemic administration may reduce overall disease activity in the short-term but adverse effects preclude its uninhibited use and it is best preserved for refractory RA and severe extra-articular complications.
- There have been reports linking glucocorticoid therapy to fetal congenital malformations, and there is little data on lactation.

Prednisone, dexamethasone, and betamethasone appear to be safe, but should be used only when necessary.

- Long-term use of glucocorticoids may be associated with a wide range of consequences, including cataracts, premature coronary artery disease, accelerated osteoporosis, muscle atrophy, and increased risk of avascular necrosis.
- Risks of infection associated with use of low dose glucocorticoids may be as great as the risks associated with anti-TNF therapy.

Disease-modifying antirheumatic drugs (DMARDs)

- All patients with active disease should be offered a DMARD early. The rationale is to prevent or reduce joint destruction. Evidence from systematic reviews suggest that early introduction of DMARDs decrease pain, swelling, and joint damage, and improves the likelihood of achieving remission.
- Guidelines now recommend that the majority of patients with newly diagnosed RA should be started on DMARD therapy within 3 months of diagnosis. However, efficacy is unpredictable and variable in duration.
- Toxicity is an important concern and this should always be discussed with patients.
- These agents are also slow-acting, sometimes taking up to 6–9 months to have maximal effect (although treatment decisions based on efficacy can generally be made in 3–4 months). The final choice of DMARD is influenced by a number of factors including, patient compliance, convenience of administration, severity of disease, presence of other medical conditions, pregnancy, monitoring requirements and frequency, and nature of adverse events.
- Both the American College of Rheumatology and EULAR have published recommendations regarding the appropriate use of DMARDs for the treatment of RA.[1,2]

Sulfasalazine and hydroxychloroquine

- Sulfasalazine (SSZ 1.0–1.5 g po bid) and hydroxychloroquine (HCQ 400 mg po qd) are sometimes used initially in RA, partly because of their relative safety and convenience. Both agents are generally well-tolerated and take effect within 1–3 months. Many clinicians would now, however, choose methotrexate first if there is evidence of early aggressive disease.
- Retinal toxicity and maculopathy with HCQ are rare. The risk increases with abnormal liver or kidney function, after a cumulative dose of 800 g, and in patients aged 70 years and over. The eyes should be checked formally by an ophthalmologist yearly and the patient informed to report any visual disturbances.

[1] Singh JA et al. 2012 update of the 2008 American College of Rheumatology recommendations for the use of disease-modifying antirheumatic drugs and biologic agents in the treatment of rheumatoid arthritis. Arthritis Care Res 2012: **64**: 625–639.

[2] Smolen JS, et al. EULAR recommendations for the management off rheumatoid arthritis with synthetic and biological disease-modifying antirheumatic drugs. Ann Rheum Dis 2010; **69**: 964–976.

Table 5.7 Pharmacotherapy of rheumatoid arthritis

Drug type	Examples
Pain relief	Simple analgesia
	NSAIDs
Disease-modifying drugs	Glucocorticoids (oral, IM, intra-articular)
	Methotrexate
	Sulfasalazine
	Hydroxychloroquine
	Leflunomide
Biological therapies	Anti-TNF: etanercept, infliximab, adalimumab, golimumab, certolizumab
	Anti B-cell: rituximab
	CTLA4 Ig: abatacept
	IL-6 antibodies: tocilizumab
For disease complications	Anemia: iron, erythropoietin
	Osteoporosis: estrogens, bisphosphonates, teriparatide
	Vasculitis: glucocorticoids, cyclophosphamide
	Amyloidosis: chlorambucil, anti-TNF therapies

- There is potential for accumulation of HCQ in the fetus during pregnancy, and for chromosomal damage, although in studies of SLE, no significant risk to the fetus has been found among women who have taken HCQ prior to conception and during pregnancy.
- Sulfasalazine has been used successfully in pregnancy. There have been case reports of congenital malformations, although the overall risk is considered very small.
- Sulfasalazine may cause leukopenia, pancytopenia, hemolysis, and aplastic anemia. Serious bone marrow toxicity is, however, uncommon. It can also induce a hepatic transaminitis.
- Sulfasalazine can rarely cause a hypersensitivity reaction characterized by liver function test abnormalities, lymphadenopathy, and rash.
- Spermatogenesis can be affected by SSZ, but it is reversible. There does not appear to be an adverse effect on female fertility.

Methotrexate
- Methotrexate (MTX 10–30 mg) is given weekly by mouth or SQ or IM injection. Toxicity, particularly stomatitis, GI disturbance, and alopecia, may be reduced by the addition of folic acid daily, without loss of therapeutic effect.
- All patients taking methotrexate should receive 1–5 mg of folic acid to reduce toxicity; higher doses of folic acid may be used to manage side effects, if necessary.

- Pneumonitis is uncommon and pulmonary fibrosis (a rare complication of MTX) should not deter the physician from using MTX in aggressive systemic and skeletal disease. Rare, life-threatening, pulmonary toxicity can occur at any time and is not necessarily related to dose or duration of treatment. A chest X-ray should be taken before MTX is started.
- Mild drug-induced hepatitis is relatively common and is often corrected by the addition of folic acid. Overt liver disease is rare. Routine liver biopsy is not necessary, being restricted to pretreatment assessment of patients with other liver disease and patients with persistent liver function abnormalities in spite of discontinuing treatment.
- Myelosuppression is rarely severe. Antifolate drugs such as trimethoprim and folate deficiency increase the risk of toxicity. Penicillins lead to decreased clearance of methotrexate, but are often used in combination without ill effect. Renal impairment reduces methotrexate clearance and may lead to toxicity; doses may need to be adjusted in patients with renal insufficiency. Pregnancy and breastfeeding are contraindications to the use of MTX. Both men and women should wait 3 months after stopping treatment before trying to conceive a child. Diminished fertility caused by MTX is reversible.
- NSAID use is not contraindicated. There is the potential for interaction and hepatotoxicity and close monitoring remains a pre-requisite for commencing therapy.
- Patients having major operations are often advised to stop treatment for 1–2 weeks either side of surgery, although there is no evidence to suggest that this reduces the risk of postoperative complications such as wound healing or sepsis, and increases the risk of a disease flare, particularly among patients who remain off of methotrexate > 4 weeks.

Leflunomide

- Leflunomide (LEF 10–20 mg po qd) is effective for the treatment of moderately active rheumatoid arthritis.
- A loading dose of leflunomide is no longer recommended; most patients may simply start taking 20 mg daily.
- Gastrointestinal side effects, including diarrhea, nausea, and transaminitis, may all occur.
- Patients with pre-existing liver disease should not be treated with leflunomide, and it should be used with caution in combination with other drugs that are also associated with hepatotoxicity (such as methotrexate).
- If liver toxicity is observed, the drug should be stopped, and washout with cholestyramine should be used to help clear the drug.
- Peripheral neuropathy has been reported, but seems uncommon.

Other DMARDs

- Other DMARDs, including oral and IM gold, D-penicillamine, azathioprine, cyclosporine, and cyclophosphamide, have largely fallen out of favor due to the availability of more effective or less toxic regimens. Combined therapy (such as MTX + HCQ + SSZ) is substantially more effective than monotherapy, particularly for patients with early disease.[1] Decisions should be based on discussion between the doctor and patient taking into account the risks and benefits. These agents, their side-effects and monitoring are detailed in Table 5.7.

Biologic Agents

- Biologic DMARDs are drugs that are directed against specific components of the immune system.
- Broadly speaking, these drugs fall into three major groups
  - Cytokine-directed strategies (anti-TNF-α, anti-IL6)
  - T-cell directed strategies (CTLA4-Ig)
  - B-cell directed strategies (anti-CD20)
- Overall, these agents are associated with a roughly equal increased rate of serious infection (i.e., infections requiring hospitalization or intravenous antibiotics)

Table 5.8 Adverse reactions of NSAIDs

Organ/complication	Occurrence	Comments
GI tract	Common	Gastritis, bleeding, and perforation. High risk in elderly and those with ulcer history
Renal	Common	Fluid retention Papillary necrosis
Hypertension	Common	Interference with drugs such as thiazide diuretics
Myocardial infarction	Increased risk in those with cardiovascular risk factors	Associated with COX-2 inhibition
Pulmonary	Not uncommon	Exacerbation of asthma Pneumonitis (naproxen)
Skin	Not uncommon	Hypersensitivity Erythema multiforme
CNS	Not uncommon	Tinnitus, fatigue, cognitive disturbance
	Rare	Aseptic meningitis
Hepatic	Uncommon	Drug-induced hepatitis
Hematological	Rare	Bone marrow dyscrasias

[1] O'Dell JR. Therapeutic strategies for rheumatoid arthritis. *N Engl J Med* 2004; 350: 2591–2602.

Table 5.9 Monitoring guidelines for DMARDs in rheumatoid arthritis

Monitoring	Other side-effects	Main toxicity	Drug
CBC and LFT every 2 weeks until dose stable and thereafter every 3 months	Stains body fluid, rash, hepatitis	Myelosuppression	Sulfasalazine
CBC and LFT every 2 weeks until dose stable. Baseline CXR. CBC and LFT every 4–6 weeks. BMP every 6 months thereafter	Hepatitis, pneumonitis, rash	Myelosuppression	Methotrexate
Ophthalmic review if visual disturbance	Visual disturbance	Macular damage	Hydroxychloroquine
CBC and urinalysis before every dose	Rash, reversible proteinuria	Myelosuppression	*Intramuscular gold
CBC and urinalysis every 2 weeks until dose stable then monthly	Rashes, proteinuria	Myelosuppression, drug-induced myastheic syndrome	*D-penicillamine
CBC every 2 weeks until dose stable then every 8 weeks. LFT every 3 months	Hepatitis	Myelosuppression	*Azathioprine
CBC every 2 weeks for 6 weeks then every 8 weeks. LFT and blood pressure every 12 weeks	Hepatitis, diarrhea, alopecia, skin allergies	Myelosuppression	Leflunomide
Serum creatinine and BP every 2 weeks until the dose has been stable for 3 months. Thereafter serum creatinine and BP monthly. CBC, LFTs monthly until dose stable for 3 months and then 3-monthly. Serum lipids 6-monthly.	Gum hyperplasia, hyperlipidemia, hyperuricemia	Hypertension, renal toxicity	*Cyclosporine (Neoral®)

CBC = complete blood count; CXR = chest radiograph; LFT = liver function tests; U+E = urea and electrolytes. (*) agents are no longer commonly used for RA.

- Patients treated with anti-TNF-α strategies are at increased risk of opportunistic infections, including tuberculosis, coccidiomycosis, cryptococcus, histoplasmosis, and aspergillus.
- Both anti-TNF-α drugs and rituximab have been associated with reactivation of Hepatitis B.
- If possible, patients should receive necessary vaccines before initiation of therapy with biologic agents; all live vaccines are contraindicated in patients actively receiving therapy with biologic DMARDs

Anti-TNF-α therapy

- TNF-α is a potent proinflammatory cytokine whose levels are elevated in RA.
- At present, there are 5 agents available for the treatment of active RA, namely etanercept (Enbrel®), infliximab (Remicade®), adalimumab (Humira®), golimumab (Simphoni®), and certolizumab pegol (Cimzia®).
- Etanercept is a recombinant human TNF receptor fusion protein. Infliximab is a chimeric human–murine anti-TNF-α monoclonal antibody, while adalimumab and golimumab are fully humanized anti-TNF monoclonal antibodies. Certolizumab pegol is a PEGylated Fab fragment of a fully human TNF-α monoclonal antibody.
- The efficacy of all TNF inhibitors is enhanced by co-administration with low dose methotrexate (e.g., 15–25 mg po/SQ/IM weekly). These agents are dosed as follows:
  - Infliximab (3–5 mg/kg) is administered by slow IV infusion at 0, 2, and 6 weeks, and every 4–8 weeks thereafter depending on response.
  - Etanercept is administered by SQ injection and can be given either once or twice weekly (i.e., 50 mg SQ weekly.
  - Adalimumab (40 mg) is given by SQ injection every 1–2 weeks.
  - Certolizumab pegol (400 mg) is administered SQ every two weeks for the first month, and then monthly afterwards.
  - Golimumab (50 mg) is also given by SQ injection every 4 weeks.
- These therapies are not without their adverse events. Serious bacterial infections have been reported, and patients with active infection should have their treatment stopped. Patients at risk of recurrent infection should not use these drugs (e.g., indwelling urinary catheter, immunodeficiency states). Other reported side-effects include demyelination, worsening of heart failure, lupus-like syndromes, and bone marrow dyscrasias.
- Reactivation of tuberculosis has been reported mainly in infliximab patients, and most commonly within 3 months of beginning of treatment. Patients should be assessed for TB risk, and guidelines for assessing risk and managing Mycobacterium tuberculosis infection in patients due to start anti-TNF therapy have been published by the British Thoracic Society (www.brit-thoracic.org.uk).
- There remains concern about the long-term safety of these drugs, especially with regard to malignancy. Debate continues about whether reports of lymphoma in RA patients on anti-TNF-α therapy reflect a real drug effect or the known increased incidence of lymphoma in RA patients. It is reassuring that an increased risk of lymphoma has not

been observed in registry studies. No increased risk has been found with other types of solid tumor malignancy, but there is an increased risk of skin cancer, and patients should undergo yearly screening.

- TNF-inhibitors are category B for pregnancy, and there have been many reports of successful pregnancies in patients on anti-TNF-α therapy.

Interleukin-6 receptor antagonists: tocilizumab (Actemra®)

Tocilizumab (4 mg/kg IV q 4 weeks), is an effective therapy for patients who fail treatment with methotrexate or TNF inhibitors. Tocilizumab may be used as monotherapy, but like the TNF inhibitors, is more efficacious when used in combination with methotrexate. Patients should be carefully monitored for liver function test abnormalities, dose-dependent neutropenia and hypercholesterolemia. Some patients may require dose adjustments, or addition of a statin for hypercholesterolemia. Diverticulitis is a relative contraindication, due to a potential risk of bowel perforation identified in clinical trials.

CTLA4-Ig: abatacept (Orencia®)

Abatacept disrupts the CD80/86 co-stimulatory signal required for T-cell activation by competing with CD28 for binding. Dosing is weight-based (<60 kg: 500 mg; 60–100 kg: 750 mg; >100 kg: 1000 mg). The drug is administered intravenously on weeks 0, 2, and 4, and then monthly afterwards, and is effective in patients who have previously failed methotrexate or TNF-inhibitors. Following an intravenous loading dose, patients may be transitioned to a subcutaneous formulation (125 mg SQ weekly). Abatacept should be avoided in patients with COPD, due to a higher risk of infection.

B cell therapy: rituximab (Rituxan®)

Rituximab is a chimeric monoclonal antibody against human CD20 that leads to rapid CD20-positive B cell depletion in the peripheral blood. Treatment with rituximab (two-1000 mg infusions, given 2 weeks apart) may lead to responses lasting for 6 months or longer. There is concern about persistent hypogammaglobulinemia in patients who receive repeated courses of this drug, and it is prudent to monitor immunoglobulin levels annually in such patients. Patients should be carefully monitored for infusion reactions, especially those with pre-existing cardiopulmonary conditions.

Janus Kinase (JAK) inhibitors: tofacitinib (Xejanz®)

Tofacitinib is the first of a new class of agents that interfere with the JAK-STAT cell signaling pathway, and the first oral biologic agent available in the United States. Tofacitinib is an inhibitor of Janus Kinase 3 (JAK-3), and inhibits the production of multiple cytokines. In clinical trials, tofacitinib appears to be effective for the treatment of moderate to server rheumatoid arthritis. Tofacitinib 5 mg po BID has been approved by the FDA for the treatment of patients with an inadequate response to methotrexate, and may be used in combination with methotrexate, or as monotherapy. Prior to initiating treatment with tofacitinib, patients should be tested for latent tuberculosis. Also, tofacitinib has been associated with an increased risk of zoster; it therefore may be prudent to consider vaccination prior to initiating therapy.

Pharmacotherapy: Take-Home Message

The number of treatment options for patients with RA can be overwhelming; although several treatment guidelines exist, one simple approach to the management of the newly diagnosed patients is the following:

- Methotrexate remains the cornerstone of therapy
- Once started, methotrexate should be titrated rapidly to therapeutic levels (as tolerated) over a few weeks.
- Combination therapy with conventional DMARDs may be as effective as TNF-antagonists for some patients
- Patients with risk factors (e.g., RF/ACPA positive, patients with erosive disease, high disease burden, high levels of disability, or persistent elevation of acute phase reactants) should be early candidates for combination or biologic therapy.
- All TNF antagonists are approximately equally effective when combined with methotrexate.
- For patients who fail treatment with TNF-antagonists, one reasonable strategy is to start with a four-month trial of either abatacept or tocilizumab. Patients who fail to respond to treatment with these agents may still respond to rituximab
- Abatacept and tocilizumab may also be reasonable treatments for patients with early rheumatoid arthritis.

Pregnancy

- Hydroxychloroquine, sulfasalazine, TNF-inhibitors, and low dose prednisone may be the best options for women during conception and pregnancy.
- Hydroxychloroquine is FDA Pregnancy Class C, but there are no clear fetal risks associated with use of this drug.
- Sulfasalazine is FDA Pregnancy Class B, but should be used with folate (800 mcg po qd), since it inhibits dihydrofolate reductase.
- Glucocorticoids are FDA Pregnancy Class B. Prednisone is inactivated by the placenta, which decreases the risk to the fetus, but prednisone use is still associated with an increased risk of cleft lip/palate and lower birth weight.
- TNF inhibitors have been linked to VACTERL (vertebral anomalies, anal atresia, cardiovascular anomalies, tracheoesophageal fistula, renal and limb anomalies), but the relationship is controversial. Etanercept and certolizumab appear to cross the placenta at a lower rate than infliximab and adalimumab.
- Methotrexate and leflunomide are both FDA Pregnancy Class X, and cannot be used during any stage of pregnancy.
- Methotrexate should be stopped at least 3 months prior to conception
- Women who have been treated with leflunomide must be treated with cholestyramine 8g po TID for 11 days, and plasma levels must be <0.02 mg/L on two tests taken 14 days apart before conception may be considered.
- Tocilizumab has been associated with an increased frequency of spontaneous miscarriage, and should be avoided.

- Rituximab is FDA Pregnancy Class C, and has been associated with a 21% first-trimester pregnancy loss, which is higher than the 10–15% loss reported in the general population, but it is difficult to know if this is a statistically significant difference.

Surgery in RA

- Damage to joints, with associated pain and loss of function remains a familiar feature of chronic RA. Surgical intervention may have a place in such situations but certain procedures (e.g., shoulder replacement) may only be effective in reducing pain and may not necessarily improve function.
- Synovectomy is less frequently performed now, although tenosynovectomy is common, and a quick and safe relief of nerve entrapment.
- Common surgical procedures include:
  - decompression of the carpal tunnel
  - reconstructive arthroplasty of hip and knee; less often the shoulder, elbow, and small joints of the hand
  - corrective arthrotomies of the metatarsals
  - stabilization of the cervical spine
  - tendon release and transfer
  - arthrodesis, particularly of the ankle joint.
- Patients should ideally be seen by a surgeon with expertise in dealing with patients with RA.

Management summary for treating RA

- Figure 5.2 summarizes the management of RA.
- There remains a need for the development of early predictors of long-term outcome in RA, allowing better patient selection for early intervention. Early functional impairment remains a crude but reliable indicator of poor prognosis.
- A high RF titer, high ESR or CRP at diagnosis, male gender, radiographic evidence of erosions, and rheumatoid nodules are features associated with aggressive disease. Thorough evaluation of early onset disease, combination therapies, and early institution of biologic agents (when appropriate) dramatically improve outcomes associated with aggressive disease.
- Of all patients with RA, 20% will have mild disease, 75% moderate disease with relapses and remissions, and 5% will have severe destructive disease.
- Patients are at risk of early cardiovascular disease. It is important to assess cardiovascular risk factors such as cholesterol, blood pressure, diabetes, corticosteroid use, smoking, etc. and modify them if possible.
- A multidisciplinary team is important in patient care and should be involved at an early stage.
- DMARD monitoring is needed to ensure patients do not suffer serious side effects.
- Patients should be involved directly in any decisions about their care.

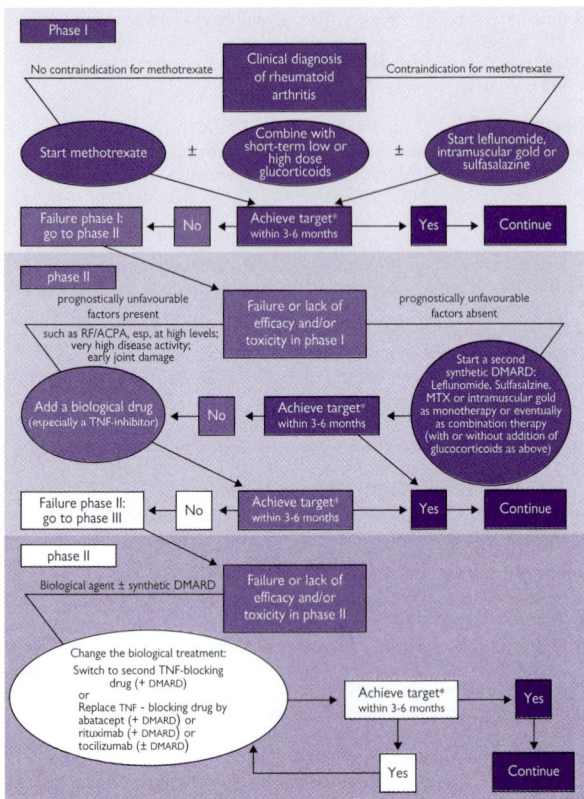

* The treatment target is clinical remission or, if remission is unlikely to be achievable, at least low disease activity

Fig. 5.2 An algorithm for the management of adult rheumatoid arthritis based on European League Against Rheumatism recommendations.

Rheumatoid factor positive polyarthritis in childhood

- This subset of juvenile idiopathic arthritis (see Chapter 9 for further details of classification) is clinically and genetically indistinguishable from adult RA. Approximately 25% of cases have a family history of seropositive RA.
- The disease usually presents as a polyarthritis (five or more joints) of the small joints of the hands and feet. In patients who present at 10 years of age or younger, there is often associated early involvement of the wrists, knees, ankles, and hindfeet as well. All other features of adult RA may be seen in children.
- Fever is rare.
- The ILAR criteria suggest that three consecutive positive tests for serum IgM RF should be taken twice over the course of 3 months before the diagnosis is made. That said, in clinical practice, the diagnosis is generally made on the basis of clinical presentation. Children are commonly ACPA-negative, although when present, these antibodies may help confirm the diagnosis. This is because transient positive titers are seen in infection. It is also important to bear in mind that RF is also found in SLE (see Chapter 10), vasculitis (see Chapter 15), hypergammaglobulinemia, and sarcoidosis (see Chapter 18). The clinical features may also appear similar to juvenile psoriatic arthropathy (see Chapter 9).
- Radiological changes with periostitis and local osteoporosis tend to occur early in the disease. One-third of cases progress to severe functional limitation within 10–15 years.
- Differences from adult RA include the problem of growth retardation, a tendency to early fusion of the carpal bones, and erosions at the distal interphalangeal joints.
- A few cases of aortic regurgitation and pericarditis have been reported. Pulmonary manifestations of RA are, however, relatively uncommon.
- In the few cases that have been followed through pregnancy, there appears to be an almost universal post-pregnancy relapse of the RA.
- Treatment of RA in children is much the same as for adults. Early introduction of a DMARD is encouraged and most centers use as first-line therapy. MTX is well-tolerated in children. Oral therapy is first-line, but SQ administration is increasingly used, and has been shown to be effective in those with poor adherence or side-effects to oral treatment. A recent study using leflunomide found high rates of clinical improvement, but not as great as with MTX.
- Cytotoxic agents tend to be spared for use in those with associated amyloidosis, vasculitis, pulmonary fibrosis, or aortic valve disease in the presence of active arthritis.
- Biologic therapy is appropriate for patients with active polyarticular disease who have been intolerant of, or not responded to, MTX.

Osteoarthritis (OA)

Introduction

Epidemiology and pathology

- Osteoarthritis (OA) is a chronic degenerative disorder characterized by cartilage loss; it is the most common condition to affect joints in humans. It is estimated that 12.1% of the population of the United States >25 years have OA, and the prevalence increases with age.
- In the elderly in the West, OA is second to cardiovascular disease as a cause of disability.
- Although there are recognized associations between OA, age, and trauma, advances in cartilage biochemistry and the recognition of crystal-associated disease have renewed interest in OA as a dynamic condition of cartilage loss (chondropathy) with a periarticular bone reaction. At present, however, OA is assessed and managed clinically as a structural rather than physiological condition, with an emphasis on late, rather than early, disease.
- OA is now viewed as a dynamic process with episodic progress. Chondrocyte dysfunction leads to metalloproteinase enzyme release causing collagen and proteoglycan degradation. Synovial inflammation is present, with production of cytokines such as IL-1 and TNF-α that also induce metalloproteinase production.
- Macroscopic changes in OA include cystic bone degeneration, cartilage loss, and growth of irregular abnormal bone at joint margins (osteophytes). Microscopic changes include flaking and fibrillation of articular cartilage with variations in vascularity and cellularity of subchondral bone, leading to sclerosis and new bone formation.
- Most surveys of OA rely on radiographic features for definition and severity. These are problematic because correlation of radiographic change with clinical status, symptoms, and function can be poor; it is best at the hip and knee, but poor in the hand and spine. The correlation between pathology and radiology is shown in Table 6.1.
- There are various subgroups of OA and these are described below in the section on clinical features.

Risk factors

- Although no gender difference occurs in mild disease, severe disease favors women and patients older than 50 years. There is also a polyarticular form of hand OA—"nodal generalized OA"—that has a predilection for perimenopausal women.
- OA of the hip is more common in Europeans than Asians or African Americans.
- The Framingham study found that 27% of those aged 63–70 years had radiographic evidence of knee OA; this increased to 44% in those over 80 years old.
- Susceptibility factors include:
  - obesity (close association with knee OA, but not hip)
  - family history (particularly nodal generalized OA)
  - high bone density such as osteopetrosis (there is a negative correlation between OA onset and low bone density)
  - trauma

- femoral dysplasia (for hip OA)
  - hypermobility (rigorous studies required, though one recent large study suggests hypermobility is protective against hand OA).
- There is increased concordance for OA in monozygotic compared to dizygotic twins.
- Smoking appears to be protective for knee OA.
- Suggested risk factors for hip OA include previous hip disease (e.g., Perthes'), acetabular dysplasia, avascular necrosis of the femoral head, severe trauma, generalized OA, and occupation (e.g., farming).
- There is little evidence to link OA with repetitive injury from occupation, except perhaps knee-bending in men.
- Longshoremen and miners have a higher incidence of knee OA.

Table 6.1 Radiographic–pathological correlates in OA

Pathological change	Radiographic abnormality
Cartilage fibrillation, erosion	Localized joint-space narrowing
Subchondral new bone	Sclerosis
Myxoid degeneration	Subchondral cysts
Trabecular compression	Bone collapse/attrition
Fragmentation of osteochondral surface	Osseous ("loose") bodies

Clinical features of OA

- The clinical features of pain and stiffness, functional impairment, and anatomical change, are interrelated but often discordant.
- There are several potential mechanisms for pain; none are completely understood. Pain may arise from inflammatory mediators or intra-articular hypertension, stimulating capsular, periosteal, and synovial nerve fibers. Pain may also arise from enthesopathy or bursitis that can accompany structural alteration, muscle weakness, and altered joint use.
- Although stiffness is a common complaint in OA, prolonged early morning stiffness should lead the clinician to consider the presence of an inflammatory arthropathy.
- Bony enlargement and deformity, crepitus, restricted movement, joint instability, and "stress" pain can also occur. Muscle weakness and wasting may be present.
- There are several subsets of OA that are worth noting. They are not absolute, and one set of characteristics may dominate the evolving disease at any one time. These subsets are:
  - primary OA:
    - Nodal generalized OA
    - Erosive ("inflammatory") OA
    - Large joint OA (knee and hip)
    - Spinal OA
  - secondary OA (see Table 6.2).

Nodal generalized OA

- This common condition is characterized by:
  - polyarticular finger involvement
  - Heberden's nodes (distal interphalangeal joint)
  - Bouchard's nodes (proximal interphalangeal joint)
  - predisposition to OA of knee, hip, and spine
  - good functional outcome in the hands
  - female preponderance
  - peak onset around the menopause
  - strong family history.
- There is a tendency to greater distal joint disease. The first carpometacarpal (CMC), metacarpophalangeal (MCP), and interphalangeal (IP) joints of the thumb are also often involved, as are the index and middle MCP.
- The more proximal joints of the hand and wrist are otherwise relatively spared.

Erosive OA

- This uncommon condition is characterized by:
  - hand interphalangeal involvement
  - tendency to joint ankylosis
  - florid inflammation (episodic)
  - radiographic subchondral erosive change.

- Unlike nodal OA, proximal and distal IP joints are equally involved and, less frequently, the MCPs.
- IP joint instability is common. Given the additional risk of ankylosis, functional impairment is more likely than nodal OA.
- The principal hallmark of the condition is subchondral erosive change that can lead to remodeling.

Large joint OA

- The knee is commonly affected and most frequently in the patellofemoral and medial tibiofemoral compartments; severe bone and cartilage loss at the latter site causes instability and the classic varus (bow knee) deformity.
- Subdivision of hip disease is usually made on the basis of local radiographic patterns. There are two principal groups:
  i. Superior pole: common pattern, often unilateral, more common in men, and likely to progress
  ii. Central (medial): less common, usually bilateral, more common in women, and less likely to progress.
- Indeterminate "concentric" radiographic patterns also exist.

Secondary OA

- Secondary OA is seen in association with a wide variety of disorders as illustrated in Table 6.2.

Natural history of OA

- Progression in the knee may take many years. Cohort studies have found that radiographic deterioration occurs in one-third.
- Progression of hip disease is variable. A Danish study found that 66% of hips worsened radiologically over 10 years, although symptomatic improvement was common.
- Hand disease is relapsing and remitting with episodic inflammatory phases associated with redness and swelling. Flares then reduce in frequency, and pain also improves.

Table 6.2 Secondary causes of OA

Trauma	Inflammatory arthritis
Metabolic/endocrine	Crystal deposition disease
Hemochromatosis	Calcium pyrophosphate
Acromegaly	Uric acid
Hyperparathyroidism	Hydroxyapatite
Ochronosis (alkaptonuria)	
Neuropathic disorders	Anatomical abnormalities
Diabetes mellitus	Bone dysplasia

The investigation of OA

- OA is a clinical and radiological diagnosis. There are no specific laboratory tests.
- Joint space narrowing may be difficult to appreciate in early OA; as the disease progresses, other findings may appear, including osteophytes, subchondral bone sclerosis, and subchondral cysts.
- Radiographs correlate poorly with symptoms and clinical function. Many older patients will have radiographic changes consistent with OA, but will be asymptomatic.
- MRI may be better at identifying early loss of articular cartilage, but this and other imaging modalities have not been well validated for the evaluation of osteoarthritis.
- Laboratory tests (including synovial fluid analysis) may be useful to exclude other causes of joint pain, such as pseudogout.
- There are potential markers of tissue destruction and inflammation that may be of use clinically in the future. A profile of several markers with genetic analysis may in the future provide an individual assessment for disease development and response to therapy. Examples of markers include:
  - cartilage oligomeric matrix protein (COMP)
  - pyridinoline and bone sialoprotein
  - metalloproteinases
  - hylauronan.

The management of OA

Successful management

Successful management centers on:
- A good history:
  - symptoms and impact on life
  - functional disability
  - functional requirements
  - patient expectation
  - psychological factors.
- A good examination:
  - extent of abnormality
  - origin of pain
  - degree of inflammation
  - instability of joint
  - muscle condition
  - other medical, soft-tissue, and neurological disease.
- A multidisciplinary approach.

Modalities for management

- There are several resources that provide specific guidance regarding the treatment of osteoarthritis. The Osteoarthritis Research Society International (OARSI) has developed evidence-based expert consensus guidelines regarding the management of osteoarthritis of the hip and knee (http:// www.oarsi.org). In the United Kingdom, the National Institute for Health and Clinical Excellence (NICE) has published evidence-based guidelines for the cost-effective treatment of osteoarthritis (http://www.nice.org.uk/ CG59). Both of these guidelines include a discussion of pharmacologic and non-pharmacologic therapies, and may help with treatment decisions.
- Exercise is an important intervention, to build muscle strength, encourage weight loss, improve endurance and joint proprioception. Advice alone is not as good as a specific program with follow-up. Evidence-based guidelines for exercise in hip and knee OA have been published.[1] In more marked disease, support splints and walking aids may be necessary.
- Education has been shown in meta-analyses to have a significant effect on pain and function, but only 20% as effective as NSAID treatment.
- Topical preparations have minimal systemic absorption, and may help patients avoid cumulative toxicities associated with polypharmacy. Topical 1% diclofenac gel (2–4 g every 6 hours) has been FDA approved for the treatment of osteoarthritis, and may be useful for treatment of symptomatic osteoarthritis in the hands and knees. Topical capsaicin (0.025% or 0.075% every 6–8 hours) may also provide significant pain relief.
- When topical therapies are not practical or efficacious, treatment often starts with acetaminophen. That said, it is only modestly more effective than placebo, and chronic use is associated with cardiovascular and gastrointestinal toxicity. Unintentional overdose is the most common cause of liver failure in the United States, and patients must be counseled to avoid other medications that may contain acetaminophen.

- NSAIDs are more effective than acetaminophen. Short-acting NSAIDs, such as ibuprofen (400 mg every 4–6 hours) are widely available, but patients may find greater levels of relief with longer acting NSAIDs, such as diclofenac (50 mg every 8 hours), naproxen (500 mg every 12 hours), or nabumetone (500–750 mg every 8–12 hours); these may be of particular use for short periods during disease flares.
- Long-term use of NSAIDs may be problematic, particularly among the elderly. The selective COX-2 inhibitors are as efficacious as standard NSAIDs, but there remains concern over cardiovascular safety; they should be used with caution and avoided in patients with cardiovascular risk factors.
- Tramadol and duloxetine may also be useful for control of the pain associated with osteoarthritis. Narcotics are associated with a high rate of discontinuation due to side effects.
- Intra-articular injections of corticosteroids are very useful in treating inflammatory disease flares, and may result in sustained symptom improvement, although response duration is variable. Many practitioners also add local anesthetic, although there is no clear evidence that this improves the efficacy of the treatment. Most data are available for knee OA. Infection is rare (< 1 in 10,000 incidence), but care should be taken to clean overlying skin, and injection through infected/psoriatic skin should be avoided. Other side effects to warn patients about are skin depigmentation and fat atrophy. It is advised that patients receive no more than 2 or 3 injections per year.
- The efficacy of intra-articular injection of hyaluronic acid derivatives (visco-supplementation) is controversial, although it may provide prolonged relief in some cases.
- Glucosamine and chondroitin sulfate are found in articular cartilage. Anecdotal evidence suggests that when given as oral supplements, these agents have an analgesic effect in mild-to-moderate OA of the knee, but this has been difficult to demonstrate consistently in controlled trials. There is little evidence for use in OA at other sites.
- Acupuncture has been shown in randomized controlled trials to be better than placebo acupuncture in improving symptoms.
- There is some evidence that avocado/soybean unsaponifiable (ASU) supplementation, evening primrose oil, and omega-3 fish oils improve pain.
- The clinician should also seek ways to reduce the impact of disability. Options include:[1]
  - occupational therapy: splints, tools, safe environment
  - treat depression, anxiety, fibromyalgia
  - coping strategies—behavioral therapy
  - patient education.
- For patients with activity-limiting osteoarthritis, joint replacement is effective at reducing pain, although function may not be restored. Arthroscopy and osteotomy may be helpful in some cases.

[1] Roddy E, Zhang W, Dohetry M et al. Evidence-based recommendations for the role of exercise in the management of osteoarthritis of the hip or knee: the MOVE consensus. Rheumatology 2005; 44: 67–73.

The crystal arthropathies

The crystal arthropathies include gout, calcium pyrophosphate deposition disease (CPPD) or pseudogout, basic calcium phosphate (BCP) associated syndromes, and calcium oxalate arthritis. These conditions will be discussed in this chapter.

Gout and hyperuricemia

Epidemiology of gout

- In its most general sense, gout is a group of conditions characterized by hyperuricemia and uric acid crystal formation. These clinical conditions include arthritis, tophaceous gout, uric acid nephrolithiasis, and gouty nephropathy. In its more commonly assumed definition, gout refers to the acute inflammatory arthropathy caused by uric acid crystal deposition.
- Gout is a relatively common condition, and is the most common form of inflammatory arthritis. Prevalence data from the United States on self-reported disease show figures of 13.6 per 1000 persons in adult men and 6.4 per 1000 persons for women. It is more common in the middle aged and elderly, and its prevalence may be increasing due to changes in lifestyle and diet.
- The risk factors for gout mirror those for hyperuricemia, and are shown in Table 7.1.

The clinical features of gout

- The first stage of the condition is usually asymptomatic hyperuricemia.
- Clinically, the first symptom is most often an acute, self-limiting, monoarticular inflammatory arthritis; up to 60–70% of attacks first occur in the big toe ("podagra"). Other frequently involved joints include the ankle, foot, knee, wrist, elbow (olecranon bursa), and the small joints of the hands. The axial large joints and spine are rarely involved. Some 70–80% of individuals will have recurrent attacks within 2 years.
- In the later stages of untreated disease, acute attacks are more often polyarticular (with shorter periods of remission), and are associated with joint damage and deformity; these later stages are associated with loss of mobility, chronic pain, and formation of tophi.
- Tophi are deposits of urate embedded in a matrix composed of lipids, proteins, and calcific debris. Tophi are usually subcutaneous, but rarely can occur in bone and other organs such as the eye. The classic sites for tophi are the pinna of the ear, bursa of the elbow and knee, Achilles tendon, and the dorsal surface of the MCP joints. Tophi are usually painless, but the overlying skin may ulcerate and become infected. Those most at risk of tophi are patients with prolonged severe hyperuricemia, polyarticular gout, and the elderly with primary nodal OA (see Chapter 6) on diuretics.
- Hyperuricemia by itself does not confirm a diagnosis of gout. Some clinicians will treat asymptomatic hyperuricemia to prevent the onset of "urate nephropathy," but this is controversial.

Table 7.1 The causes of hyperuricemia and risk factors for gout

Primary gout	Male gender
	Age <40 years
	Obesity
	Family history
	Alcohol use and purine rich foods
	Renal insufficiency
	Hypertension
Inherited metabolic syndromes	X-linked HPRT deficiency (Lesch–Nyhan) X-linked raised PRPP synthetase activity Autosomal recessive G6P deficiency (von Gierke's disease)
Uric acid overproduction	Cell lysis—tumor lysis syndrome, myeloproliferative disease, hemolytic anemia, psoriasis, trauma; Drugs—alcohol, cytotoxic drugs, warfarin
Uric acid underexcretion	Renal failure
	Drugs—alcohol, salicylates, diuretics, laxatives, cyclosporine, levodopa, ethambutol, pyrazinamide
Lead toxicity	Renal impairment and altered purine turnover

HPRT = hypoxanthine guanine phosphoribosyltransferase—a salvage enzyme converting hypoxanthine back to precursors and therefore competing with its conversion to xanthine and then uric acid. PRPP = phosphoribosylpyrophosphate synthetase—a component enzyme in purine ring synthesis. G6P = glucose 6 phosphatase. G6P deficiency leads to increased activity of amidophosphoribosyltransferase and purine formation.

Diagnosis of gout

- Synovial fluid analysis remains the single most important diagnostic study. The diagnosis is made by the presence of typical, negatively birefringent, needle-shaped crystals seen with a polarized light microscope. The crystals may be extra- or intracellular. The absence of crystals does not rule out the diagnosis.
- Serum uric acid levels may be normal during an acute attack and may not reflect pre-attack levels. They cannot be used to exclude the diagnosis during an acute attack. Uric acid levels are of value in assessing the patient once the acute attack has subsided, either to establish the presence of hyperuricemia or to monitor the effectiveness of therapies that lower serum urate.
- Radiographs are often normal during the early phase of the disease, except for the presence of soft tissue swelling. They are, however, useful for excluding other conditions such as trauma or infection (see Table 7.2). Later in the disease, radiographs may demonstrate tophi near joints, tissue swelling, joint erosions, periosteal new bone formation, and joint deformity. Once these changes occur, gout may be misdiagnosed as RA (see Chapter 5) in some cases.
- Dual-Energy Computed Tomography (DECT) can differentiate urate from calcium, and may be useful to confirm a diagnosis of gout when arthrocentesis is not practical.
- Causes of hyperuricemia should always be considered.

The management of gouty arthritis

- The efficacy of any public health improvement measure for the prevention of gout has yet to be proven. It is reasonable to suggest that avoiding excess weight gain and alcohol, controlling hypertension, and avoiding exposure to diuretics and lead, may have some effect on decreasing the incidence of the condition.
- The management of gout otherwise should be seen as two phases: treatment of the acute attack, and treatment of chronic or tophaceous gout. The principal therapies for acute gout are NSAIDs, colchicine, and steroids. Many treatments are empiric rather than evidence based.
- Traditionally indomethacin has been the NSAID of choice in acute gout, but has no advantage over other NSAIDs. With treatment, symptoms should subside within 3–5 days.
- NSAIDs are contraindicated in renal insufficiency and should be used with caution in the elderly (who are often also taking aspirin) or those with GI risk factors. Evidence shows that NSAIDs decrease pain, swelling, and duration of attack. There is no evidence for the use of selective COX-2 inhibitors in gout.
- Colchicine can be very effective in acute gout, especially when treatment is started at the first sign of symptoms (i.e., a "pill-in-the-pocket" strategy). Oral colchicine, given at 0.6 mg BID to TID for 5 days is very useful and can be well tolerated. It is often given in addition to NSAIDs (although there is no evidence to support this) or when NSAIDs are contraindicated. The 5-day dosage may be repeated for an acute attack after 72 hours. IV colchicine is not used due to the potential for bone marrow suppression. There are no randomized controlled trials comparing colchicine to NSAIDs.
- Steroid regimens range from oral prednisone at tapering doses from 20–50 mg daily for an average of 10 days, to IM triamcinolone 60 mg once only. A study comparing IM triamcinolone with indomethacin found no significant difference in time to recovery.
- Intra-articular steroids are useful if only one or two joints are affected. In a case series from 1999, injection of triamcinolone acetonide into affected joints resolved all symptoms within 48 hours.
- Corticosteroids should not be used if there is a possibility of septic arthritis.
- Drugs that decrease serum uric acid levels are the standard therapy for prophylaxis against repeated gout attacks, but should not be started after just one isolated attack. Allopurinol, a xanthine oxidase inhibitor, is the drug most commonly used, and the drug of choice in the presence of nephrolithiasis, or tophi. The drug should not be started during an acute attack of gout, as it is likely to make the situation worse. Allopurinol should be initiated at 100 mg/d (or lower, in patients with renal insufficiency), and slowly titrated. Patients may require doses anywhere between 100–900 mg daily to achieve normal serum uric acid levels (i.e., < 5 mg/dL). The dose should be adjusted down in renal impairment. The onset of action of allopurinol is rapid, with effects seen as early as 4 days to 2 weeks.

Table 7.2 Clinical conditions that can mimic gouty arthritis

CPPD disease (pseudogout)
BCP arthritis
Cellulitis
Infectious arthritis
Trauma
Rheumatoid arthritis
Psoriatic arthritis
Erythema nodosum
Reactive arthritis

- Allopurinol can lead to a hypersensitivity reaction with rash and fever. Rarely a severe reaction is seen with hepatitis, nephritis, and toxic epidermal necrolysis. In patients with mild to moderate intolerance, allopurinol can be reintroduced at very low levels, e.g. 100 mg, and built up slowly using desensitization regimens. Allopurinol can interfere with the metabolism of azathioprine and warfarin, augmenting their potential side effects. During its introduction a patient may also experience an acute flare of gout. This may be treated with NSAIDs and/or low dose colchicine. Prior to treatment with allopurinol, Koreans, Han Chinese, and Thai patients should be screened for the presence of the HLA B*5801 allele, which is associated with an increased risk of hypersensitivity reactions.
- Some patients may respond to a combination of allopurinol and a uricosuric agent (such as probenecid) when either alone has been ineffective. Uricosuric drugs should be avoided in patients with renal insufficiency or history of nephrolithiasis.
- Febuxostat (40–80 mg po QD) is a non-purine xanthine oxidase inhibitor that has been approved by the Food and Drug Administration in the United States for the chronic management of hyperuricemia in patients with gout. Unlike allopurinol, febuxostat does not need to be adjusted based on renal function; it therefore may be especially appropriate for patients who are allergic to allopurinol or have severe renal insufficiency. Febuxostat 80 mg daily is more effective than allopurinol.
- Pegloticase (8 mg IV every 2 weeks) may be considered for patients who are refractory to conventional therapies. Premedication with antihistamines and corticoisteroids is mandatory, and treatment must be discontinued if pre-infusion serum uric acid levels begin to increase, which indicates the presence of anti-pegloticase antibodies that are associated with infusion reactions. Because of the importance of monitoring serum uric acid, this drug should not be combined with other urate-lowering agents.

- In patients who are unable to take allopurinol or a uricosuric drug, daily low-dose oral colchicine may be useful in preventing attacks. It is usually given in doses of 0.6 mg po BID. Serious side effects can still occur at this dose. This low-dose regimen may also be useful as prophylaxis against acute flares during the introduction of allopurinol.
- Fenofibrate is an established treatment for many lipid disorders. It also has the ability to decrease serum urate by increasing renal uric acid clearance. It may have a role (off label) in patients resistant or intolerant to other agents. It should be avoided in hepatic and biliary disease, hypothyroidism and pregnancy. Side effects may include arthralgias and myalgias.
- Increasing intake of (low-fat) dairy, and decreasing intake of organ meats and alcohol, may help reduce the risk of gout attacks.
- Patients with uric acid stones are best managed with adequate hydration, urinary alkalization, and allopurinol. This regimen is also effective in preventing calcium oxalate stones.
- Finally, gouty tophi may be amenable to surgical removal.

Khanna D. et al., "2012 American College of Rheumatology Guidelines for the Management of Gout. Part 1. Systemic Nonpharmacologic and Pharmacologic Therapeutic Approaches to Hyperuricemia" Arthritis Care Res 2012; 64 (10): 1431–1446.

Plate 1 MR scan of the neck showing loss of height and signal affecting several discs with multisegmental spondylotic bars, compression of the cord from protrusion of the C5/6 disc and myeloppathic changes (high signal) in the cord.

Plate 2 Patterns of radiographic abnormality in chronic SAI: sclerosis and cystic changes in greater tuberosity.

Plate 3 Dactylitis, nail changes, and DIP joint arthritis in psoriatic arthritis.

(a)

(b)

Plate 4 (a) Normal nailfold capillaries. (b) Nailfold capillaries in scleroderma showing avascular areas and dilated capillaries in an irregular orientation (original magnification 65x).

Plate 5 Diffuse arm and hand swelling in chronic regional pain syndrome (reflex sympathetic dystrophy).

Plate 6 Slight flexion of fourth and fifth fingers as a result of an ulnar nerve lesion at the elbow. The area of sensory loss is indicated by the dotted line.

Plate 7 Psoriatic spondylitis: Non-marginal and "floating" (non-attached) syndesmophytes.

Plate 8 Spondylolysis. The defect in the pars interarticularis (black arrows) may only be noted on an oblique view. The patient has had a spinal fusion (open arrows).

(a)

(b)

Plate 9 Testing passive hip flexion and rotational movements (a) and hip abduction (b). The pelvis should be fixed when testing abduction and adduction.

Plate 10 Bone scintigraphy showing osteonecrosis of the left femoral head (on the right-hand side as this is an anterior view). Photopenia (an early sign) corresponds to ischemia.

Plate 11 The "patellar tap" test. Any fluid in the suprapatellar pouch is squeezed distally by the left hand. The patella is depressed by the right hand. It will normally tap the underlying femur immediately. Any delay in eliciting the tap or a feeling of damping as the patella is depressed suggests a joint effusion.

Plate 12 Injection of the glenohumeral joint via the anterior route

Plate 13 Injection of the subacromial space.

Plate 14 Injection of tennis elbow (lateral humeral epicondylitis/enthesitis).

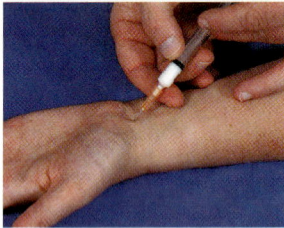

Plate 15 Injection of the carpal tunnel to the ulnar side of Palmaris longus tendon.

Plate 16 Nodules associated with joint diseases. (a) RA: typically over extensor surfaces and pressure areas. (b) Chronic tophaceous gout: tophi can be indistinguishable clinically from RA nodules though may appear as eccentric swellings around joints (image provided courtesy of Dr. R. A. Watts). (c) Multicentric reticulohistiocytosis: nodules are in the skin, are small, yellowish-brown, and are often around nails. (d) Nodal OA: swelling is bony, typically at PIPs and DIPs.

Plate 17 Bone scintigraphy (⁹⁹ᵐTc MDP) of a 65-year-old man with widespread bone pain and weakness suspected to have metastatic malignancy. Undecalcified transiliac bone biopsy confirmed severe osteomalacia. There was coincidental Paget's disease (arrowed lesions).

Plate 18 Increased growth of the left lower limb due to chronic knee inflammation in (RF-) JIA.

Plate 19 Lupus pernio presenting as a bluish-red or violaceous swelling of the nose extending onto the cheek.

Plate 20 Nailfold capillaries, demonstrating normal capillary loops. Magnified 300x. Photograph used with the kind permission of Graham Dinsdale, Tonia Moore, and Ariane Herrick.

Plate 21 Nailfold capillaries, demonstrating abnormal capillary loops, including capillary loop dilatation and dropout. Magnified 300x. Photograph used with the kind permission of Graham Dinsdale, Tonia Moore, and Ariane Herrick.

Calcium pyrophosphate dihydrate (CPPD) disease

- CPPD disease is the second most common form of crystal arthropathy. Our understanding of the pathophysiology of CPPD remains rudimentary, and consequently no specific therapies for this arthropathy exist.
- Several clinical syndromes are associated with CPPD the features of the condition are heterogeneous, sometimes mimicking other rheumatic conditions. Definite associations with CPPD and chondrocalcinosis (i.e., calcification of fibro- and hyaline cartilage typically at the knee and wrist) include:
  - hypomagnesemia
  - hypophosphatasia
  - hemochromatosis
  - Wilson's disease
  - hyperparathyroidism.
- Possible associations include:
  - gout
  - ochronosis
  - hypocalciuric hypercalcemia
  - diabetes mellitus
  - X-linked hypophosphatemic rickets.
- These crystals are also found in the synovial fluid of patients with both acute and chronic arthritis. They are associated with advanced age, chondrocalcinosis, and a characteristic pattern of severe joint degeneration.
- There are several presentations of CPPD that afford at least some form of classification based on clinical features. It is not easy to categorize all cases, but the classification serves to point out the heterogeneity of the condition in acute, chronic, inflammatory, and noninflammatory arthritis (see Tables 7.3, 7.4).

Laboratory tests

- CPPD disease is defined by the presence of positively birefringent, rhomboid crystals on examination of synovial fluid under polarized light microscopy. The crystals may be intra- or extracellular. These crystals may be difficult to visualize; therefore, the absence of CPPD crystals in synovial fluid does not necessarily rule out CPPD disease.
- Radiographs of the affected joints may not be helpful in establishing the diagnosis. The presence of chondrocalcinosis increases the likelihood of CPPD disease. Radiographic clues that may help to distinguish CPPD from OA include:
  - axial involvement
  - sacroiliac erosions
  - cortical erosions of the femur
  - osteonecrosis of the medial femoral condyle.

Table 7.3 The clinical presentations of CPPD disease

Type	Description	Frequency	Features
A	Pseudogout	25%	Acute pain and swelling, often amonoarthropathy of the knee, wrist or shoulder. Rare in small joints
B	Pseudorheumatoid	5%	Polyarthritis. Synovitis. Joint flares out of phase with each other
C and D	Pseudo-osteoarthritis: C with attacks D without acute attacks	50%	Acute attacks on chronic symptoms
E	Asymptomatic	?	Incidental chondrocalcinosis
F	Pseudoneurotrophic	Rare	Severe joint destruction and neuropathy
Others	Tophaceous CPPD deposits		Spinal CPPD: 'Crowned dens syndrome' deposits around the atlantoaxial joint. Spinal stenosis. Cervical myelopathy
			Tendon and bursa deposits

- Patients under the age of 60 years should be screened for secondary CPPD disease, i.e. serum calcium, magnesium, alkaline phosphatase, ferritin, iron, and iron binding capacity.

Management of CPPD disease

- NSAIDs are the most commonly used therapy, but must be used with caution as the majority of affected patients are elderly.
- Joint aspiration and intra-articular corticosteroids are of benefit in acute flares of pseudogout. The role of oral steroids remains unclear.
- Low-dose oral colchicine (0.6 mg QD-BID) may reduce the frequency of acute attacks in pseudogout.
- Rest, splinting, and eventual joint replacement may be helpful.
- Other therapies that have been tried include:
  - oral magnesium carbonate
  - intra-articular glycosaminoglycan polysulfate
  - intra-articular corticosteroids
  - IM gold or hydroxychloroquine for type B ("pseudorheumatoid") disease.

Table 7.4 Factors that may trigger acute pseudogout

Intercurrent illness, e.g., chest infection
Direct trauma to the joint
Surgery, especially parathyroidectomy
Blood transfusion and parenteral fluids
Institution of thyroxine replacement therapy
Joint lavage

Basic calcium phosphate (BCP) associated disease

- BCP crystals include hydroxyapatite, octacalcium phosphate, and tricalcium phosphate.
- These crystals are associated with several rheumatic conditions as shown in Table 7.5.
- The treatment of these conditions is as per CPPD disease (see previous section), with NSAIDs and colchicine principally.
- Calcium hydroxyapetitie crystals are not visible under plain or polarized light microscopy, but may be visualized by staining with alizarin red.

Table 7.5 BCP associated conditions

Articular disease	Milwaukee shoulder syndrome (severe degenerative arthropathy, more common on the dominant side and in elderly women)
	Osteoarthritis (synovial fluid crystals found in up to 60% of OA patients)
	Erosive arthritis
	Mixed crystal deposition
Periarticular	Pseudopodagra. Calcific tendonitis and bursitis

Calcium oxalate arthritis

- This is an unusual form of arthritis. The crystals are positively birefringent and bipyramidal on polarized light microscopy.
- Radiographs and laboratory tests are not diagnostic.
- Treatment is as for CPPD disease.
- Several conditions are associated with calcium oxalate arthritis (Table 7.6).

Table 7.6 Conditions associated with calcium oxalate arthritis

End-stage renal disease on dialysis
Short bowel syndrome
Diet rich in rhubarb, spinach, ascorbic acid
Thiamine deficiency
Pyridoxine deficiency
Primary oxalosis: recessive trait
Early renal failure (age 20s)
Arthritis
Tendonitis

The spondyloarthridities

Introduction

- This set of diseases is also referred to as the "spondyloarthropathies". Using the name "spondyloarthritis" emphasizes the inflammatory nature of these syndromes.
- The seronegative spondyloarthridities are classically characterized by some combination of axial and peripheral joint manifestations:
  - Axial: sacroiliitis and inflammatory back pain
  - Peripheral: asymmetric arthritis, enthesitis, dactylitis
- These diseases may also be accompanied by:
  - extra-articular disease
  - anterior uveitis
- The group is made up of several conditions that often overlap. Five major diseases are recognized by the European Spondyloarthropathy Study Group (ESSG). These are:
  - ankylosing spondylitis
  - psoriatic arthritis
  - reactive arthropathy
  - enteropathic arthritis
  - undifferentiated spondyloarthritis.
- The diagnosis "undifferentiated spondyloarthritis" includes subsets of cases in which features such as dactylitis, uveitis, or sacroiliitis exist without the full criteria for a diagnosis.
- In addition, we recognize a juvenile enthesitis related arthritis.
- Some physicians suggest that other diseases that may be associated with sacroiliitis should also be classified as a spondyloarthritis. These diseases include Behçet's disease, Whipple's disease, and SAPHO (Synovitis-Acne-Pustulosis-Hyperostosis-Osteitis) syndrome.
- Pathological changes are mainly at the insertion of tendons and ligaments into bone (i.e., *enthesis*), and extra-articular changes may also develop in the eye, aortic valve, lung, and skin.

Diagnostic criteria and clinical subsets

- There is a general consensus that most criteria are too restricted given the wide spectrum of disease. For example, radiographic evidence of sacroiliitis in the absence of symptoms, or unilateral sacroiliitis with only dactylitis or uveitis, would be excluded by most criteria and yet could be part of the spondyloarthritis spectrum.
- Most clinical criteria require the presence of radiographic sacroiliitis, which make them less sensitive for detecting early disease.
- To address these shortcomings, the Assessment of Spondyloarthritis International Society (ASAS) classification criteria were developed (Table 8.1 and 8.2).
- The ASAS criteria allow patients to be classified as having spondyloarthritis before the onset of radiographic sacroiliitis, and solidify the use of MRI as the standard-of-care modality for detecting sacroiliitis.
- A variety of symptoms and signs are present, and Table 8.3 highlights the differences between these conditions.
- The specific expression of disease is a product of inter related genetic and environmental factors. The precise link between triggers such as infection and pathogenesis, and indeed the exact role of the HLA B27 molecule remains a mystery.
- The HLA B27 molecule has an association with the spondylo-arthropathies ranging between 50–95%. Interpretation of a positive result is complicated by the presence of this allele of the HLA B gene in up to 5–10% of the normal population. It may be useful to assess symptomatic first-degree relatives of HLA B27+ probands with ankylosing spondylitis (AS), for whom the risk of developing the same disease is approximately 1 in 3.
- There are a number of interesting observations in the study of HLA B27, which include the following:
  - HLA B27 is inherited as an autosomal co-dominant characteristic: 50% of first-degree relatives of probands with HLA B27 possess the antigen.
  - 5–10% of HLA B27 positive individuals develop AS over time and 20% of individuals with B27 develop a reactive arthropathy after contact with agents such as chlamydia or salmonella.
  - Only 50% of patients with psoriatic or enteropathic spondylitis are HLA B27 positive.
  - Only 50% of non-Caucasians with AS are HLA B27 positive. This is considerably less than the prevalence of HLA B27 among Caucasians with AS (95%).
  - Relatives of probands with both sacroiliitis and HLA B27 frequently remain disease free.
  - Concordance in identical twins is 70% vs 13% in non-identical twins.
  - Uveitis is a common accompaniment of AS. HLA B27 is found in up to 40% of cases of uveitis, even in the absence of underlying rheumatic disease.

Table 8.1 Assessment of Spondyloarthritis International Society (ASAS) classification criteria for axial spondyloarthritis

Classification requires the following:

1. Chronic back pain (≥3 months)
2. Age of onset < 45 years
3. Sacroiliitis on imaging + 1 clinical feature, OR HLA-B27 + 2 clinical features

Clinical features

1. Inflammatory back pain
2. Arthritis
3. Enthesitis
4. Dactylitis—sausage-like fingers
5. Uveitis
6. Psoriasis
7. Crohn's disease/ ulcerative colitis
8. Good response to NSAIDs
9. Family history of spondyloarthritis
10. HLA-B27-positive
11. Elevated C-reactive protein

Radiological features of sacroiliitis:

1. MRI features of sacroiliitis (i.e., bone marrow edema)
2. Radiographic sacroiliitis

The ASAS classification criteria have a sensitivity of 82.9%, and a specificity of 84.4%

Rudwaleit M, et al. *Ann rheum Dis* 2009; 68: 777–783.

Table 8.2 Assessment of Spondyloarthritis International Society (ASAS) classification criteria for peripheral spondyloarthritis

Classification requires the following:
 1 clinical feature + 1 associated feature, OR
 2 clinical features

In either case, at least one clinical feature must be arthritis, ethesitis, or dactylitis.

Clinical features

1. Arthritis (typically asymmetric, affecting predominantly the lower extremities)

2. Enthesitis

3. Dactylitis

4. Inflammatory back pain

5. Family history of spondyloarthritis

Associated features:

1. Uveitis

2. HLA-B27

2. Preceeding genitourinary or gastrointestinal infection

3. Psoriasis

4. Inflammatory bowedl disease

5. Sacroiliitis on imaging

The ASAS classification criteria have a sensitivity of 77.8%, and a specificity of 82.8% for peripheral spondyloarthritis

Rudwaleit M, Curr Opin Rheumatol 2010; 22: 375–80.

Table 8.3 Comparison of the seronegative spondyloarthridities

Feature	AS	REA	PA	EA
Sex	More ♂	♂ = ♀	♂ = ♀	♂ = ♀
Age onset (years)	20–30	Any age	Any age	Any age
Onset	Gradual	Sudden	Variable	Gradual
% HLA B27 positive	95		20 (50 if sacroiliac disease is present)	
Sacroiliitis	Always	Often	Often	Often
Peripheral joint disease	Lower limb > upper	Usually lower limb	Usually lower limb	Usually lower limb
Enthesitis	Present	Present	Present	Present
Uveitis	Common	Not common	Not common	Not common
Conjunctivitis	Not seen	Not common	Not seen	Not seen
Urethritis	Not seen	Rare	Not seen	Not seen
Skin disease	Not seen	Rare	Very common	Rare
Mucosal disease	Not seen	Not seen	Not seen	Not common

AS, ankylosing spondylitis; REA, reactive arthritis; PA, psoriatic arthritis; EA, enteropathic arthropathy.

Ankylosing spondylitis

Epidemiology

- Few clinicians rely solely on the criteria; most would consider the diagnosis of ankylosing spondylitis (AS) in any case of symptomatic inflammatory back pain with radiographic evidence of sacroiliitis.
- The modified New York criteria for AS, shown in Table 8.4, are better at capturing well-established disease; many patients with early AS would not meet the radiologic criteria, which requires unequivocal evidence of sacroiliitis on a plain radiograph.
- The difficulty comes in recognizing early disease or subtle radiological change. There is often an insidious onset of back pain and morning stiffness that tends to improve with exercise. MRI is more sensitive than plain radiographs for detecting sacroiliitis, but occasionally, sacroiliitis is a chance finding in the absence of pain.
- Patients are typically <40 years of age with a male to female ratio of approximately 3:1.
- The condition occurs more frequently in Caucasian populations. In American Indians, where HLA B27 prevalence is high, AS is particularly frequent, whereas the condition is less common in African-Americans, and rarer still in Sub-Saharan Africans, reflecting the declining prevalence of HLA B27 in these groups.
- Prevalence estimates in Caucasians range from 0.05–0.23% in adults. This may be an underestimate as people with mild symptoms may not seek medical advice.
- As previously stated, HLA B27 typing has led to greater understanding of the spondyloarthropathies, but should not be considered a diagnostic test or necessary for the diagnosis of AS. Up to 5% of Caucasian patients with AS are negative for HLA B27.

Clinical features of AS

- The principal feature of the condition and allied diseases is *enthesitis*, i.e., fibrosis and ossification of ligament, tendon, and capsule insertions into bone (the entheses), mainly in the region of the discs and sacroiliac joints.
- Synovitis also occurs, typically in the larger peripheral joints (hips and knees in particular). 20–40% of patients have some degree of peripheral joint disease at some stage during their illness, moreso in women than in men. Approximately 50% of patients with adult AS will develop hip arthritis and some of these will need surgery.
- The standardized mortality ratio is 1.5; this increased mortality is due to cardiac valve and respiratory disease, amyloidosis, and fractures.
- Like other forms of chronic disease, AS patients have a significant risk of having to alter or give up work.
- Although recognized as typical of as, few patients progress to the classical late "bamboo spine." When the spine does fuse (with "syndesmophytes" bridging the gap between vertebral bodies) microfractures can occur leading to acute episodes of severe pain and

Table 8.4 Diagnostic criteria: Modified New York Criteria

Clinical criteria:

Low back pain and stiffness for >3 months improving with exercise but not relieved by rest

Limitation of lumbar spine movements in sagittal and frontal planes

Limitation of chest expansion relative to normal values for age and sex

Radiological criteria:

Greater than or equal to Grade II bilateral sacroiliitis

Grade III or IV unilateral sacroiliitis

Combined diagnostic criteria:

Definite AS if 1 radiological and 1 clinical criterion

Probable AS if 3 clinical criteria or a radiological criterion without signs or symptoms satisfying the clinical criteria

Van der Linden et al. Evaluation of diagnostic criteria for ankylosing spondylitis: a proposal for modification of the New York Criteria. Arthritis Rheum, 1984; 27: 361–8.

spondylodiscitis, a term given to collapse of the vertebral end-plate and destruction of the disc–bone border.

- This process is usually self-limiting, requiring rest and analgesia for up to 3 weeks. Most spinal disease is limited to chronic low-grade pain and stiffness with clinical evidence of a symmetrical reduction in spinal mobility.
- Patients may have insertional tendonitis at several other common sites including the Achilles tendon, intercostal muscles, plantar fascia, and dactylitis of the hands and feet.

Extra-articular disease in AS

- Constitutional features of fatigue, weight loss, low-grade fever, and anemia are common. Fatigue as opposed to pain or stiffness can be the most troublesome symptom for many patients.
- Iritis occurs in up to 40% of cases but has little correlation with disease activity in the spine. There are no known triggers for this condition and although self-limiting, topical or systemic steroids may be required in severe cases. Iritis is usually unilateral.
- Upper lobe, bilateral pulmonary fibrosis is a recognized feature of the disease. Occasionally the fibrotic area is invaded by aspergillus with changes mimicking tuberculosis. Treatment of the fibrosis is of not effective. Pleuritis can occur as a consequence of insertional tendonitis of the costosternal and costovertebral muscles. Fusion of the thoracic wall leads to rigidity and reduction in chest expansion. Ventilation is maintained by the diaphragm; however, there is a threefold increased risk of death from a respiratory cause compared with a normal population.

- Cardiac involvement includes aortic incompetence, cardiomegaly, and conduction defects. Of the 20% of patients with aortic valve disease, the majority are clinically undetectable.
- Neurological complaints are not a feature of AS, although nerve root entrapment or spinal cord/cauda equine compression can occur as a result of spinal fusion or fractures.
- Primary renal involvement is uncommon and if present may be due to coexistent medical conditions, NSAID use, or renal amyloidosis.
- Osteoporosis is an under-recognized finding. Estimates of prevalence range from 20–60%, increasing with age and disease duration, and disease is largely confined to the axial skeleton. Bone density scanning may be inaccurate in the lumbar spine due to the presence of syndesmophytes late in the disease. Studies suggest that bone loss occurs early and during the acute inflammatory stage of the disease and that further bone loss, long-term, is rarely seen. Micro-fractures may occur with trauma but the classical vertebral compression and wedge fractures of osteoporosis are rarely seen. Further work needs to be done to establish the need for, and efficacy of, current osteoporosis therapies for patients with AS.

Diagnostic evaluation of AS

- There is little correlation between any of the inflammatory markers and disease activity or clinical symptoms.
- Radiological evaluation is the most helpful form of investigation. Plain anteroposterior view radiographs are of the most value, but may not show early changes. A false positive result is common due to projection artifacts. Early changes include loss of the subchondral sclerotic line. Changes may initially be asymmetric. Later findings include the more classical findings of subchondral sclerosis, erosions, and finally ankylosis. Radionuclide scanning may be sensitive but is non-specific and may be more confusing than helpful. CT provides excellent views of the SI joints (in exchange for a higher radiation dose). MRI may demonstrate joint erosions, and also bone edema and fatty change in marrow that are not detected by CT or plain radiographs.
- The main radiological features of 'primary' AS and that associated with inflammatory bowel disease are:
  - symmetrical sacroiliac changes
  - ascending spread of disease
  - facet joint involvement
  - squaring of vertebrae
  - syndesmophytes
  - ossification
  - osteitis pubis.
- It is said that AS associated reactive arthritis or psoriatic arthropathy (PsA), i.e., secondary AS, tends to differ by being far less severe radiologically, with often asymmetrical sacroiliac disease and random spinal involvement.
- It is important to differentiate syndesmophytes from osteophytes. Syndesmophytes are vertical; osteophytes are horizontal, and occur in association with disc-space narrowing.

- AS should be distinguished from diffuse idiopathic skeletal hyperostosis (DISH). The two conditions are compared in Table 8.5.

Disease status and prognostic indicators in AS

- There are validated self-administered instruments defining disease status in AS. Since one lacks the advantage of valuable laboratory tests, it is helpful that there is a good correlation between the self-reporting of symptoms and observed clinical status of patients with AS.
- Instruments for assessing disease status include indexes produced by the Royal National Hospital for Rheumatic Diseases, Bath, UK, namely the Bath Ankylosing Spondylitis Functional Index (BASFI), Disease Activity Index (BASDAI) (see Table 8.6), Metrology Index (BASMI), and Radiology Index (BASRI).
- It is difficult to define outcome for individual patients when considering prognosis. The main predictive factors in AS appear to be:
  - early hip involvement
  - an ESR > 30
  - poor initial response to NSAIDs
  - early loss of lumbar spine mobility
  - presence of dactylitis
  - oligoarticular disease
  - onset < 16 years
  - low social–educational background
  - sporadic disease rather than familial.

Table 8.5 Differentiating diffuse idiopathic skeletal hyperostosis (DISH) and ankylosing spondylitis (AS)

Feature	DISH	AS
Age of onset (years)	Usually > 50	Usually < 40
Kyphosis	No	Yes
Reduced mobility	Occasionally	Very often
Pain	Common	Very common
Reduced chest expansion	No	Common
Radiological findings:		
Hyperostosis	Yes	Yes
Sacroiliac joint erosions	No	Yes
ALL ossification	Yes—common	No
PLL ossification	Yes—occasionally	No
Syndesmophytes	No	Very common
Erosive enthesitis	No	Very common
Non-erosive enthesitis	Very common	Common

ALL, anterior longitudinal ligament; PLL, posterior longitudinal ligament.

Table 8.6 Bath Ankylosing Spondylitis Disease Activity Index (BASDAI)

The assessment comprises 6 questions with an analogue score answer of 0 ('none') to 10 ('very severe') for each on a 10 cm scale.

The questions are:

1. How would you describe the overall level of fatigue/tiredness you have experienced?

2. How would you describe the overall level of AS neck, back or hip pain you have had?

3. How would you describe the overall level of pain/swelling in joints other than neck, back, or hips you have had?

4. How would you describe the overall level of discomfort you have had from any areas tender to touch or pressure?

5. How would you describe the overall level of discomfort you have had from the time you wake up?

6. How long does your morning stiffness last from the time you wake up? (for this score the 10 cm scale is divided evenly so that 30 mins lies at 2.5 cm, 1 hr at 5 cm, 1 and a half hours at 7.5 cm, and 2 or more hours at 10 cm).

The score is calculated by adding each of the measures for question 1 to 4 to the mean of the sum of questions 5 and 6, and then dividing the whole by 5. The maximum score therefore is 10.

The treatment of ankylosing spondylitis

- General principles include the following:
  - patient education
  - exercise
  - physical therapy and hydrotherapy
  - avoid smoking
  - NSAIDs for spinal disease
  - self-help groups.
- Emphasis is placed on the need to maintain posture and physical activity. Extension exercises are important as the natural history of the disease is toward flexion and loss of height. Physical therapy and rehabilitation provide benefit in the short term but it remains unclear about long-term benefits. Spa treatment has been shown to improve function for up to 9 months, with subsequent reduction in health resource use. Spa therapy is expensive and not widely available.
- Fatigue may be a major concern, hampering exercise. In some cases, low-dose amitriptyline at night may ameliorate this problem.
- For the majority of patients, NSAIDs remain the treatment of choice. The majority will be taking diclofenac or naproxen. Indomethacin was widely used but less so now because of its GI side effects.
- Preliminary data suggest that continuous use of NSAIDs (such as ketoprofen or celecoxib) slow radiographic progression of disease over a 2-year period. Compared to non-selective NSAIDs, COX-2

inhibitors have fewer GI side effects and are equally effective at providing symptomatic relief, but have fallen out of favor. Celecoxib is the only COX-2 still available in the United States.

- Sulfasalazine has been shown in meta-analysis to be efficacious when compared with placebo for peripheral joint disease only. However, improvement in symptoms and quality of life is often not dramatic and sulfasalazine has a small role to play, perhaps mainly in peripheral inflammatory disease.
- Mixed results have been found with MTX. A Cochrane meta-analysis concluded that there is insufficient evidence to support the use of MTX. Benefit may be limited to patients with peripheral disease.
- Joint inflammation can be managed in acute, severe cases with intra-articular corticosteroids, as can dactylitis and tendonitis by local steroid infiltration. Care should be taken injecting around tendons, as rupture can occur. Injection around the Achilles tendon is not recommended. Systemic steroids are rarely used, though there is evidence that low dose IV therapy can produce a short-lived improvement in symptoms.
- Infliximab, etanercept, adalimumab, and golimumab have been used in spinal and peripheral disease with good results in clinical outcome measures. Inevitably some patients require joint replacement, most commonly at the hip. Response to such surgery is usually excellent provided there are not major periarticular contractures secondary to ankylosis.
- Surgery for spinal deformity is possible but carries considerable anesthetic and surgical risk and should be carried out in specialist centers.
- Topical steroid eye drops should be used to treat uveitis. If the symptoms persist for more than 3 days an ophthalmological opinion should be sought. Infliximab and etanercept have been used to treat resistant iritis.
- Any associated psoriasis, inflammatory bowel disease, or concern over reactive inflammation secondary to an infection should be treated accordingly.
- There is no treatment for pulmonary fibrosis associated with AS. Given the added potential concern of reduced chest expansion, patients should be advised not to smoke in an attempt to avoid further lung disease.
- Nevertheless, it is important to remember that the majority of patients have some level of functional impairment due to their disease, and many will lead full, active lives.

Psoriatic arthritis

Epidemiology and clinical features

- The association between psoriasis and an inflammatory arthropathy is well-recognized. It may affect any peripheral joint as well as the axial skeleton and sacroiliac joints. Epidemiological studies support the notion of a distinct disease as opposed to the random finding of coexisting common conditions such as psoriasis and RA. Psoriasis affects 1–2% of the population, and 10–40% of these develop arthritis.
- The condition affects women and men equally, usually between the ages of 20–40.
- RF can be present in up to 10% of patients with psoriasis, 90% remaining seronegative, and most patients with psoriatic arthritis run a benign course. In about 20% of cases there is a chronic, progressive, and deforming arthropathy with an often asymmetrical pattern, including distal interphalangeal joint involvement, and specific radiological features that can distinguish it from RA.
- Nail lesions may be the only clinical feature that can identify patients with psoriasis who are destined to develop arthritis. These lesions occur in 90% of patients with psoriatic arthritis (PsA) and in 40% of patients with psoriasis alone. A comparison between PsA and RA (see Chapter 5) is made in Table 8.7. The joint symptoms most commonly occur after the diagnosis of psoriasis, but may predate or occur simultaneously in a minority.
- The clinical patterns of psoriatic arthritis are:
  - distal, involving the distal interphalangeal joints (DIP)
  - asymmetric oligoarthritis
  - symmetrical polyarthritis, indistinguishable from RA
  - spondylarthropathy
  - arthritis mutilans
- Arthritis mutilans is a classic (but uncommon) manifestation of psoriatic arthritis. Bone resorption leads to collapse of the soft tissue in the digits, creating "telescoping fingers." This can also be seen in severe RA.
- The radiological features associated with PsA which help to differentiate it from RA include:
  - absence of juxtaarticular osteoporosis
  - DIP disease
  - "whittling" (lysis) of terminal phalanges
  - asymmetry
  - "pencil-in-cup" deformities
  - ankylosis
  - periostitis
  - spondylitis.
- The patterns of arthritis may change over time in > 60% of patients.
- It is not clear though if the patterns of disease have any prognostic significance and the changes and prognosis are variable.
- The frequency of spinal involvement can vary between 2% in isolated back disease, to 40%, when associated with peripheral arthritis.

Table 8.7 Comparison of psoriatic arthritis and rheumatoid arthritis

Feature	Psoriatic arthritis	Rheumatoid arthritis
Sex ratio	F = M	F > M
Symmetry of joint disease	Less common	Very common
DIP involvement	Common	Uncommon
Spine involvement	Common	Uncommon
Skin/nail changes	Common	Uncommon
Enthesopathy	Common	Uncommon
Ankylosis	Common	Uncommon
Osteopenia	Uncommon	Common

- Dactylitis, swelling of the whole finger, occurs in over one-third of patients. Tenosynovitis and enthesitis are also common, particularly at the plantar fascia insertion and Achilles tendon.
- Hyperuricemia, probably related to high skin cell turnover, is not uncommon. In patients with psoriatic arthritis, the possibility of gout should be kept in mind.
- The 2006 CASPAR criteria for the classification of psoriatic arthritis are sometimes used to establish the diagnosis of psoriatic arthritis, although they were not designed for this purpose (Table 8.8).
- The CASPAR criteria allow subjects to be classified as having psoriatic arthritis based on the presence of dactylitis or enthesitis in the absence of true arthritis. The CASPAR criteria also allow subjects to be classified as having psoriatic arthritis with only a family history of psoriasis, as long as other criteria are met.

Treatment of PsA

- This should include the treatment of the skin as well as the joints and many patients are also under the care of a dermatologist.
- Patient education, physiotherapy, occupational therapy, and surgery all have a role to play akin to that already described above for RA and AS.
- Initial treatment in mild cases is with NSAIDs, adding a DMARD if inflammation and joint damage persist. The reader is referred to the section on the Evaluation and Treatment of Rheumatoid Arthritis in Chapter 5 for further details on specific agents. Sulfasalazine and leflunomide may be used with some effect; there are anecdotal reports of "flares" of skin psoriasis with hydroxychloroquine, glucocorticoid taper, and TNF-inhibitors. The most commonly used agent is MTX; it also can have a dramatic effect on the skin disease. Sulfasalazine may also be efficacious. Only physical therapy, NSAIDs, TNF inhibitors, and direct steroid injections appear to be consistently effective for axial arthritis.

- Oral and IM steroids should be avoided, but intra-articular steroids may be used. Psoriatic plaques are colonized by bacteria, and injection through a plaque should be avoided for fear of introducing infection. Steroid taper may lead to a flare of pustular psoriasis.
- Patients with severe and unresponsive disease can be offered cyclosporine A and retinoids.
- Etanercept, infliximab, adalimumab, and golimumab are FDA approved for the treatment of PsA and have positive effects on skin as well as joint disease. The doses required to treat psoriatic arthritis may be higher than the doses used to treat RA. Patients treated with etanercept 50 mg twice weekly, adalimumab 50 mg weekly, or adalimumab 40 mg weekly have a higher response rate than patients treated with standard RA doses, although the higher doses may be accompanied by a higher risk of complications, such as infection.

Table 8.8 The Classification Criteria for Psoriatic Arthritis (CASPAR)

≥3 points required to meet criteria for psoriatic arthritis
2 points: A personal or family history of psoriasis
1 point: Typical psoriatic nail dystrophy
1 point: Absence of rheumatoid factor (RF)
1 point: Dactylitis (on exam or by history)
1 point: Juxta-articular bone formation on plain radiographs

Taylor W, et al. Classification criteria for psoriatic arthritis: development of new criteria from a large international study. Arthritis Rheum 2008; 54: 2665–2673.

Reactive arthropathy

Clinical presentation

- Reactive arthritis is an aseptic inflammatory arthritis triggered by an infectious agent outside the joint.
- Spondyloarthritis can be defined as reactive if urethritis/cervicitis (sexually transmitted reactive arthritis or SARA) or diarrhea (gut associated reactive arthritis or GARA) are present. The features of the spondyloarthridities can vary in the reactive subgroup from one patient to another, and in the same patient at any given time in the course of the disease.
- The onset of reactive arthritis may be acute, with fever, weight loss, and diffuse polyarticular involvement. More often, however, there is limited joint synovitis and a low-grade, or absent, fever.
- Mucocutaneous features include painless balanitis circinata of the glans penis, and pustular psoriasis of the palms or feet (keratoderma blennorhagica); these can be associated with a more severe outcome.
- Conjunctivitis is observed early. Uveitis is less frequent early in disease, often occurring in recurrent disease and between episodes of arthritis.
- Acute diarrhea may precede the musculoskeletal symptoms by up to 1 month. The GI symptoms may be so mild that they are ignored by the patient and often the provoking agent has cleared from the gut before the joint symptoms arise. Several triggering agents have been isolated from stools and these include *Shigella*, *Salmonella*, *Clostridium*, and *Yersinia*. Chronic diarrhea does not appear to be associated with reactive arthritis. However, the demarcations can be blurred and some patients may have inflammatory bowel-associated arthropathies, or silent inflammatory lesions that appear to manifest as 'reactive-like' and are best described as undifferentiated spondyloarthropathy.
- Urethritis, prostatitis, or cervicitis may be present at prompt suspicion of infection. Rigorous investigation is required to ensure pathogenic mycoplasma and ureaplasma are identified and eradicated. The most common nongonococcal urethritis is due to Chlamydia.
- Recurrent or repeated infections do not always lead to a recurrence of arthritis and may occur in the absence of further sexual intercourse. There are some important differential diagnoses outside the spondyloarthridities that include HIV-associated arthritis, Lyme disease, parvovirus arthropathies, and Behçet's disease (see Chapter 18).

Diagnosis and treatment of reactive arthritis

- The inflammatory nature of the condition can be confirmed by the presence of an elevated ESR and CRP. For therapeutic decisions in some cases, but mainly for epidemiological purposes, many tests can be done looking for a causative agent. Most screens are negative and in this sense there is merit in just taking a close history and limited investigation rather than a full diagnostic work-up. If required, the clinician should request stool, urine, and blood cultures, urethral and vaginal swabs, and aspirate a swollen joint looking for cells, crystals, and infection. It may be helpful to enlist the expertise of colleagues in infectious diseases for the assessment of sexually acquired infections.

- The use of monoclonal antibodies, or DNA and RNA hybridization, in the search for products of triggering agents, is limited to research purposes. Likewise, tests for detecting antibodies to bacteria have no specific place in current clinical practice and do not have a predictive value on outcome.
- In the early stages of disease there are no radiological signs except in a very small number of cases where changes in the sacroiliac joints may be seen and probably predate presentation.
- There is no specific cure. NSAIDs and local corticosteroid injections are the mainstay of therapeutic intervention. If symptoms persist longer than 6 months and there is clinical evidence of ongoing synovitis and joint destruction then a disease-modifying agent such as sulfasalazine, MTX, or TNF inhibitors should be considered.
- Taking account of all symptoms, the bulk of patients are in complete remission at the end of 2 years, the majority within 6 months. The metatarsophalangeal joints and the heel often remain sites of persistent pain, and balanitis and keratoderma may persist, acting as markers of potential poorer prognosis. Other factors that may be predictive of poor outcome include oligoarthritis of the hip, persistently elevated ESR, poor response to NSAIDs, dactylitis, and involvement of the lumbosacral spine.
- Aseptic urethritis and early conjunctivitis resolve quickly and spontaneously. Antibiotic therapy will clear underlying infections but this may not have any effect on the duration of disease.
- Uveitis should be treated in the usual way with topical steroid drops and a referral to an ophthalmologist if there has been no response within 3 days.
- Patient education, particularly in the context of food hygiene and of prevention of exposure to sexually acquired infection, is important. Contact tracing is vital in cases of sexually transmitted infection.

Enteric arthropathy

Clinical presentation

- The arthropathies of ulcerative colitis and Crohn's disease have many similarities and the combination of peripheral and axial skeletal disease, enthesopathies, mucocutaneous, and ocular disease fits neatly into the diagnostic realm of the spondyloarthropathies.
- The exact pathology is unknown, but is thought to be due to impairment of the gut-mediated immunity and increased bowel permeability, allowing bacteria to pass through the bowel wall into the circulation.
- Mono- or asymmetrical oligoarthritis can be coincident with the onset of bowel disease or arise during the course of the disease. There is a close association between exacerbation of bowel and peripheral joint disorders, and enteropathic arthritis (EA) tends to remit after removal of diseased bowel tissue. The knees and ankles are most commonly involved.
- In contrast to peripheral arthritis, sacroiliitis is not clearly associated with either the onset or exacerbation of the bowel disease and may be present for years prior to the onset of colitis or ileitis.
- Other nonarticular features to look for include:
  - uveitis (in about 10%)
  - erythema nodosum
  - pyoderma gangrenosum
  - aphthous stomatitis.
- Arthropathy associated with inflammatory bowel disease often improves with treatment of the bowel symptoms. Intra-articular steroids, sulfasalazine, and MTX can be used in resistant cases. NSAIDs should be used with caution as they can cause a flare of Crohn's disease. Anti-TNF-α therapies used in treatment of Crohn's disease may also improve joint symptoms.
- Enteric arthropathy may exist in patients with minimal or no gut symptoms. Presence of an asymmetric arthritis associated with oral ulcerations or erythema nodosum should trigger a colonoscopy with blind biopsies to evaluate for the presence of inflammatory bowel disease or Behçet's disease.

Undifferentiated spondyloarthritis

Epidemiology and clinical presentation

- Undifferentiated spondyloarthritis is one of the most common spondyloarthridities, with a prevalence approaching 2%.
- Undifferentiated spondyloarthritis is used to describe patients who meet some of the clinical features associated with the spondyloarthridities, but not enough to be classified as one of the diseases described in this chapter.
- Using ESSG criteria, the diagnosis of undifferentiated spondyloarthritis may be entertained if the patient has one of the following two major criteria (in the absence of psoriasis, inflammatory bowel disease, or other evidence of one of the other forms of spondyloarthritis):
  - Inflammatory back pain (onset <40 years old, insidious onset, symptoms ≥3 months, morning stiffness, improvement with exercise)
  - Asymmetric synovitis (predominantly of the lower extremities)
- Most of these patients are young men with inflammatory lower back pain and/or an asymmetric oligoarthritis, and are HLA-B-27 positive. Dactylitis and extra-articular manifestations are less common among patients with this diagnosis.
- In general, radiographic evidence of sacroiliitis is mild. Clear evidence of sacroiliitis on plain radiographs may indicate that the patient is evolving towards a diagnosis of ankylosing spondylitis. A small number of patients may eventually develop clear evidence of psoriatic arthritis.

Diagnosis and treatment

- Diagnosis is based on clinical features. Although most patients are HLA-B27 positive, inflammatory markers may not be elevated, and cannot be used to exclude this diagnosis.
- Early identification and treatment of patients who are destined to evolve into ankylosing spondylitis may be key to preventing morbidity associated with this disease. How to identify patients at highest risk for progression, however, is not clear.
- MRI typically demonstrates evidence of sacroiliitis before changes on visible on plain radiographs, and may be useful for identifying which patients merit treatment with TNF-α inhibitors.
- For other patients, non-steroidal anti-inflammatory agents remain the mainstay of therapy. Methotrexate, sulfasalazine, and leflunomide may also play a role in the treatment of undifferentiated spondyloarthritis, although this has not been well established.

SAPHO

Epidemiology and clinical presentation

- SAPHO is a relapsing and remitting illness that primarily affects young adults. The prevalence of SAPHO is unknown, but may be around 1/10,000.
- The acronym describes the components of this disease: Synovitis, Acne, Pustulosis, Hyperostosis, and Osteitis. Older names for this syndrome include:
  - Acne arthritis
  - Pustulotic arthro-osteitis
  - Sternoclavicular hyperostosis
  - Acne-associated spondyloarthropathy
- Palmoplantar pustulosis is the most common skin finding in SAPHO, and is found in over half of patients with this diagnosis. Other skin lesions associated with SAPHO include psoriasis vulagris, severe acne, psoriasis, hidradenitis suppurativa, acne conglobata, pyoderma gangrenosum, and Sweet's syndrome. It is important to note, however, that skin lesions may be subtle: 16% of patients may have no skin findings at all.
- Hyperostosis, particularly of the sternoclavicular joints, is likely the result of recurrent osteitis. This osteitis is aseptic, and does not respond to antibiotics. That said, 15% fo patients with chronic recurrent multifocal osteomyelitis have infection with *Proprionibacterium acnes,* although the significance of this finding is not completely clear.
- The synovitis most commonly affects the anterior chest wall; 63% of patients will have involvement of the steronoclavicular joints. Peripheral joint involvement may be either symmetric or asymmetric.
- Because of its association with psoriasis, SAPHO is often classified as a form of spondyloarthropathy. It is also interesting to note that 10% of patients with SAPHO are HLA-B27 positive.

Diagnosis and treatment

- This syndrome has four major subtypes:
  - Osteoarticular manifestations of severe acne
  - Osteoarticular manifestations of palmoplantar pustulosis
  - Hyperostosis with or without dermatosis
  - Chronic recurrent multifocal osteomyelitis involving the axial or peripheral skeleton, with or without dermatosis
- To diagnose SAPHO, infectious causes of osteomyelitis must be excluded.
- Plain radiographs of the anterior chest wall may demonstrate lytic lesions and sclerosis in the sternoclavicular heads.
- Involvement of the sternoclavicular heads may be more clearly demonstrated with a Technitium-99 bone scan.
- Treatment includes non-steroidal anti-inflammatory agents as a first line therapy. Methotrexate is the most commonly used steroid sparing

agent, although low-dose glucocorticoids, methotrexate, sulfasalazine, colchicine, and cyclosporine have all been used.
- Intravenous pamidronate may be particularly effective for the treatment of osteitis. TNF-α blockade with etanercept and infliximab has also been used with some success.
- The overall prognosis is felt to be better than that associated with the other spondyloarthridities, although this is difficult to prove.

Spondyloarthridities in childhood

Epidemiology and clinical presentation

- This umbrella term covers a heterogeneous group of diseases associated with HLA B27 that affect children under the age of 16 and produce a spectrum of symptoms in adulthood.
- The disease group includes:
  - enthesitis and arthritis syndrome
  - juvenile ankylosing spondylitis
  - juvenile reactive arthritis
  - juvenile psoriatic arthritis(JPsA)
  - arthritis associated with inflammatory bowel disease
- Using the ILAR classification, this spectrum of diseases is called enthesitis-related arthritis (ERA).
- Incidence is estimated at 1.44 per 100,000 children. Prevalence has increased over the last 30 years.
- IgM RF and antinuclear antibodies are not found. 90% patients will be HLA B27 positive.
- The diagnosis is often more difficult in childhood as symptoms of back pain and radiological changes are uncommon. The diagnosis rests more often on the presence of lower limb large joint arthritis with enthesopathy, acute uveitis, psoriasis, or bowel pathology, and may be difficult to separate from JIA. The reader is referred to Chapter 9 for a description of the classification criteria for childhood arthropathies.
- Apart from an increased incidence of peripheral disease and rare axial symptoms, juvenile onset spondyloarthridities resemble the adult forms. This lack of early axial disease may lead to initial misdiagnosis as oligoarticular JIA.
- The Rome and New York criteria for the diagnosis of adult AS have not been validated in children; nevertheless, a small proportion of children fit these criteria and is considered to have juvenile AS. Approximately 5–8% of children attending rheumatology clinics have AS. This compares with 75% having JIA. Juvenile AS commonly presents with lower limb large joint arthritis (often knees and ankles) with the early course often episodic. It also appears to differ from adult AS in the precocious destruction of the hip joint. The condition is reported more often in men than women, and 50% of cases go on to develop AS in adult life.
- Enthesitis and arthritis syndrome usually affects the feet and can be disabling. The disease is usually episodic, but some cases are chronic, resulting in bony erosions and joint ankylosis. Over 70% patients with enthesitis syndrome will fulfill diagnostic criteria for AS after 5–10 years from onset.
- Childhood reactive arthritis and enteropathic arthropathy are essentially similar to adult disease.

JPsA

- JPsA is defined in the ILAR criteria as either arthritis in the presence of psoriasis, or arthritis and at least 2 of:
  - dactylitis
  - nail abnormalities (pitting or onycholysis)
  - family history of psoriasis confirmed by a dermatologist in at least one first-degree relative.
- The incidence of JPsA is estimated at 3 per 100,000, with a prevalence of 15 per 100,000.
- Oligo- or polyarthritis may occur and can affect large or small joints, the spine, and sacroiliac joints. Anterior uveitis is seen in 10–20%.
- JPsA, traditionally grouped with the spondylarthropathies, has greater clinical and laboratory similarity to JIA; important dissimilarities with the spondylarthropathies include a lack of association with HLA B27, and AS as an outcome.
- JPsA is also more common in girls than in boys.

Treatment of JPsA

- The principles of treatment include education, physical therapy, splints, orthotics, NSAIDs, and intra-articular corticosteroids for peripheral arthritis. Oral corticosteroids may be used for severe arthritis or enthesitis.
- In the presence of significant axial disease, polyarthritis, or persistent oligoarthropathy, sulfasalazine may be started (initially at 12.5 mg/kg/day, increasing weekly over 1 month to 50 mg/kg/day in 2–3 divided doses). However sulfasalazine may be no better than placebo, as seen in recent trials.
- MTX has shown little effect in spondyloarthropathy patients without JPsA. MTX and cyclosporine have been used successfully in the treatment of JPsA alone or in combination.
- Infliximab, etanercept, and adalimumab have been used and appear to be as effective as in adult spondyloarthropathy treatment. They have also been used to treat uveitis.

Prognosis in juvenile spondyloarthropathy

Remission rates vary widely in studies, with estimates of 10–20% in remission at 10 years. A large proportion of children will therefore have persisting disease in adult life, with associated disability.

Juvenile idiopathic arthritis (JIA)

Introduction

- The classification of childhood onset arthritis has seen several changes over recent years. In this chapter, we will discuss juvenile arthritis using headings and criteria from the International League of Associations for Rheumatology (ILAR). The terms *juvenile rheumatoid arthritis* and *juvenile chronic arthritis* were discarded in the ILAR classification. The term *juvenile idiopathic arthritis* was adopted to indicate arthritis present for at least 6 weeks and currently of no known cause in a patient <16 years. It is a diagnosis of exclusion.
- JIA is one of the most common chronic disorders of childhood, with an estimated US incidence of 11.7 per 100,000, and prevalence of 0.5 cases per 1,000 children.
- The categories of JIA are:
  - systemic onset arthritis
  - oligoarthritis (4 or fewer joints) ("persistent" or "extended")
  - polyarthritis (rheumatoid factor positive and negative)
  - juvenile psoriatic arthritis
  - enthesitis related arthritis
  - undifferentiated arthritis.
- Where features of other rheumatic diseases are particular to childhood, these are discussed at the end of the relevant chapter.
  - rheumatoid factor positive polyarthritis (see Chapter 5)
  - psoriatic arthritis and enthesis related arthritis (see Chapter 8)
  - SLE (see Chapter 10)
  - back pain (see Chapter 20).
- The classifications were derived for research purposes and are not primarily meant as diagnostic criteria. For a review of classification of JIA we recommend Hofer *et al.* (2002).[1] For an overview of the spectrum of pediatric and adolescent rheumatology we recommend Davies and Copeman (2006).[2]

General management principles in juvenile rheumatic diseases

- Early, aggressive treatment is generally advocated to prevent disability and improve prognosis. The advent of anti-TNF-α in particular has greatly improved outcomes associated with these diagnoses.
- A multidisciplinary approach is essential. Allied health professionals provide help with patient and family education, exercise, activities of daily living (home and school), maintenance of psychological well-being in patient and family, and advice on financial and disability support.
- Monitoring of height and weight is needed, and appropriate nutritional advice given if needed.
- Ophthalmic input is required if uveitis is present.

[1] Hofer M, Southwood T. Classification of childhood arthritis. Best Practice and Research in Clinical Rheumatology 2002; 16: 379–96.
[2] Davies K, Copeman A. The spectrum of paediatric and adolescent Rheumatology. Best Practice and Research in Clinical Rheumatology 2006; 20: 179–200.

- The dose of corticosteroid should be kept to the lowest possible to reduce the development of growth retardation. That said, higher doses of steroid are often required than in adults to gain initial control of disease. Bone density scanning (DEXA) should be considered and calcium and vitamin D should be given. Bisphosphonates should only be given under the guidance of a specialist.
- A close connection with the child's school is needed. Fatigue is a common symptom and may require changes to the child's school timetable. It is important to continue education as much as possible during hospital admissions.
- Excellent communication skills are required to explain often complex treatments to patient and family. Coming to terms with a chronic disease is a difficult process and again will need a close working relationship between members of the multidisciplinary team.
- The onset of adolescence brings new challenges. It is important to encourage the patient to be more active in decisions about disease management. Adolescence is a time of huge emotional and physical changes, and a chronic illness can make these changes more difficult. Discussion of personal issues such as sexuality, smoking, and alcohol require a good rapport with the patient. Parents should be encouraged to help develop the patient's independence in making treatment decisions, though this can be a long process. Adolescence is also the time to introduce the subject of transition from care by pediatric to adult health professionals. This is a gradual process and should be managed sensitively.

Oligoarthritis (previously termed pauciarticular JRA)

- This is the most commonly encountered subset of the childhood chronic arthritides, accounting for 40–50% of all JIA.
- The condition is more common in boys than girls (4:1) and peaks between the ages of 1–3 years, though it can appear in the teenage years. Overall, the disease affects an estimated 30 per 100 000 children.
- ILAR classification criteria require the presence of arthritis affecting 1–4 joints during the first 6 months of disease. The persistent subtype affects no further joints in the disease course. The extended subtype affects a total of >4 joints after the first 6 months of disease.
- Certain other distinct characteristics include:
  - a single swollen joint in the lower extremity (knee or ankle) in a child who otherwise seems to be in good health
  - chronic anterior uveitis (more common in girls)
  - presence of antinuclear antibodies
  - unique immunogenetics.
- The ILAR classification has the following exclusion criteria:
  - family history of psoriasis in at least one first- or second-degree relative
  - family history consistent with medically confirmed HLA B27 associated disease in at least one first- or second-degree relative.
  - a positive rheumatoid factor test on 2 occasions at least 3 months apart
  - HLA B27 positive male with onset of arthritis >6 years of age.
  - Presence of systemic arthritis (see next section).
- The etiology of the condition is unknown. Several lines of evidence indicate that genetic factors (HLA associations) are involved in disease susceptibility.

Clinical features

- JIA is always a clinical diagnosis of exclusion. There are no specific signs, symptoms, or laboratory tests. Nevertheless, the clinical picture is often quite recognizable (as above), and usually milder than conditions such as reactive or infective arthritis.
- Constitutional symptoms of fever, malaise, weight loss, and anorexia are not part of oligoarthritis. If present, this virtually excludes the diagnosis.

Joints

- Joint swelling, rather than pain, is the more common complaint. Stiffness may occur but rarely seems to limit function. Two-thirds of cases present with single joint disease, and a further 30% with 2 joints involved. There may be associated juxta-articular muscle atrophy. The child may simply present with a limping gait.
- The joints most commonly involved are the knee, ankle, and elbow. Disease in 1 or 2 small joints of the hand is uncommon but can be seen and does not predict progression to polyarticular disease. Shoulder and hip involvement are very rare; disease here should

prompt a search for another condition. Occasionally patients may develop disease of the temporomandibular joint and cervical spine.

- A period of 2–5 years of active arthritis is a typical course for the condition. A patient who remains pauciarticular for 5 years is unlikely to progress to polyarticular disease. A minority of cases will progress but the criteria for judging this likelihood remains unclear; that said, some 40% of patients with concomitant uveitis develop polyarticular disease and, therefore, risk factors for uveitis might be considered partly as criteria for risk of polyarticular disease.
- Leg length discrepancy can occur due to unequal limb growth, which commonly occurs in children with persistent knee inflammation. When disease begins before 3 years of age there is a risk of the affected limb being longer. Flexing the knee on the affected side compensates for the discrepancy and this in turn will exacerbate any flexion contractures.
- Disease onset after the age of 9 years may result in a shorter affected limb; this is a consequence of early epiphyseal closure.
- Synovial cysts occur and respond to intra-articular steroid injections (which may have to be given under general anesthetic).They can rupture, presenting as acute intense limb pain and swelling.
- Over 80% of children suffer little or no musculoskeletal disability after 15 years follow-up.

Eyes
- Uveitis (iridocyclitis) is the most serious complication of oligoarticular JIA. Up to 30% of cases develop a chronic, insidious, and potentially sight-threatening uveitis (most often anterior chamber).
- Slit-lamp examination is crucial in children diagnosed with oligoarticular JIA.
- The disease course does not necessarily follow the arthritis, and can be relapsing and remitting.
- The risk of uveitis is associated with the mode of onset of arthritis and not the later extent of articular disease.
- Risk factors include:
  - female gender (female to male ratio up to 7.5:1)
  - young onset disease (mean age 4 years)
  - oligoarthritis
  - positive antinuclear antibody.
- The uveitis is commonly asymptomatic; only 25% of patients complain of redness in the eye, pain, or visual disturbance. Up to two-thirds of patients have bilateral disease though not necessarily at the same time. As such, regular ophthalmic examination is required, even in the absence of symptoms (see Table 9.1).
- Uveitis and arthritis develop at different times. Uveitis may predate arthritis in up to 10% of cases. Otherwise, it is usually detected within 7 years (mean 2 years) of the onset of arthritis.
- The main determinants of poor outcome of uveitis are the extent of initial disease at presentation, and uveitis documented before the onset of arthritis. Early intervention is probably the single most important factor in determining outcome.
- Chronic asymptomatic uveitis persisting into adulthood is recognized.

- Treatment is with topical corticosteroids. Oral corticosteroids may be used for severe disease but concerns remain regarding growth retardation. Methotrexate is most frequently used, but azathioprine, cyclosporine, and anti-TNF-α therapies may also be effective.

Diagnostic evaluation of oligoarthritis

- There are no diagnostic procedures.
- The acute-phase reactants are usually mildly raised.
- A persistent high ESR, with no other evidence of inflammation on other laboratory tests, might suggest the rare, congenital disorder hyperfibrinogenemia. A high ESR should prompt a search for infection, occult inflammation, or malignancy, e.g., leukemia.
- ANA are present in 40–75% of children. There is no evidence that ANA precede the development of the condition, or that titers correlate with disease activity.
- Rheumatoid factor is rare; positive in <5% of cases.
- Plain radiographs are valuable for assessing joint damage; however, the expertise of a pediatric radiologist familiar with normal variants of skeletal development should be sought.
- Clinical assessment and investigation should seek to exclude the common conditions of childhood rheumatic disease (see Table 9.2).

Treatment of oligoarthritis

- Approximately half of patients with oligoarticular JIA will have persistent disease or functional joint problems 10 years after diagnosis.
- The main principles are the maintenance of normal joint function during active disease, and the early treatment of ocular inflammation. A team approach is required.
- Initially NSAIDs are given (ibuprofen or naproxyn most often).
- Intra-articular steroid injections may be useful in several situations:
  - the very young (unable to take oral medication)
  - marked persistent joint swelling
  - synovial cysts causing limitation of movement.
- Cases with prolonged disease or extension to polyarticular disease require more aggressive treatment. MTX is the drug of choice.

Table 9.1 Uveitis surveillance: recommended frequency of slit-lamp examination

Condition	Frequency
Systemic onset	Yearly
Oligoarthritis and rheumatoid factor negative	
Onset before age 7:	ANA positive: every 2–3-months for 4 years, then every 6-months for 3 years, then yearly
	ANA negative: every 6-months for 7 years, then yearly
Onset after age 7:	Every 6-months for 4 years, then yearly

Table 9.2 The differential diagnosis of oligoarthritis

Condition	Examples
Monoarticular disease	Septic arthritis
	TB
	Trauma/hemarthrosis
	Patellofemoral pain
	Pigmented villonodular synovitis (requires tissue biopsy)
	Foreign-body synovitis
	Thalassaemia/sickle cell/hemophilia
Short-lived inflammatory arthropathy	Lyme disease
	Viral arthritis
	Reactive arthritis
	Post-streptococcal arthritis
The spondylarthropathies	
Pain conditions	Hypermobility/regional pain syndromes
	Complex regional pain syndromes
	Avulsion fractures
	Aseptic (avascular) necrosis
	Enthesitis
	Osteoid osteoma/bone pain

- Anti-TNF therapy is increasingly used, especially in cases unresponsive to MTX. These agents should only be used under specialist pediatric supervision.
- Abatacept, a CTLA-4 inhibitor, is approved for patients who fail anti-TNF-α therapy.
- Motor development and activity is very important. There should always be assessment of growth, development, and social interaction. Physical therapy makes an important contribution to the overall management of the condition.
- Joint surgery is rarely necessary.
- Uveitis can be more of a therapeutic challenge than the joint disease. Corticosteroid eye drops and mydriatics to prevent synechiae (fibrous bands that adhere the iris to the lens) are the typical initial regimen in mild disease. More severe disease requires oral prednisone. MTX and anti-TNF-α therapies may also help eye disease.
- Surgery may be necessary for cataracts, keratopathy, or glaucoma.

Systemic arthritis (previously systemic onset JRA)

- Systemic onset disease accounts for approximately 5–10% of juvenile arthritis.
- There is an equal sex incidence in systemic onset disease.
- The peak age of onset is 5 years.
- The nonarticular features of the condition make a viral etiology an attractive hypothesis, but there is little evidence for this.
- HLA studies demonstrate genetic heterogeneity with no clear associations.

Clinical features

- While arthritis is required to confirm the diagnosis, true joint inflammation may not be present at the onset of disease; some patients have developed inflammation as late as 9 years after the onset.
- The ILAR classification criteria require the presence of arthritis with, or preceded by, a daily fever of at least 2 weeks duration in association with one or more of the following: an erythematous evanescent rash, generalized lymphadenopathy, hepatomegaly and/or splenomegaly, and serositis (see Table 9.3).
- Most patients have arthritis at disease onset, and 50–60% will develop chronic persistent symptoms. In >75% of cases, the wrists, knees, and ankles are involved. Hip involvement occurs in about 50% of cases and is almost always bilateral, and associated with polyarticular disease. Hip and wrist joints are the most common sites of progressive destructive arthropathy, and one-third of patients with hip involvement will require hip arthroplasty. Tenosynovitis of the carpus and tarsus is common, and of the small joints, the hands are often affected more than the feet.
- Fever is the one extra-articular feature essential to making the diagnosis. The fever pattern is described as quotidian, often rising to 39°C before falling rapidly to normal, and typically in the late afternoon or early evening following a regular daily pattern. The patient often appears toxic during the fever, with chills and rigors, severe arthralgias and myalgias, and very often a rash. The fever should be present for at least 2 weeks and quotidian in character for at least 3 days to satisfy the diagnosis. Fever may persist for months even with treatment.
- The rash of systemic arthritis is a salmon-pink color, most prominent over the chest, abdomen, back, and intertrigenous areas. The rash is usually macular, though occasional urticarial, with individual lesions 3–5 mm in diameter that may coalesce into larger ones. It has a tendency to come and go with the fever spike.
- Hepatomegaly, splenomegaly, and lymphadenopathy are common findings and usually asymptomatic. Mild elevation in serum transaminases occurs frequently and is usually not significant clinically. This makes assessment of potentially hepatotoxic medications difficult. Chronic liver disease does not occur. It is, however, a feature of adult onset Still's disease. Very rarely, an acute fulminant liver failure occurs

Table 9.3 Clinical features of systemic arthritis

Frequency	Feature
Very common	Spiking fever (with chills and sweats)
	Evanescent rash
	Myalgias
	Arthralgias—oligo/polyarthritis—usually after first 6 months from onset
	Growth abnormalities
Common	Generalized lymphadenopathy
	Hepatosplenomegaly
	Polyserositis
	Anorexia
	Weight loss
Rare	Myocarditis
	Coagulopathy
	Eye disease
	CNS involvement
	Hematophagocytic syndrome
	Primary pulmonary disease
	Renal disease
	Amyloidosis

with encephalopathy, disseminated intravascular coagulation, and bleeding.
- This syndrome is associated with considerable morbidity and mortality, treatment being supportive with corticosteroids and cyclosporine.
- Involvement of the serosal surfaces is one hallmark of systemic arthritis. Pericarditis, pleuritis, and sterile peritonitis are recognized manifestations of the disease; pericarditis is by far the more common of these. Most children will have echocardiographic evidence of pericarditis during systemic flares, but <15% will be symptomatic. Rarely, the patient may have myocarditis, suggested clinically by persistent tachycardia, cardiomegaly, and congestive heart failure. There should always be a high index of suspicion in these cases as the mortality rate is high. Valvular disease is almost never seen. This may help to separate systemic arthritis from acute rheumatic fever with myocarditis.
- Abnormalities of growth are often as a consequence of hypercatabolism, poor nutrient intake, and concomitant use of corticosteroids. Suppression of disease activity and adequate nutrition are the most effective therapy. Growth hormone supplementation

is reserved for patients whose growth is persistently below the third percentile on height charts and before epiphyseal fusion has occurred.

- Among the rarer features, CNS manifestations are dominated by irritability and lethargy during fever spikes; renal involvement may occur as a complication of treatment or indicate the onset of amyloidosis; and ocular involvement is distinctly unusual relative to other forms of JIA, though asymptomatic uveitis does occur.
- Amyloidosis is a serious complication of all subtypes of JIA and is associated with significant morbidity and mortality. The most common cause of death with amyloidosis is renal failure (80% of cases in most series), followed by infection (10% of cases). Secondary amyloidosis is rare if inflammation can be controlled.
- Macrophage activation syndrome may be seen in association with systemic onset JIA. This is characterized by fever, hepatosplenomegaly, bruising, and encephalopathy. Acute phase reactants (particularly the ferritin) are highly elevated.

Differential diagnosis

- The differential diagnosis of systemic arthritis should always be kept in mind and looked for as many infectious and post-infectious disorders, other inflammatory diseases, and malignancy have similar clinical manifestations. In particular, Kawasaki's disease and other forms of vasculitis should be excluded, as well as the fever syndromes.
- Features that may raise suspicion of another diagnosis include:
  - leukopenia, thrombocytopenia
  - child looks ill even during afebrile episodes
  - bony tenderness
  - "hard" hepatosplenomegaly/lymphadenopathy
  - recent antibiotic use
  - monoarthritis
  - persistent diarrhea
  - marked weight loss.

Diagnostic evaluation of systemic arthritis

- There are no specific diagnostic tests.
- Characteristic hematological abnormalities include anemia, thrombocytosis, and leukocytosis; the latter two abnormalities are hallmarks of the condition, so much so that normal counts raise suspicion about the diagnosis.
- Acute phase markers are usually increased; the ESR, CRP, gammaglobulins, and serum complement (this may help to differentiate the disease from SLE). The ESR may be normal or elevated in the hematophagocytic syndrome complicating systemic arthritis.
- Hypoalbuminemia may be multifactorial in etiology (poor diet, reduced synthesis, intestinal leak), but should prompt the search for proteinuria, which, if "heavy," could suggest amyloidosis and the need for renal or rectal biopsy, or scintigraphy using iodinated serum amyloid-P to detect deposits.
- Most children are seronegative for ANA and RF. No antinuclear antibody specificities have been consistently identified.

The following tests are suggested for all patients in the initial diagnostic investigation of systemic arthritis:
- Complete blood count and differential
- Renal and liver function tests
- Coagulation screen
- Serum immunoglobulins
- Serum albumin
- Antinuclear antibody titer
- Blood cultures
- Chest radiograph
- Plain radiographs of selected affected joints
- Abdominal and pelvic ultrasound
- Electrocardiograph
- Ocular slit lamp examination.

The following tests should also be considered:
- Muscle enzymes
- Rheumatoid factor
- Viral serology—parvovirus, adenovirus etc.
- Antistreptolysin antibody titers
- Serum IgD
- Urine homovanillic and vanillylmandelic acid
- Joint aspiration (for monoarthritis)
- Tissue biopsy (including bone marrow aspirate)
- Echocardiogram
- Upper gastrointestinal barium series
- Isotope bone and/or gallium scan.

Table 9.4 Radiological abnormalities seen in systemic jia

Feature	Percentage
Soft tissue swelling	80%
Joint space narrowing	50%
Growth abnormalities	50%
Erosions	40%
Subluxation	20%
Ankylosis	20%
Joint destruction	15%
Protrusio acetabulae	10%
Periosteal new bone	10%

The treatment of systemic arthritis

- The general approach to the management of the arthritis assumes the same principles as oligoarthritis.[1] However, there is increased drug-related toxicity in systemic JIA. This is seen with salicylates, NSAIDs, and DMARDs.
- Initial control of fever, joint pain, and serositis should be with NSAIDs; ibuprofen (60 mg/kg/day in 6 divided doses) indomethacin (1–2 mg/kg/day in 2 divided doses) are commonly used. The dose should be decreased in the presence of severe hypoalbuminemia as the drugs are protein-bound. NSAIDs should be tried for at least 1 week before being deemed to have failed. Indomethacin is particularly useful for pericarditis; otherwise, this may respond to pulsed methylprednisolone, as does myocarditis.
- When NSAIDs fail to control symptoms, regular or pulsed corticosteroid treatment is indicated. Steroids will control symptoms but they do not limit the duration or alter the prognosis of the disease and should be used judiciously. The daily dose should be at 1–2 mg/kg/day in divided doses.
- If symptoms persist past 4–8 weeks, MTX should be added, although MTX is not as effective in this situation as in oligoarticular JIA. Patients who have evidence of severe systemic disease (including anemia, high fevers, severe serositis, malnutrition, or macrophage activating syndrome) should be treated simultaneously with glucocorticoids.
- If the patient does not respond, consideration should be given to the use of IL-1 or TNF-α blockade.
- Anakinra may be particularly effective for the treatment of systemic arthritis, even among patients who have previously failed other therapies. Anti-TNF-α therapies may be effective in systemic JIA with persistent polyarthritis, but studies imply that infliximab may be more effective than etanercept.
- Tocilizumab, an IL-6 receptor inhibitor, has also been approved for treatment of systemic onset JIA patients older than 2 years.
- Significant cardiac compromise from effusion may require pericardiocentesis.
- Most patients with systemic onset JIA will experience one of three disease courses: monocyclic (11%), polycyclic (34%), or unremitting (55%).

[1] Weiss JE, Ilowite NT. Juvenile idiopathic arthritis. *Pediatr Clin N Am.* 2005; 52: 413–442.

Rheumatoid factor negative polyarticular JIA (previously polyarticular onset JRA)

General points

- There are two subtypes; rheumatoid factor (RF) negative (80%) and factor positive (20%).
- The arthritis usually affects 5 or more joints within the first 6 months of disease. There must be no psoriasis in the patient or in any first-degree relative.
- Polyarticular onset occurs in about 25% of all patients with JIA.

Clinical manifestations

- There are three clinical subsets that have been recognized (Table 9.5):
  - Early onset oligoarthritis, which is asymmetric, and associated with ANA-positivity and a high risk of uveitis. This form has an average age of onset <6 years old, and tends to affect girls more than boys.
  - Symmetric synovitis with a predilection for the MCPs and tenosynovitis of the wrists and ankles. The average age of onset is 7–9 years old.
  - Dry synovitis, which is associated with stiffness, and leads to flexion contractures and joint destruction. Carpal fusion and tendonopathies are common in the hands, leading to classical features such as boutonniere and swan-neck deformities. Flexion contracture is the first manifestation of elbow involvement, and the shoulders are commonly affected. This form often responds poorly to treatment.
- Cervical spine involvement is common with features akin to RA; apophyseal joint fusion, instability, and risk of cord compression. There is often fusion of the apophyseal joints of C3–C5 leaving rigid segments that sublux above and below. Atlantoaxial subluxation, seen in RF-positive arthritis and juvenile ankylosing spondylitis, is rare in RF-negative polyarthropathy.
- Temporomandibular joint involvement is common, leading to reduced growth and micrognathia. Dental malocclusion may require surgery when growth is completed. Growth disturbance is also common, and occurs in proportion to the degree and duration of inflammation.

Laboratory tests

The laboratory features are nonspecific in RF-negative polyarthritis. The ESR, CRP, leukocyte count, and platelet count can be elevated or normal. A low red cell count is unusual and should prompt a search for an alternative diagnosis. In patients with a prior diagnosis of RF-negative polyarticular JIA, radiographs of the joints should be obtained yearly.

Treatment

- The management of this condition involves a common approach as discussed in the first two sections of this chapter, with adaptations according to the different subtypes shown.

Table 9.5 Proposed subclassification of RF-negative polyarthritis

Subclassification	Percentage of cases	Characteristics
1. Early onset oligoarthritis	About 40%	Female preponderance
		Most cases in very young (<3 years of age)
		Possible increased risk of eye disease
		Severe polyarthritis
2. Symmetric synovitis	15%	Mild pain
		Thick pannus
		Equal in sexes
		Functional impairmen late
		Tenosynovitis common
3. Dry synovitis	15%	Little joint swelling
		Progressive stiffness
		Chronic muscle wasting
		Often referred late in to onset

- Treatment should start with a trial of an NSAID for 4–8 weeks, moving to a second NSAID for the same period of time if the first fails. Ibuprofen, naproxyn, and diclofenac are commonly used.
- In nonresponders to NSAIDs, intra-articular steroid injections may be necessary. Topical steroids should also be used from the onset with eye disease.
- DMARDs should also be introduced immediately, since NSAIDs alone are unlikely to induce remission.
- **Methotrexate is the first-line drug of choice**. Sulfasalazine may be used if there are features of spondyloarthropathy. Treatments should be continued for at least 6 months following remission. The TNF-α inhibitors are used for patients intolerant of or unresponsive to, methotrexate.
- In all cases, surgery and rehabilitation play an important role in management, and physical therapy and occupational therapy advice should be employed early.

Rheumatoid factor positive polyarticular JIA

General points

- The RF should be checked on 2 occasions, 3 months apart. RF positive disease tends to occur most often in girls; it follows a pattern similar to adult RA (see Chapter 5).
- Rheumatoid factor positive polyarticular JIA accounts for 5% of all cases of JIA.

Clinical manifestations

- This form of JIA is a symmetric polyarthritis that has a predilection for the wrists, MCPs, and PIPs.
- Rheumatoid nodules may be found around the elbows or other joints.
- Associated symptoms include tenosynovitis, low grade fever, hepatosplenomegaly, lymphadenopathy, serositis, and pericardial effusions.
- Uveitis is uncommon. Keratitis and dry eyes may be seen.

Laboratory tests

As in adult rheumatoid arthritis, children with this diagnosis may have non-specific evidence of inflammation (including anemia, neutrophilia, throm-bocytosis, and elevated acute phase reactants). Many children will also have cyclic citrullinated peptide antibodies. ANA testing may be useful to distinguish this diagnosis from SLE.

Treatment and prognosis

- Treatment strategies are similar to those used for rheumatoid-factor negative polyarticular JIA.
- Early immunosuppression with methotrexate or other agents is key to preventing the long-term consequences of this disease.
- Only 6% of patients with rheumatoid-factor positive polyarticular JIA achieve remission at 10 years.

Juvenile psoriatic arthritis

General points
- Juvenile psoriatic arthritis has only recently been recognized in children.
- As in adults, the arthritis may predate the rash by 15 years or longer.
- Juvenile psoriatic arthritis accounts for 2–15% of children with JIA.

Clinical manifestations
- Juvenile psoriatic arthritis is an asymmetric arthritis associated with dactylitis. It rarely involves the sacroiliac joints.
- This diagnosis is affects more girls than boys, and up to 20% of patients develop an asymptomatic chronic uveitis.
- Examination of the nails for evidence of pitting may provide evidence of psoriasis in a patient who otherwise has no evidence of skin disease.

Laboratory tests
There are no specific laboratory findings associated with juvenile psoriatic arthritis. Because the joint complaints can predate the onset of psoriasis, it is probably underdiagnosed.

Treatment and prognosis
- Treatment strategies are similar to those used for rheumatoid-factor negative polyarticular JIA.
- Methotrexate is the treatment of choice.
- Because this is a relatively new subset of JIA, the long-term prognosis associated with this diagnosis is largely unknown.

Enthesitis related arthritis

General points

- Enthesitis is tenderness at the point of insertion of a tendon, ligament, joint capsule, or fascia into bone.
- Enthesitis related arthritis is diagnosed if at least two of the following criteria are present:
    - Sacroiliac joint tenderness or inflammatory lumbosacral pain
    - HLA-B27 positive
    - Acute onset anterior uveitis
    - History of a spondyloarthritis in a first degree relative.
- This diagnosis assumes that the patient has no evidence of another form of JIA. The patient is assumed to be rheumatoid factor-negative, with no family history of psoriasis (in a first-degree relative).

Clinical manifestations

- This diagnosis has a predilection for males; 70% of patients with this diagnosis are boys. The age of onset is generally between 10–12 years.
- This form of JIA presents with a peripheral oligoarthritis; axial involvement is a late finding.
- Uveitis may be present in up to 25% of patients.

Laboratory tests

Although 70% of patients with enthesitis related arthritis are HLA-B27 positive, there are no truly specific laboratory findings associated with this diagnosis.

Treatment and prognosis

- Treatment strategies are similar to those used for rheumatoid-factor negative polyarticular JIA.
- This form of arthritis is associated with poor outcomes, with greater levels of chronic disability and chronic pain than that associated with other forms of JIA.
- A persistently elevated ESR and/or hip arthritis are risk factors for the development of sacroiliitis.
- Female gender, family history of ankylosing spondylitis, and polyarthritis are all poor prognostic factors.

Chronic, infantile, neurological, cutaneous, & articular syndrome (CINCA)

- Closer scrutiny of pediatric inflammatory arthropathies has led to the description of syndromes that can be distinguished from systemic JIA. Among these syndromes is chronic, infantile, neurological, cutaneous, and articular syndrome (CINCA), which is distinguished from JIA by in its involvement of the central nervous system. The pathophysiology of this condition is unknown; no immune complex, autoantibody, or immunodeficiency has been found.
- CINCA is also known as neonatal onset multisystem inflammatory disease (NOMID)
- The first symptoms are often present at birth, generally after an uneventful pregnancy. Three-quarters of neonates (the rest usually within 6 months of birth) have a nonpruritic urticarial rash that resembles that of Still's disease. Intermittent flares of the condition are associated with fever and enlargement of the lymph nodes and spleen.
- Central nervous system and sensory anomalies are important manifestations of CINCA. Chronic meningitis may result in recurrent headaches and seizures. There may also be transient episodes of hemiplegia.
- Sensory anomalies are progressive. These include perceptive deafness and optic atrophy. Other eye involvement includes uveitis, chorioretinitis, keratitis, and conjunctivitis.
- The skull tends to have an increased cranial volume and there is delay in closure of the anterior fontanelle, and sometimes calcification of the falx and dura.
- Joint involvement is variable but most often involves the knee. The main finding is an overgrowth of the epiphyseal plate, resulting in bony enlargement. Progressive contractures, loss of movement, and function ensue. There is progressive growth retardation and, despite normal growth hormone profiles, a height below the third percentile is very frequent.
- Common morphological changes are also found. These include skull enlargement (often frontal bossing), a saddle-back nose, clubbing of the fingers and toes, and short and thick hands and feet.
- CINCA is caused by a mutation in the cold-induced autoinflammatory syndrome 1 (CIAS1) gene, which encodes cryopyrin. This protein forms part of the inflammasome, which leads to the activation of interleukin-1 β. Other CIAS1 mutations lead to other cryopyrinopathies, including familial cold autoinflammatory and Muckle-Wells syndromes.
- Blockade of the interleukin-1 receptor with anakinra results in dramatic improvement in the signs and symptoms associated with CINCA, but relapse occurs rapidly after treatment is stopped.
- Other forms of immunosuppression, including high dose corticosteroids, may be only moderately effective.

Still's disease

- This condition has similar clinical and laboratory features to systemic JIA. 75% of cases range between the ages of 16–35 years at onset.
- The fever pattern is identical and 90% of cases develop the typical rash.
- One feature not seen in juvenile disease is the complaint of sore throat during fever spikes. Pulmonary and ocular disease seem to be more common in adult onset Still's disease, and cardiac involvement less so.
- Patients with a chronic articular course do not do well. Several factors predict a poor outcome in terms of progressive articular damage.
  - a polyarticular onset
  - axial arthritis
  - need for steroids within 2 years of onset of disease
  - history of childhood arthritis
  - rash
- The treatment of Still's disease should follow the same lines as that for systemic JIA.

Systemic lupus erythematosus (SLE)

Introduction

- Systemic lupus erythematosus (SLE) is a complex clinical syndrome characterized by autoimmune-mediated, systemic inflammation that can affect multiple organs. This rubric encompasses a wide range of clinical manifestations of greatly varying severity.
- It is important to remember that there are variations in the incidence of clinical features between ethnic groups. With this in mind, the physician needs a keen sense of awareness of a variety of multisystem pathologies and to appreciate that SLE has taken on the mantle of syphilis as the great mimic of other conditions.
- The American Rheumatism Association (ARA), now the American College of Rheumatology (ACR), published its revised criteria for the classification of SLE in 1997 (see Table 10.1). As stated in other sections of this book, criteria are for the classification of the disease for epidemiological and research purposes mostly, and not as a diagnostic tool. In practice, however, these criteria have often been used as a guide to establish a clinical diagnosis.
- In 2011, the Systemic Lupus International Collaborating Clinics (SLICC) group undertook a revision of the ACR Classification Criteria, to reflect our current understanding of this disease (see Table 10.2).
- The new criteria expand the use of immunologic criteria, which now allow the use of the direct Coombs test and hypocomplementemia to establish a classification of SLE.
- The new criteria require the presence of at least one immunologic and one clinical criterion to establish a classification of SLE; a classification of SLE could not be made based on immunologic criteria alone.
- The SLICC Revision of the ACR Criteria have better sensitivity than the 1997 ACR Criteria (94% versus 86%), and result in fewer misclassifications. The specificity of these criteria are roughly equivalent (92% versus 93%).

Table 10.1 1997 ACR Classification Criteria for SLE SLE may be diagnosed if 4 or more of the 11 criteria are present either serially or simultaneously.

1	Malar rash	
2	Discoid rash	
3	Photosensitivity	
4	Oral ulcers	
5	Arthritis	
6	Serositis:	Pleuritis or pericarditis
7	Renal disorder:	Persistent proteinuria of >0.5 g/24 h or cellular casts
8	Neurological disorder (having excluded other causes):	Seizures or psychosis
9	Hematological disorders:	Hemolytic anemia or
		Leukopenia <4.0 × 10^9/liter on 2 or more occasions
		Lymphopenia <1.5 × 10^9/liter on 2 or more occasions
		Thrombocytopenia <100 × 10^9/liter
10	Immunological disorders:	Anti-ds DNA antibody
		Anti-Sm antibody
		Positive antiphospholipid antibodies
11	Antinuclear antibody in raised titer	

Table 10.2 Systemic Lupus International Collaborating Clinics (SLICC) Revision of the ACR Classification Criteria for SLE SLE may be diagnosed if 4 criteria are present (including at least one clinical and one immunologic criterion). SLE may also be diagnosed in a patient with biopsy-proven lupus nephritis in the presence of ANA or dsDNA.

Clinical Criteria	Acute or subacute cutaneous lupus
	Chronic cutaneous lupus
	Oral/nasal ulcers
	Non-scarring alopecia
	Inflammatory synovitis
	Serositis
	Proteinuria ($\geq$500 mg/24 hr) or red blood cell casts
	Neurological disorder*
	Hemolytic anemia
	Leukopenia (<4000/mm^3) or lymphopenia (<1000/mm^3)
	Thrombocytopenia (<100,000/mm^3)
Immunologic Criteria	Antinuclear antibody (ANA)
	Anti-ds DNA antibody
	Anti-Sm antibody
	Antiphospholipid antibody†
	Low complement (C3, C4, or CH50)
	Direct Coombs test (in absence of hemolytic anemia)

*Neurologic disorders include seizure, psychosis, mononeuritis multiplex, myelitis, peripheral or cranial neuropathy, cerebritis (acute confusional state)

†Evidence of antiphospholipid antibodies include lupus anticoagulant, false-positive test for syphilis, anticardiolipin antibodies, or medium-high titer anti-β2 glycoprotein†

The clinical features of SLE

Lupus is 10–20 times more common in women than men, and most likely to develop between the ages of 15–40 years. There are several nonspecific features that are also found in many other chronic diseases. Of these, lethargy and fatigue are often the most disabling. Weight loss and persistent lymphadenopathy can also be seen in association with SLE.

Musculoskeletal

- Morning stiffness and polyarticular, symmetric arthralgias or arthritis occur in 90% of cases. In most cases, symptoms outweigh objective clinical signs, and overt joint damage from synovitis (e.g., erosions) occurs in less than 10% of patients.
- Reversible subluxation of joints without erosive disease (Jaccoud's arthropathy) can also occur in both the hands and feet.
- Avascular necrosis occurs in 5–10% of patients; most cases being associated with previous steroid use. The risk of avascular necrosis increases dramatically among patients using greater than 20 mg of prednisone daily.
- Myalgias are common, but true myositis in < 5%, and myopathy may be a consequence of steroid treatment.

Skin

Approximately half of patients diagnosed with SLE will have the classic "butterfly" rash of the nasal bridge and malar bones. The cutaneous manifestations of SLE are listed in Table 10.3.

Cardiovascular disease

- Pericardial disease is the most common component of heart involvement in lupus. Most cases are clinically silent; a mild pericarditis is more common than a clinically significant pericardial effusion. On echocardiography, pericardial thickening is seen more frequently than pericardial effusions.
- Although SLE can lead to life-threatening pericardial effusions or constrictive pericarditis, these manifestations are quite rare.
- Myocarditis is often asymptomatic, and may be present in 8% to 25% of patients. Clinical myocarditis (defined by combinations of tachycardia, dysrhythmias, a prolonged PR interval on electrocardiography, cardiomegaly, and congestive cardiac failure) is considerably less common. Histological studies suggest that a mild non-specific perivascular inflammatory infiltrate is a common feature.
- Corticosteroid therapy, although indicated for inflammatory cardiac disease, is itself an added risk factor for atherosclerosis given its propensity to induce hypertension, hypercholesterolemia, and obesity.
- Systolic murmurs are common. The classic endocarditis described by Libman and Sachs rarely causes clinically significant lesions. Any valve vegetations identified in a patient who is febrile should raise the possibility of bacterial endocarditis.
- Women with SLE have a 5–6% increased risk of coronary heart disease compared to the general population. This risk is increased 50% in women 35–44.

Table 10.2 Cutaneous manifestations of SLE

Frequency of occurrence	Feature
Common (20–50%)	Malar rash
	Photosensitive rash
	Chronic discoid lesions
	Nonscarring alopecia
Less common (5–20%)	Mucosal ulcers
Occasional (5%)	Periorbital edema
	Bullous lupus
	Severe scarring alopecia
	Subacute cutaneous lupus
	Leg ulcers
	Panniculitis
	Cutaneous vasculitis

Pulmonary disease

- Because of the tendency for disease to be subclinical, chest radiographs and pulmonary function tests invariably indicate a greater degree of involvement than is evident clinically, and patients may present quite late in the disease process following a history of slow onset non-productive cough and increasing shortness of breath on exertion. Pulmonary function tests typically show both diminished total lung capacity and peak flow rates.
- Pleuritic pain/pleuritis is present in up to 60% of cases.
- Pleural effusions are a feature in one-third of patients but they are usually small and clinically insignificant.
- Interstitial fibrosis, pulmonary vasculitis, and pneumonitis are found in up to one-fifth of lupus patients, but pulmonary hemorrhage is rare.
- Pulmonary hypertension is found in approximately 10% of patients with SLE, and is associated with Raynaud's phenomenon, vasculitis, and antiphospholipid antibodies.
- There is great interest in antiphospholipid antibodies and thrombotic events in lupus. Patients presenting with pleuritic pain and/or pulmonary hypertension should be investigated for the presence of pulmonary emboli and antiphospholipid syndrome.

Renal involvement

- Assessment of blood pressure for hypertension, urine for protein, blood, and casts, and the serum creatinine is an essential part of regular monitoring. Symptoms suggesting renal failure rarely become obvious until substantial damage has occurred. If early disease is suspected, the physician should consider a spot urine protein/creatinine ratio, which is more accurate than urine dipstick and more convenient than the conventional 24-h urine collection for protein and creatinine. The glomerular filtration rate and renal function may also be assessed by nuclear medicine techniques.

- Renal biopsy should be considered when > 500 mg proteinuria is detected. It must also be remembered that a renal biopsy has complications in itself.
- In 2003, the International Society of Nephrology (ISN) and Renal Pathology Society (RPS) released a new classification of lupus nephritis designed to standardize definitions. The 2003 ISN/RPS classification of lupus nephritis replaced the 1982 modified World Health Organization classification.
  - Class I: Minimal mesangial lupus nephritis
  - Class II: Mesangial proliferative lupus nephritis
  - Class III: Focal lupus nephritis (< 50% of glomeruli)
    - Class III (A): Active lesions
    - Class III (A/C): Active and chronic lesions
    - Class III (C): Chronic inactive lesions
  - Class IV: Diffuse lupus nephritis (≥ 50% glomeruli), divided into diffuse segmental (IV-S) or global (IV-G) lupus nephritis:
    - Class IV (A): Active lesions
    - Class IV (A/C): Active and chronic lesions
    - Class IV (C): Chronic inactive lesions
  - Class V: Membranous lupus nephritis
  - Class VI: Advanced sclerosing lupus nephritis (≥90% globally sclerosed glomeruli without evidence of activity)
- Chronic, inactive lesions (glomerulosclerosis) are a poor prognostic feature.
- Although no uniform standard exists, we would recommend that lupus patients with microscopic hematuria and/or proteinuria with a decreased glomerular filtration rate should be considered for renal biopsy. However, biopsies should be read at centers experienced with the assessment of lupus nephritis.

Hematopoietic involvement

- A high ESR is a common finding.
- A normochromic, normocytic 'anemia of chronic inflammation' is present in up to 70% of patients with lupus. Renal failure, NSAID-induced gastric bleeding, Coombs' positive and microangiopathic hemolysis, and red cell aplasia, are factors that may contribute to the anemia.
- Leukopenia and lymphopenia are common abnormalities of the white cell count in 50% and 80% of patients respectively. A leukocytosis is rare, suggesting infection or steroid therapy.
- There are several forms of clinical thrombocytopenia. Chronic, indolent, and uncomplicated thrombocytopenia (<100 × 10⁹/liter) is not uncommon, particularly among SLE patients with antiphospholipid antibodies. A rarer acute and life-threatening severe thrombocytopenia is also recognized. This requires aggressive therapy initially with high-dose systemic steroids, and patients may require intravenous

immunoglobulin. Some patients may also present with what initially appears to be an idiopathic thrombocytopenia (ITP), later followed by other manifestations of lupus.

Nervous system disorders

- Features of neurological disease range from cognitive impairment (in up to 50% of patients) to psychoses and seizures (in 5–10% of patients over the course of their disease). Thromboembolic disease associated with antiphospholipid antibodies can cause major cerebrovascular damage (see Chapter 10).
- Approximately 10% of patients will develop a sensory (or less often sensorimotor) peripheral neuropathy. Cranial nerve involvement is less common.
- Up to 70% prevalence of psychiatric illness has been quoted in the literature. However, this includes anxiety and depression, rarely separated in studies from the nonspecific stresses associated with debilitating and often painful disease, as opposed to the disease per se. This said, it does emphasize the degree of the problem and that depression must be assessed and managed seriously in lupus.
- Although it is accepted that corticosteroids can induce psychiatric symptoms, in general it is felt the drugs given in lupus are not responsible for most of the psychiatric manifestations observed.
- Examination of the cerebrospinal fluid in neuropsychiatric disease should be performed as part of the initial evaluation of a new neurologic finding.
- Electroencephalography is often nonspecific. Positron emission CT (SPECT and PET) is neither specific for, nor well correlated with, central nervous system involvement. MRI with gadolinium is more sensitive than CT in detecting the small vessel vasculopathy associated with SLE.
- Memory issues are common among patients with SLE, and may not indicate the presence of active neurologic disease.

Other clinical features

Other clinical features are listed in Table 10.4.

Table 10.4 Other clinical features of SLE

Vascular	Raynaud's phenomenon
	Cutaneous vasculitis
	Digital ulcers and gangrene
Gastrointestinal	Hepatomegaly (25%)
	Abdominal serositis (10–20%)
	Splenomegaly (10%)
	Mesenteric vasculitis (rare)
	Pancreatitis (rare)
Immunologic	Hypergammaglobulinemia (60%)

Antiphospholipid (antibody) syndrome and SLE

- Antiphospholipid antibodies include the lupus anticoagulant, anticardiolipin antibodies, and anti-β_2 glycoprotein-I antibodies.
- Antiphospholipid antibodies are present in up to one-third of patients with SLE.
- Although the presence of antiphospholipid antibodies alone is not sufficient to make this diagnosis, half of patients with SLE and antiphospholipid antibodies will eventually demonstrate evidence of hypercoagulability.
- The manifestations of SLE-associated antiphospholipid syndrome include:
  - venous and arterial thrombosis
  - thrombocytopenia
  - cerebral disease
  - recurrent fetal loss
  - pulmonary hypertension
  - livedo reticularis.
- Some patients with antiphospholipid antibodies develop renal impairment (e.g., hypertension or proteinuria) due to multiple small thrombi.

Further details, including management, may be found in Chapter 11.

Pregnancy and SLE

- There is a disparity in the literature about whether pregnancy is associated with an increased risk of lupus flare. However, pregnancy does not appear to worsen the long-term outcome of SLE
- Active disease greatly increases the risk of miscarriage and preterm birth.
- A major complication is preeclampsia. Preexisting renal disease may be an important risk factor.
- SLE is associated with an increased rate of fetal death late in pregnancy and overall approximately 10% of lupus pregnancies result in fetal loss.
- Anti-Ro antibodies are associated with fetal heart block and neonatal lupus.
- Obstetric ultrasound should be performed every trimester. If the mother has anti-Ro antibodies, fetal echocardiogram should be performed weekly, from the 16th week to the 32nd week of gestation. If the mother lacks anti-Ro antibodies, biweekly fetal echocardiograms should be performed, starting with the 26th week of gestation.
- The antiphospholipid antibody syndrome and its associated complications during pregnancy is discussed in Chapter 10.
- Drug safety in pregnancy is discussed in Chapter 5.

Diagnosis and investigation of SLE

- The majority of investigations are aimed specifically at end-organ disease. Investigation in the form of radiographs, CBC, coagulation screen, ESR, CRP, and renal and liver biochemistry, urinalysis, and blood pressure may lead to other tests, e.g., of hemolysis or pleuritic pain. The physician is directed to autoantibody and complement tests (see Table 10.4).

- There are a variety of circulating autoantibodies to a range of nuclear, cytoplasmic, and plasma membrane antigens. Most patients (98% or more) will have antinuclear antibodies. Approximately 60% have elevated titers of dsDNA antibodies (detected by the immunofluorescent Crithidia test or by specific ELISA or radioimmunoassay). Some patients have varying combinations of antibody profile that may change over the course of the disease. The antibodies, their prevalence and clinical association are shown in Table 9.4.

- Lupus is associated with deficiencies of the early classical pathway of complement (e.g., C1q, C1r, C1s, C2). The overall consequence is decreased clearance and increased deposition of complexes. Reduced levels of complement C3 and C4 are common in SLE.

- A subset of patients will be "serologically active but clinically quiescent," meaning they will have low complement levels and raised dsDNA titers but no signs of active disease. Patients should always be treated on the basis of symptoms rather than blood tests alone.

- Some individuals may have high levels of RF and features of an erosive RA type disease. This "overlap" syndrome is sometimes called *rhupus*. The mix of clinical features and autoantibodies is not peculiar to SLE, and all the autoimmune rheumatic diseases are subject to the phenomenon of "overlap" or "undifferentiated" disease. In this situation, a number of clinical features and antibodies common to several diseases are present. Treatment is determined by the end-organ disease that is present. The concept of "mixed connective tissue disease" as a specific diagnosis, rather than "undifferentiated" disease remains controversial, since most patients eventually declare themselves as either SLE or scleroderma.

- When this term is used, mixed connective tissue disease refers specifically to patients who have high-titer antibodies to RNP. These patients can have features of both SLE and scleroderma, with a tendency to develop Raynad's phenomenon and pulmonary fibrosis.

- The assessment of disease activity is central to patient management. Several global activity indices have been produced that correlate well and are reliable. Awareness of changes in lupus activity, whether improvement of disease or not, is an essential part of decision making and drug treatment. Global scoring systems such as the Systemic Lupus Erythematosus Disease Activity Index (SLEDAI) and the British Isles Lupus Assessment Group (BILAG) activity index are of some value, both in the context of clinical trials and long-term follow-up of patients.

Table 10.4 Autoantibodies of systemic lupus erythematosus used in clinical practice

Autoantibody		Prevalence (%)	Associations
Intracellular:	DNA	40–90	Renal disease
	Histone	30–80	Drug-induced lupus
	Sm	30 (Africans, Caribbeans), 10 (Caucasians)	
	UI RNP	20–30	
	rRNP	5–15	
	Ro/SS-A	25–40	Sjögren's syndrome, cutaneous lupus, congenital heart block
	La/SS-B	10–15	Ro/SS-A
Cell membrane:	Cardiolipin	20–40	Pregnancy loss, thrombosis
	Red cell	< 10	Hemolytic anemia
	Platelets	< 10	Immune thrombocytopenia
Extracellular:	RF	25	
	Complement C1q	50	Renal disease

- Equally constructive is the concept of an index of damage as distinct from disease activity. For example, a patient with shortness of breath may have an active but reversible pneumonitis or an irreversible fibrosis; the distinction between disease activity and damage is important since the treatments are different. The SLICC (Systemic Lupus International Collaborating Clinics) damage index has been developed as a method of recording damage in patients with SLE. The reader is referred to two articles by Gladman et al.[1,2] as the background for the current scoring system.

[1] Gladman DD et al. Senitivity to change of 3 systemic lupus erythematosus disease activity indices: international validation. *Journal of Rheumatology*, 1994; 21: 1468–71
[2] Gladman DD et al. The development and initial validation of the Systemic Lupus International Collaborating Clinics/American College of Rheumatology damage index for systemic lupus erythematosus. *Arthritis and Rheumatism*, 1996; 39: 363–9

Drug-induced lupus erythematosus (DILE)

- Many drugs have been implicated in causing DILE. Those definitely and most commonly associated with DILE are:
  - minocycline
  - hydralazine
  - procainamide
  - isoniazid
  - quinidine
  - methyldopa
  - chlorpromazine
  - sulfasalazine
  - anti-TNF inhibitors
- Hydralazine-associated DILE is considered to be dose dependent, while procainamide-associated DILE may be time-dependent.
- Up to 90% of cases taking procainamide develop a positive antinuclear antibody (ANA) and 30% of these develop DILE.
- Renal, central nervous system, and skin features of SLE are rare in DILE. Other features of SLE such as articular and serosal disease are common.
- In the majority of cases, the condition subsides after drug withdrawal. There is no contraindication to using these drugs in idiopathic SLE.

The treatment of SLE

- Several general measures are important:
  - rest as appropriate
  - avoid overexposure to sunlight
  - sunblock should be SPF 30 or greater, and should protect against both UVA and UVB
  - control cardiovascular risk factors.
- Initial evaluation should include an assessment of risk for glucocorticoid induced osteoporosis. Most patients should take calcium and vitamin D. Patients on prednisone >5 mg daily should be offered a bisphosphonate (assuming not contraindicated e.g., premenopausal women, renal insufficiency) as prophylaxis against steroid-induced osteoporosis.
- Vaccinations, apart from "live" vaccine (e.g., varicella, MMR, yellow fever, live polio) in patients on immunosuppressive drugs, are not contraindicated, but the degree of response differs from the healthy individual.
- Estrogen contraceptive pills should be avoided in those with antiphopholipid antibodies, very active disease, or nephrotic syndrome. Progesterone-only or other methods of contraception can be used. Many patients tolerate hormone replacement therapy (HRT) but use in the menopause is controversial: there is a 20% increase in SLE flares among women taking HRT.

Reduction of cardiovascular disease risk factors

- Management of traditional risk factors (smoking, hypertension, diabetes, obesity)
- Statins for hypercholesterolemia
- Aspirin if antiphospholipid antibodies are present
- Tighter control of SLE disease activity.

Table 10.5 outlines the common therapies used to treat the various clinical manifestations of SLE. The management of SLE as an acute rheumatological emergency is discussed in Chapter 21.

Standard therapies for SLE

SLE is generally treated with glucocorticoids in combination with a steroid-sparing agent, such as the drugs listed below. The initial dose of glucocorticoids should reflect the severity of the disease manifestations; in severe cases of lupus nephritis or neuropsychiatric lupus, for example, it is not uncommon to treat with high dose intravenous methylprednisolone (e.g., 1000 mg daily for three days) prior to starting treatment with oral prednisone at 1 mg/kg/day. Low dose glucocorticoids are also sometimes used as part of a chronic remission-maintenance regimen, although this strategy may increase the long-term risk of cardiovascular events and osteoporosis.

The steroid sparing agent is often selected based on the predominant disease manifestations (e.g., hydroxychloroquine for serositis, methotrexate for arthritis, mycophenolate mofetil for glomerulonephritis), with cyclophosphamide and belimumab reserved for patients with the greatest disease activity.

Hydroxychloroquine

All patients with SLE should receive treatment with hydroxychloroquine (400 mg daily). It is especially effective for the treatment of serositis, arthralgias, and cutaneous manifestations of SLE; in addition, chronic use leads to a reduction in flares, delays onset of renal and neurologic involvement, and potentiates response to mycophenolate mofetil. Patients taking hydroxychloroquine should have a yearly examination to look for evidence of retinopathy.

Cyclophosphamide

Intravenous cyclophosphamide (750 mg/m^2 BSA monthly for six months) is often used for the treatment of severe SLE flares. Intravenous hydration and mesna (300 mg/m^2 administered both prior to the infusion and four hours after the start of the infusion) may be helpful to prevent bladder toxicity; leuprolide injections (3.75 mg IM 2 weeks prior to each cyclophosphamide treatment) may help preserve fertility in women. Lower dose cyclophosphamide regimens (EuroLupus) have chiefly been validated in Caucasian populations, and their efficacy for African American patients is less clear.

Azathioprine

Milder forms of SLE may respond to treatment with azathioprine (1.5–2.5 mg/kg/day). Unlike other drugs commonly used for SLE, azathioprine and hydroxychloroquine are not contraindicated during pregnancy.

Mycophenolate mofetil (MMF)

MMF (1.0–1.5 g twice daily) has become the treatment of choice for lupus nephritis, with the possible exception of rapidly-progressive glomerulonephritis, for which cyclophosphamide should still be considered. When used for remission induction of lupus nephritis, rates of remission, relapse, and infection are superior to those achieved by treatment with cyclophosphamide followed by azathioprine maintenance therapy. MMF was not associated with amenorrhea; bone marrow suppression is uncommon

Belimumab (Benlysta®)

B lymphocyte stimulator (BLyS, also known as BAFF) is required for the development of mature plasma B-cells. Belimumab (Benlysta®), a monoclonal antibody that targets BLyS, has been approved by the United States Food and Drug Administration for the treatment of SLE among patients with moderate to severe disease. Belimumab 10 mg/kg administered intravenously on days 0, 14, 28 and every 28 days afterwards has been demonstrated in two randomized clinical trials to decrease disease activity and increase time to first flare when added to standard-of-care therapies. Patients should receive premedication with acetaminophen and diphenhydramine, and the drug should be administered over 1 hour.

Patients with anti-dsDNA antibodies and low serum complements are the most likely to respond to therapy. Belimumab should not be used for the treatment of lupus nephritis, since it has not been well studied for this indication.

Other therapies for SLE

Rituximab

Encouraging results were seen initially in open label series using this anti-CD20 monoclonal antibody in patients with active systemic disease who had failed, or only had partial response to, conventional treatments. However, randomized placebo-controlled trials have failed to demonstrate that rituximab was beneficial to patients with moderate-to-severe SLE. Additionally, progressive multifocal leukoencephalopathy has been reported in association with rituximab therapy, leading to a black box warning.

Rituximab may be appropriate for the treatment of immune-mediated thrombocytopenia associated with SLE, or for patients with truly refractory disease, who have failed all other therapies, but likely does not have a role in the routine treatment of SLE.

Autologous hemopoietic stem cell transplantation (HSCT)

HSCT is used to treat hematological diseases, but has been used in patients with severe refractory SLE. The procedure is effective in inducing remission, and is curative in <50% in non-blinded studies. Mortality is high and long-term effects are unknown. New autoimmune conditions have been reported after HSCT. It is currently used only in those with life-threatening SLE.

High dose intravenous cyclophosphamide (50 mg/kg daily for 4 days) without stem cell transplant has been explored for the treatment of several autoimmune diseases. Although this option allows patients to avoid the toxicity associated with HSCT, it appears to be no more effective than standard-dose intravenous cyclophosphamide regimens.

Other agents

- Pooled immunoglobulin (IVIG 0.4 g/kg IV daily for five days) may be of use in severely ill patients not responding to other therapies, and perhaps moreso in situations where sepsis is the trigger and is life-threatening. It may have a role in drug-resistant membranous and membranoproliferative nephritis, and has been used in severe autoimmune thrombocytopenia and hemolytic anemia with good effect.
- The efficacy of anti-TNF-α therapy in SLE is at present not clear. 16% of RA patients on these therapies develop double-stranded DNA antibodies, and 0.2% develop a transient lupus-like syndrome. A small, open label study has shown benefit in lupus nephritis and lupus arthritis, but with a high proportion of complications.

Table 10.5 Recommendations for drug use in SLE

Symptom	Drug	Regimen
Arthralgias/fever	NSAIDs (caution with renal disease)	No special recommendation
	Hydroxychloroquine	Hydroxychloroquine 400 mg daily; ophthalmic examination yearly, although the risk of untoward events is low.
Malar/discoid rash	Prednisone, hydroxychloroquine, sunscreen	
Arthritis/serositis/myositis	Prednisone, methotrexate, azathioprine, leflunomide	20–40 mg daily for 2–4 weeks, then reducing dose 5 mg steps each week. Require bone prophylaxis against osteoporosis if dose remains at 7.5 mg or above for more than 3 months.
Autoimmune anemia or thrombocytopenia (ITP)	Prednisone, azathioprine, IVIG	60–80 mg prednisolone daily for 2 weeks, reducing in 10 mg steps per week after depending on response. 2.5 mg/kg azathioprine.ITP might also require immunoglobulin or splenectomy
Renal	Prednisone, mycophenolate, azathioprine, cyclophosphamide	Severe disease may require monthly IV steroid and cyclophosphamide for 6 months then 2–3 monthly for 2 years
Central nervous system	Prednisone, azathioprine	Up to 80 mg daily of prednisone (1 mg/kg/day)
Raynaud's disease	See Chapter 13	

Prognosis and survival in SLE

- Many studies of the duration of disease and survival rates are confounded by inadequate attention paid to the ethnic group, age of onset, and socioeconomic status of individual patients. The number of patients lost to follow-up is also high. With the division of patients into those with or without overt nephritis, it is reasonable to state a 5-year survival in lupus of 90%. At 15 years, only 60% of those with nephritis will be alive compared with 85% of those patients without renal disease.

- Overall, men have a worse prognosis than women; men with SLE have increased mortality, and are more likely to develop nephrotic syndrome, renal failure, and myocardial infarction than women with SLE.

- A bimodal mortality curve is considered to exist. Patients who die within 5 years usually have very active disease, requiring high doses of immunosuppressives. Those patients dying later tend to do so from cardiovascular disease, renal disease, and possibly infection.

- The combined effect of the disease and its treatment is to render the immune system prone to infection. It is often difficult to apportion responsibility to one or other. The possibility of infection must always be kept in mind and treated aggressively as outcome from sepsis can be very poor.

- Controlling risk factors for cardiovascular disease is important.

- Lupus itself increases the risk of malignancy. However, immunosuppression is also associated with an increased risk of malignancy.

Childhood SLE

- This is a rare disease with an estimated incidence of 0.4 per 100,000. There are several features of childhood SLE that differ from the adult disease, although the main features and treatment are similar. General management strategies (i.e., not including pharmacological agents) for child welfare are the same as those employed in the management of all pediatric arthritides—see Chapter 9.
- The overall prepubertal male to female ratio is 3:1, suggesting a higher male frequency in childhood SLE as compared to that seen in adults; the ratio reverts to the more classic adult ratio of 9:1 post-puberty.
- The disease is more common and severe in those of African-American and Asian origin.
- The main features at presentation are arthritis, myalgias, fever, and rash (all features with a frequency of approximately 60–80% of cases at diagnosis). Malar rash is present in 30% of cases at diagnosis, and renal disease at onset of disease is high (up to 60%). True myositis with proximal weakness occurs in <10% of cases. Neuropsychiatric disease is present in up to 40% cases.
- Avascular necrosis is more common in children than adults with SLE (10–15% of cases), and is more common in SLE than other pediatric autoimmune rheumatic diseases where prolonged high-dose steroids are used.
- Raynaud's phenomenon is less common in childhood lupus and occurs in 10–20% of patients.
- As in adult disease, hydroxychloroquine and NSAIDs can be used for mild skin and joint disease.
- Oral or IV corticosteroids are given for disease not responding to the above measures, or in moderate-to-severe multisystem disease.
- Growth retardation secondary to corticosteroids is a major concern, and the lowest possible dose of steroid should be used. Bone protection with calcium and vitamin D should also be given.
- Cyclophosphamide, azathioprine, methotrexate and mycophenolate mofetil are used as in adult disease. Case reports of successful autologous stem cell transplantation have been described.
- The 10-year survival for SLE in childhood is currently estimated at 85%.

Neonatal SLE

- This is a rare condition found in the newborn and characterized by subacute cutaneous lupus skin lesions, hemolytic anemia, hepatitis, thrombocytopenia, and congenital heart block (CHB).
- It is associated with placental transmission of maternal Ro and La antibodies.
- The noncardiac manifestations resolve within 1 year. Cardiac involvement often requires early pacemaker insertion, and mortality in the first 3 years of life is up to 30%.
- In women with anti-Ro/La antibodies, there is a 5% chance of their first child being born with CHB; this rises to 15% with subsequent pregnancies.
- Fetal monitoring with echocardiography in the antenatal period is essential.
- Maternal use of hydroxychloroquine prior to and during pregnancy appears to decrease the risk of either cardiac or cutaneous neonatal lupus.

The antiphospholipid (antibody) syndrome (APS)

Introduction

The antiphospholipid syndrome (APS) was first described in the 1980s, and is characterized by arterial and venous thrombosis (with or without pregnancy morbidity) in the presence of anticardiolipin (aCL) antibodies or the lupus anticoagulant (LAC). It can be primary, or secondary to other autoimmune diseases, most commonly systemic lupus erythematosus (see Chapter 10).

APS can affect almost any organ system, and presents to many medical specialties, including rheumatology, dermatology, neurology, and cardiology. Classification criteria were produced in 1999, and updated in 2006 to reflect the use of anti- β_2 glycoprotein-1 for diagnosis (see Table 11.1).

Table 11.1 Classification criteria for the antiphospholipid syndrome

Clinical Criteria	
Vascular thrombosis	1 or more clinical episodes of arterial, venous or small vessel thrombosis in any tissue or organ, confirmed by objective criteria. Histopathology should show thrombosis without significant inflammation in the vessel wall.
Pregnancy morbidity	1 or more unexplained deaths of a morphologically normal fetus at or beyond 10 weeks gestation
	OR
	1 or more premature births of a morphologically normal neonate at or before 34 weeks gestation due to pre-eclampsia, eclampsia or placental insufficiency
	OR
	3 or more unexplained, consecutive, spontaneous abortions before 10 weeks gestation, excluding maternal anatomical or hormonal abnormalities, and excluding maternal and paternal chromosomal causes.
Laboratory criteria	Medium/high titer of IgG and/or IgM isotype anticardiolipin antibody in blood on 2 or more occasions at least 12 weeks apart using standard assays.
	Lupus anticoagulant present in plasma on 2 or more occasions at least 12 weeks apart.
	Anti-β_2 glycoprotein-I IgG or IgM in blood on 2 or more occasions at least 12 weeks apart using standard assays.

Adapted from Miyakis S. *et al.* International consensus statement on an update of the classification criteria for definite antiphospholipid syndrome (APS). *J Thrombosis Haemostasis* 2006; 4: 295–306.

Epidemiology and pathology

- Antiphospholipid (APL) is the overall term used. Patients may be classified in terms of the antibody present: anticardiolipin (aCL), lupus anticoagulant (LAC), or anti-β_2 glycoprotein-I.
- Antibodies are directed at protein–phospholipid complexes. Recently antibodies to β_2-glycoprotein I (β_2GPI) have been found to be the main target antigen involved in the binding of anticardiolipin antibodies to anionic phospholipids.
- Case control studies estimate the prevalence of aCL in the normal population to be 1–4%. Prevalence in those >65 years increases to 12–50% depending on the study. Prevalence of aCL and LAC in SLE patients is estimated at 20–40% and 10–20% respectively. These differences arise due to treatment history and the lack of uniformity of assay methods. Ethnicity also plays a role in the frequency and clinical importance of these antibodies.
- The LAC and aCL antibody tests are the most useful antibodies for identifying patients with the syndrome. The LAC test cannot be performed reliably if a patient is receiving heparin or oral anticoagulant. LAC is most strongly associated with both thrombosis and adverse pregnancy outcomes. The two tests can be discordant in up to 40% of cases and their unrelated behavior in the course of disease and in the individual patient means that both assays may be required to identify cases of APS.
- Apart from a clinical suspicion leading to a request for antiphospholipid antibody assays, a clue to their presence lies in finding a prolonged clotting time in assays for the 'internal pathway'-clotting cascade.
- The specificity of antiphospholipid antibodies probably differs in various disorders. Studies suggest that LAC and high titers of IgG aCL antibodies are associated with greater risk of thrombosis; the risk is much lower in patients with infection-related or drug-induced antibodies, which tend to be of the IgM isotype. 10% of patients with APS only have antibodies to β_2GPI. There is evidence that β_2GPI titer and simultaneous presence of aCL or LAC are associated with disease severity.
- The differential diagnosis of unexplained thrombosis includes genetic causes (e.g., protein C and S, and antithrombin III deficiencies, factor V Leyden and prothombin mutations) and drugs (including estrogen, thalidomide, IVIG). However, these are usually associated with recurrent venous thrombosis. Most striking about APS is the feature of thrombosis in the setting of thrombocytopenia. The main differential diagnosis is thrombotic thrombocytopenic purpura (TTP) and heparin induced thrombocytopenia (HIT). TTP is a microvascular disorder most often associated with neurological features of confusion, seizures, and changes in consciousness level that can mimic the catastrophic form of APS.
- Only a third of all patients with aPL ever experience thrombosis. After the first thrombotic event (either arterial or venous), recurrence is common, but can be prevented by treatment with warfarin.

Clinical features of APS

Table 11.2 summarizes the main clinical features of APS and some of the less common findings.

Thrombosis

- Antiphospholipid antibodies are paradoxically associated with thrombosis rather than hemorrhage.
- Vessels of all sizes, venous or arterial, may be affected without evidence of an inflammatory infiltrate (i.e., vasculitis). This distinction is important not only in trying to understand the pathogenesis of the disorder but also in the choice of treatment. Unlike most clotting disorders, arterial thrombosis is a major feature of APS. The antibodies should be sought particularly in the younger stroke patient where they may account for up to 20% of cases.
- Widespread thrombosis is the feature of life-threatening 'catastrophic antiphospholipid syndrome'. In this situation the patient may present with acute medical collapse, severe thrombocytopenia, multi-organ failure (notably cerebral and renal), and adult respiratory distress syndrome.

Thrombocytopenia

This is common but usually not severe enough to cause bleeding. ACL antibodies have been found in up to 30% of cases of presumed immune thrombocytopenic purpura (ITP). Some patients also develop a concomitant Coombs' positive hemolytic anemia (Evan's syndrome).

Fetal loss

Recurrent spontaneous pregnancy loss is a common complication of APS. This can occur either as recurrent early loss or intrauterine fetal demise. Screening for the antibodies in the general population is not of value. Previous pregnancy history is of importance in determining the significance of a positive antibody titer.

Other features of APS

- Transverse myelopathy, though rare, has a strong association with the presence of antiphospholipid antibodies. Chorea has also been observed
- APS may be associated with multiple cardiovascular complications including accelerated atherosclerosis, valvular heart disease, and intracardiac thrombi. However, cardiac manifestations of APS result in significant morbidity for only 5% of patients. In a European cohort, myocardial infarction was the presenting feature of APS in 3% of patients, and was seen during follow-up in 5.5%. The prevalence of aCL in patients with myocardial infarction is estimated at 5–15%; however screening is not indicated, except in younger patients, those with other symptoms and signs of APS, and those with a family history of autoimmune disease. Mitral and aortic valve thickening and dysfunction are sometimes seen on echocardiography, but significant morbidity is uncommon.

Table 11.2 Clinical features of the antiphospholipid syndrome

Feature	Subgroup	Frequency
Major features:		
Thrombosis	Deep vein thrombosis	38.9%
	Pulmonary embolism	14.1%
	Arterial thrombosis, legs	4.3%
	Arterial thrombosis, arms	2.7%
	Stroke	19.8%
	Transient ischemic attack	11.1%
	Valve thickening/dysfunction	11.6%
	Livedo reticularis	24.1%
Fetal manifestations	Early loss (<10 wks)	35.4%
	Late loss (≥10 wks)	16.9%
	Live birth	47.7%
	Premature birth	10.6%
Thrombocytopenia		29.6%
Associated features:	Leg ulcers, livedo reticularis, thrombophlebitis	
	Heart valve lesions and myocardial infarction	
	Transverse myelitis, chorea,	
	Pulmonary hypertension	
Less common findings:	Splinter hemorrhages, digital gangrene, leg ulcers	
	Amaurosis fugax, retinal artery and vein occlusion	
	Renal artery stenosis/thrombosis	
	Ischemic bone necrosis	
	Addison's disease	

Cervera R. et al. Antiphospholipid syndrome: Clinical and immunologic manifestations and patterns of disease expression in a cohort of 1000 patients. *Arthritis Rheum* 2002; 46: 1019–1027.

Treatment of APS

Treatment of APS is summarized in Table 11.4.

- Studies suggest that lifelong and oral anticoagulation is an effective therapeutic option in the secondary prevention of thrombosis. Care should be taken to maintain the INR between 2 and 3.
- Mild thrombocytopenia need not be treated. Severe cases (<50 × 10⁹/ liter) should be treated with oral corticosteroids. In those failing to respond, gamma-globulin, danazol, and splenectomy have been used with varying success.
- The presence of antiphospholipid antibodies in pregnancy, in the absence of a history of thrombosis or fetal loss, is not an indication for anticoagulation. We would, however, recommend the use of aspirin (81 mg) in these settings.
- Prophylactic heparin after surgery for DVT prophylaxis is recommended.
- Women with APS on warfarin should be converted to standard heparin or low-molecular-weight heparins prior to conception, although the reader should be aware that the latter may not be licensed for this purpose. Aspirin should also be introduced.
- Other advances have been the realization that high-dose immunosuppression is unwarranted and that combined care between rheumatology, obstetrics, and hematology, with judicious monitoring and timely intervention, has a significant impact on outcome in pregnancy.

Table 11.3 The treatment of APS

Clinical situation		Treatment
Asymptomatic		Observation and/or low-dose aspirin
Thrombosis	Deep venous—1st event	Lifelong warfarin (INR 2–3)
	1st stroke	Lifelong warfarin (INR 2–3) and/or low-dose aspirin
	Transient ischemia	Low-dose aspirin
	1st non-cerebral arterial event	Warfarin (INR 2–3) and aspirin
	Recurrent arterial/ venous event	? warfarin (INR 3–4) or LMWH, or add aspirin
	Catastrophic APS	IV heparin
		IV methylprednisolone pulse
		Plasmapheresis OR IVIG
Pregnancy	No previous history	Observation and/or low-dose aspirin
	Recurrent first trimester or second/ third trimester fetal loss	Low-dose aspirin and heparin prophylaxis
	Previous thrombosis	Low-dose aspirin and therapeutic LMWH
	Repeat fetal loss despite heparin and aspirin	Consider hydroxychloroquine and prednisone 10 mg, in addition to the above
Thrombocytopenia	Mild (100–150 count)	Observe
	Moderate (50–100)	Observe
	Severe (<50)	Corticosteroids (as ITP), IVIG, immunosuppression (e.g., rituximab)

LMWH = low molecular weight heparin

Catastrophic APS (CAPS)

Introduction

- This rare variant of APS affects small vessels and visceral organs and was first described in 1992. It is an important and serious condition that can present to many medical specialties.
- It can present in previously asymptomatic patients.
- CAPS is associated with other autoimmune conditions such as SLE (see Chapter 9), RA (see Chapter 5) and SScl (see Chapter 12).
- The trigger is an infection in 20% cases. Other precipitating factors include trauma/surgery, malignancy, warfarin withdrawal in a patient with APS, pregnancy, and oral contraceptives.
- Despite these risk factors it is estimated that 45% cases have no known trigger.
- Mortality is greater than at 50% and many patients will require critical care.

Clinical features

- Rapid onset, diffuse peripheral and central thrombosis occurs leading to:
  - arterial and venous occlusion in the extremities
  - intra-abdominal organ infarction including renal failure (i.e., antiphospholipid-associated nephropathy)
  - pulmonary emboli and adult respiratory distress syndrome
  - small vessel cerebrovascular disease
  - aortic and mitral valve defects and myocardial infarction
  - other thrombotic complications such as ovarian, testicular, adrenal and retinal vessel occlusion.
- Livedo reticularis, gangrene, and purpura are visible markers of the disorder on the skin.
- Bone marrow infarction and ARDS have also been reported.
- Classification criteria have recently been produced.[1]

Laboratory features

These include:
- Moderate to severe thrombocytopenia
- Hemolysis with schistocytes
- Disseminated intravascular coagulation
- High levels of IgG aCL antibodies or presence of lupus anticoagulant

The differential diagnosis

The clinician should consider the following conditions
- Thrombotic thrombocytopenic purpura (red cell fragments more numerous than in CAPS)
- Heparin induced thrombocytopenia
- HELLP syndrome (hemolysis, elevated liver enzymes and low platelets)

---

[1] Cervera R, Font J, Gomez-Puerta JA et al. Validation of the preliminary criteria for the classification of the catastrophic antiphospholipid syndrome. Ann Rheum Dis, 2005; 64: 1205–1209.

- Hemolytic–uremic syndrome
- Cryoglobulinemia
- Vasculitis
- Disseminated intravascular coagulation
- Sepsis
- Paroxysmal nocturnal hemoglobinuria

Treatment and prognosis

- Treatment should always include an attempt to identify and to address the precipitating event, as well as supportive care.
- In addition, IV heparin and high-dose corticosteroids should be considered.
- Life threatening CAPS should also be treated with plasmaphersis versus intravenous immunoglobulin (for 5 days at a dose of 0.4 g/kg/day).
- Case reports exist in single patients describing the use of prostacyclin, cyclosporin A, defibrotide, fibrinolytics, and rituximab.
- 25% of survivors will develop further APS-related events.
- Recurrence of CAPS is very rare.

Sjögren's syndrome (SS)

Epidemiology and pathology

- Sjögren's syndrome (SS) is a chronic autoimmune disease of unknown etiology, characterized by lymphocyte infiltration of exocrine glands resulting in xerostomia and keratoconjunctivitis sicca.
- The condition may be primary, associated with specific extraglandular (systemic) disease, or secondary, in association with a number of other autoimmune rheumatic diseases, including RA (see Chapter 5) and SLE (see Chapter 10).
- Sjögren's syndrome is also strongly associated with the development of lymphoma.
- The syndrome affects women more than men in a ratio of 9:1, and tends to occur at 40–50 years of age. It can, however, occur at any age.
- Population prevalence is estimated at 0.1–0.5%.
- The triggering of autoimmunity and the development and continuation of an autoimmune response remain a great source of interest in SS. The links between environmental stimulus and immunogenetics, and the studies of humoral and lymphocyte activity may help to untangle the mechanisms whereby immunological dysregulation can lead to malignant transformation of B cells involved in the immune process.
- Epstein–Barr and retroviruses have been implicated in pathogenesis.
- HLA DR3 is strongly associated with SS.
- Antibodies to the ribonucleoprotein complexes Ro and La are found and are thought to be formed when these antigens are exposed on the surface of apoptotic cells.
- RF and antinuclear antibodies are also common and patients may be erroneously diagnosed with RA.
- Recently discovered autoantigens in SS include fodrin and muscarinic acetylcholine receptor M3.

Two sets of classification criteria for primary SS are listed in Tables 12.1 and 12.2.

- To satisfy classification criteria for primary SS using the American-European Consensus Group (AECG) criteria, focal lymphocytic sialoadenitis (with a focus score of 1 or greater), or antibodies to Ro and/or La must be present.
- The 2012 American College of Rheumatology criteria emphasize the use of objective, rather than subjective, findings.
- Patients with a history of head and neck radiation, hepatitis C infection, HIV/AIDS, sarcoidosis, amyloidosis, graft-versus-host disease, and IgG4-related diseases are excluded by ACR criteria from participating in studies of Sjögren's syndrome, due to the presence of overlapping clinical features that may interfere with objective measures.

Table 12.1 Classification criteria for primary Sjögren's syndrome. For classification purposes, 4 of 6 criteria must be present.

Criteria	Comment
Ocular symptoms	Dry eyes > 3 months, sense of sand/gravel in eyes, or use of tear substitutes >3 times/day
Oral symptoms	Dry mouth > 3 months, recurrent swollen salivary glands, frequent use of liquid to swallow
Ocular signs	Schirmer's test
	Corneal and conjunctival staining
Oral signs	Parotid scintigraphy
	Sialography
	Salivary flow
*Focal lymphocytic sialadenitis	Focus score (# lymphocyte aggregates per 4 mm²) must be ≥1
*Antibodies to Ro/La	

*One of these two criteria must be positive for this diagnosis.
Vitali C, et al. Classification criteria for Sjögren's syndrome; a revised version of the European criteria proposed by the American-European consensus group. Ann Rheum Dis, 2002; 61: 554–8.

Table 12.2 American College of Rheumatology 2012 Classification Criteria for Sjögren's Syndrome. For classification purposes, two of the three must be present

Criteria	Comment
Serology	1. Ro or La positive, or 2. RF-positive and ANA ≥1:320
Focal lymphocytic sialadenitis	Focus score ≥1/ 4mm²
Keratoconjunctivitis sicca	Requires ocular staining score of ≥3

Shiboski SC, et al. American College of Rheumatology Classification Criteria for Sjögren's Syndrome: a data-driven, expert-consensus approach in the Sjögren's International Collaborative Clinical Alliance Cohort. Arthritis Care and Research 2012; 64: 475–487.

Clinical manifestations of SS

Glandular disease

- The initial manifestations can be non-specific and 8–10 years can elapse before the diagnosis is established.
- Typical initial features of "sicca" syndrome include subjective dry eyes (xerophthalmia) in >50% at presentation, dry mouth (xerostomia) in 40%, and parotid/salivary gland enlargement in 25%. The prevalence of these manifestations increase with the duration of disease. There may be concurrent corneal and conjunctival damage (keratoconjunctivitis sicca), and dental caries from poor tear and salivary flow, respectively.
- A number of other conditions can lead to a dry mouth or parotid/salivary gland swelling, and these should be borne in mind during assessment.
- Dry eyes may be aqueous-deficient (lacrimal gland disease, drugs, tear duct obstruction, reflex hyposecretion) or evaporative (Meibomian gland dysfunction, lip aperture disorder, low blink rate, corneal surface inflammation, vitamin A deficiency).
- The most common causes of dry eye disease are blepharitis or meibomian gland dysfunction. Prior LASIK surgery may also contribute to dry eyes.
- Dry mouth may be associated with diseases that affect the salivary gland, including Sjögren's, IgG4-related diseases, head and neck radiation, hepatitis C, HIV/AIDS, sarcoidosis, and lymphoma.
- Multiple drugs may also cause dry mouth.
- Some causes of parotid gland enlargement include:
  - Lymphoma
  - Neoplasia (rare)
  - HIV/AIDS
  - Hepatitis C
  - Sarcoid
  - IgG4-related sialoadenitis
  - Sialoadenosis (due to alcoholism, diabetes, bulimia, malnutrition)

Extraglandular (systemic) disease

Extraglandular disease is seen in one-third of patients with primary SS. The main symptoms are fatigue, low-grade fever, myalgias, and arthralgias (see Table 12.3).

Joints

Joint pain is common; radiographs rarely reveal erosive changes. In contrast to SScl (see Chapter 12), Raynaud's in SS is not associated with digital ulceration and infarcts.

Skin

- The skin may be involved with itchy annular erythema, alopecia, and hyper/hypopigmentation. A hypersensitivity vasculitis may also develop.
- Vascular involvement in SS affects small and medium-sized vessels. The most common manifestations are purpura, urticaria, and skin ulceration. Skin vasculitis in SS is more benign and treatment with corticosteroids is not always needed.

Table 12.3 The incidence of extraglandular manifestations of primary Sjögren's syndrome

Condition	Frequency (%)
Arthralgias/arthritis	37
Raynaud's phenomenon	16
Cutaneous vasculitis	12
Pulmonary disease	9
Lymphadenopathy	7
Peripheral neuropathy	7
Renal disease	6
Autoimmune hepatitis	2
Lymphoproliferative disease	2
Myositis	1

Note: The true frequency of extraglandular manifestations among subjects who meet 2012 ACR classification criteria for Sjögren's syndrome may be higher

Pulmonary disease

Pulmonary function abnormalities are seen in 25% of patients, but they are not usually clinically significant. Interstitial lung disease may occur in patients with Sjögren's syndrome, who may present with cough and dyspnea. Non-specific interstitial pneumonia (NSIP) is the pattern most commonly associated with Sjögren's syndrome, and is associated with a good prognosis. Lymphocytic interstitial pneumonia (LIP), bronchiolitis, and amyloidosis are relatively uncommon.

Renal disease

- Interstitial nephritis may occur in patients with Sjögren's syndrome, and may respond to treatment with glucocorticoids.
- Distal (Type I) renal tubular acidosis is seen in up to 25% of patients with Sjögren's syndrome. This is generally associated with a mild metabolic acidosis, but patients may present with hypokalemia due to potassium wasting.
- Glomerulonephritis is rare and seen mainly in those with SS/SLE overlap. Membranoproliferative glomerulonephritis and membranous nephropathy are the forms of glomerular disease most commonly associated with Sjögren's syndrome.

Gastrointestinal and hepatobiliary disease

- Dysphagia due to dryness of the pharynx and esophagus is common. Chronic atrophic gastritis may occur due to lymphocytic infiltration similar to that seen in the salivary glands.
- Subclinical hyperamylasemia may be observed

- There may be a close link between "autoimmune cholangitis" of SS and primary biliary cirrhosis (PBC). Sicca syndrome is found in approximately 50% of cases of PBC.
- Transaminitis may be due to hepatitis C. Hepatitis C can cause a Sjögren's-like disease often in association with a "mixed" (type II) cryoglobulinemia.

Neuromuscular disease

- Peripheral sensory neuropathy is the most common neuromuscular feature of SS, and may require measurement of epidermal nerve density by skin biopsy to confirm the diagnosis.
- Mononeuritis multiplex as a consequence of vasculitis is well recognized as is the isolated involvement of cranial nerves, particularly the trigeminal and optic nerve. A peripheral sensory neuropathy is also seen. Specific involvement of the central nervous system remains a controversy. Multiple sclerosis-like syndromes may be seen.
- Myalgias are common; myositis is rare, but responds to immunosuppression (see Chapter 13, Polymyositis).

Lymphoproliferative disease ⚠

- Patients with SS have approximately a 16-fold increased risk of developing a lymphoma, compared to age, sex, and race-matched normal controls. The lymphomas are primarily B cell in origin, usually expressing the monoclonal IgM-κ, and of two major types, either highly undifferentiated, or well-differentiated immunocytomas.
- The clinical picture is diverse. The approach to therapy should be determined by the stage and histological grade of the disease.
- The salivary glands are the main site of lymphomatous change. The presence of lymphadenopathy, organomegaly, or persistent, painful, and continuously enlarged salivary glands, in the absence of infection, should raise suspicion and warrants biopsy. Other organs and systems may be affected, including the reticuloendothelial system, lungs, kidneys, and GI tract.
- Risk factors include monoclonal gammopathy, cryoglobulins, hypocomplementemia and major salivary gland swelling.

Cardiovascular system ⚠

Anti-Ro and La antibodies cross the placenta and can cause fetal congenital heart block. Babies of mothers with these antibodies have a 1 in 50 risk of heart block. If there is a prior history of congenital heart block during a previous pregnancy, this risk increases to 20%. Fetal heart rate monitoring in specialist centers is needed. Oral dexamethasone given to mothers early following detection of heart block may reverse the condition. Neonatal lupus is also seen, its most common manifestation being a florid rash.

Other pathology in SS

- Over 50% of patients have antithyroid antibodies and altered thyroid biochemistry without necessarily overt clinical symptoms.

- Nonbacterial interstitial cystitis due to an intense inflammation of the mucosa can cause frequency, nocturia, and perineal pain.
- Mild normochromic, normocytic anemia is common. Leukopenia is seen in 15–20% of patients with SS. The ESR is often raised, but the CRP usually normal.

Other autoimmune diseases

In a recent retrospective case review of 114 patients with primary SS, 33% had an additional autoimmune disease, 6% two diseases, and 2% three diseases. Hypothyroidism was most common condition seen.

Investigation of SS

- Common laboratory findings in primary SS are detailed in Table 12.4.
- To evaluate the glandular component of the disease, various tests are used. Setting a cut-off point between the normal and abnormal individual is difficult.
- Salivary flow rates (sialometry) can be measured for whole saliva or separate secretions from different salivary glands, with or without stimulation. Patients with overt SS have decreased flow rates. This technique can be confounded by concomitant use of drugs with anticholinergic properties.
- Anatomical changes in the ductal system can be assessed by radio contrast sialography. This can, however, be painful and there is some controversy about its sensitivity and specificity.
- Scintigraphy, with uptake of ^{99}Tc, may provide a functional evaluation of all the salivary glands by observing the discharge of radioactivity form the glands after administration of lemon juice or candy. Scanning has a high sensitivity but low specificity. Neither sialography nor scintigraphy are suggested as routine investigations.
- Schirmer's test is used for the evaluation of tear secretion. Strips of filter paper 30 mm in length are slipped beneath the inferior eye-lid by a fold at one end of the strip. After 5 min, the length of paper that has been made wet by the tears is measured; wetting of <5 mm is a strong indication of diminished tear secretion.
- Ocular surface staining may be used to evaluate the tear film and demonstrate areas of damage on the ocular surface, including devitalized tissue. Ocular surface staining may be used to monitor response to treatment of dry eye over time.
- A labial gland biopsy is often essential to the establishment of a diagnosis of SS, particularly when the patient lacks anti-Ro or anti-La antibodies.
  - Because there is a (small) risk of sensory nerve damage, the biopsy should be performed by a surgeon with experience in the technique.
  - The surgical approach is critical: a shallow incision through the lamina propria of the inner lip is the preferred technique, since it allows direct visualization of the glands.
  - Elliptical wedge and punch biopsies may not provide enough glands, and are associated with a higher risk of nerve injury.
  - At least 4–6 glands must be harvested, since the pathologic process is focal.
  - Biopsies should not be performed if there is mucosal inflammation overlying the biopsy site or there is a past history of therapeutic head and neck irradiation.
  - Focal lymphocytic sialadenitis is scored in terms of the number of lymphocytic foci (i.e., aggregates of 50 or more lymphocytes), which surround ducts or blood vessels and are adjacent to histologically-normal acini.
  - The pathologist must measure the total surface area of the gland in order to calculate a focus score.

- A score of 1 or more foci per 4 mm^2 is compatible with SS. However, focal lymphocytic sialadenitis can also be seen in hepatitis C, HIV, graft versus host disease and patients with autoimmune disease in the absence of sicca.
- Other possible findings include non-specific chronic sialadenitis, sclerosing chronic sialadenitis, and MALT lymphoma, which are not specific for a diagnosis of Sjögren's syndrome. Sclerosing chronic sialadenitis is particularly common among the elderly.
- Detection of germinal center-like lesions is associated with a higher risk of progression to non-Hodgkin's lymphoma.

Table 12.4 Common laboratory findings in primary SS

Finding		Frequency (%)
General	Anemia	20
	Thrombocytopenia	13
	Leukopenia	16
	Raised ESR	22
	Monoclonal gammopathy	22
	Hypergammaglobulinemia	22
Cryoglobulinemia		9
Serology	ANA	74
	Rheumatoid factor	38
	Ro/SS-A	40
	La/SS-B	26
	ANCA	6
	Antimitochondrial	5

Garcia-Carrasco M, et al. Primary Sjögren syndrome: Clinical and immunologic disease patterns in a cohort of 400 patients. Medicine 2002; 81: 270–80.

Note that the frequency of Ro-positivity among subjects who meet the 2012 American College of Rheumatology Classification Criteria for Sjögren's syndrome is closer to 80%.

Treatment of SS

Table 12.5 summarizes the treatment options for Sjögren's syndrome.

Other treatments

- There is no evidence that azathioprine, low dose steroids, cyclosporine, infliximab or methotrexate are useful.

Table 12.5 The treatment of Sjögren's syndrome

Condition	Treatment
Dry eyes	Artificial tears
	Topical cyclosporine drops
	Punctal occlusion (plugs)
	Treatment of Meibomian gland dysfunction (with warm compresses)
Dry mouth	Frequent sips of water and good oral hygiene
	Sugar free lozenges/lemon drops
	Artificial saliva
Chromic erythematous candidiasis	Topical treatments should be sugar-free, to avoid worsening of dental carries
Sicca manifestations	May improve with the cholinergic agent pilocarpine (side effects include flushing/sweating) or cemiveline (fewer side effects)
Vaginal dryness	Patients may respond to propionic acid gels. Rigorous treatment of infection. Advice on lubricants etc. if there is pain with intercourse
Salivary gland	Acute suppurative parotitis should initially be treated with intravenous antibiotics, which much cover broadly for S. aureus (including MRSA) and anaerobes. Patients who exhibit an adequate response may be transitioned to oral antibiotics
Arthralgia	Hydroxychloroquine 200–400 mg/day (see Drugs in RA, for monitoring)
Systemic vasculitis	Necrotizing vasculitis and glomerulonephritis— prednisone and/or cyclophosphamide. Cryoglobulinemic vasculitis—rituximab. Leukocytoclastic vasculitis—may be refractory to immunosuppressive therapy.
Liver disease	Cholestasis may respond to ursodeoxycholic acid 10–15 mg/kg/day
Chronic erythematous candidiasis	Topical nystatin, miconazole, or ketoconazole
Interstitial lung disease	Prednisone

- Hydroxychloroquine normalizes ESR and immunoglobulin levels, but has no effect on salivary flow rates. Many clinicians use it to treat fatigue, myalgias, and arthralgias.
- Rituximab may improve salivary flow rates and diminish fatigue in patients with Sjögren's syndrome.
- Oral interferon alpha improves salivary flow but long-term use may be limited.

Systemic sclerosis and related disorders

Epidemiology and diagnostic criteria

- Scleroderma is a spectrum of rare disorders ranging from limited to generalized, nonsystemic to systemic, and environmental to autoimmune rheumatic disease. Systemic scleroderma (systemic sclerosis) predominantly affects women and is associated with production of collagen, widespread microvascular damage, and inflammation.
- The spectrum of scleroderma and scleroderma-like syndromes includes:
  - Raynaud's phenomenon—primary, secondary
  - Scleroderma (localized)—morphea, linear, *en coup-de-sabre*
  - Scleroderma (systemic)—limited cutaneous, diffuse cutaneous, scleroderma sine scleroderma
  - Chemical induced—environmental, occupational, drugs
  - Scleroderma-like disease (see Table 13.1)—metabolic, immunological, localized sclerosis, and visceral disease.
- There is no single diagnostic test for systemic sclerosis (SSc) although there are specific autoantibodies. For the purpose of separating it from other autoimmune rheumatic diseases and identifying case profiles, preliminary criteria were developed in 1980 by the American Rheumatism Association. These criteria have a 97% sensitivity and specificity for definite SSc, but are less sensitive for the largest subset of patients with limited cutaneous disease, failing to identify 10% of such cases.
- At minimum, a patient must have Raynaud's, a scleroderma-specific autoantibody, and abnormal nailfold capillaries to consider a diagnosis of SSc.
- Currently the most widely used classification of SSc (see Table 13.2) defines two subsets divided into limited cutaneous (lcSSc) and diffuse cutaneous (dcSSc). Over 60% of cases are in the 'limited' subset, where visceral involvement is late, some 10–30 years after onset of Raynaud's.
- The term *limited cutaneous* is now preferred to CREST (calcinosis, Raynaud's, esophageal dysphagia, sclerodactyly, telangiectasia), although this acronym is a useful reminder of the common characteristics of lcSSc.
- DcSSc is more serious, of rapid onset, and associated with organ failure often within the first 5 years of presentation.
- Clearly, these models will continue to change and develop as knowledge of pathogenesis advances and immunological findings are matched to clinical subsets.
- Several chemical agents have been implicated in the development of scleroderma, including:
  - silica
  - organic chemicals:
    - aliphatic hydrocarbons—vinyl chloride, naphtha
    - aromatic hydrocarbons—benzene, toluene
  - drugs: hydroxytryptophan, carbidopa, fenfluramine, bleomycin.

Table 13.1 Scleroderma-like syndromes

Metabolic/ inherited	Carcinoid syndrome	Scleroderma-like lesions can be found with malignant carcinoid; their presence is associated with a poor prognosis
	Acromegaly	Associated with skin puffiness that can mimic early scleroderma. Acromegaly-skin also associated with increase in sebum and sweat absent in SSc.
	Phenylketonuria	Phenylalanine-restricted diet may improve skin changes.
	Amyloidosis	Plaques from direct dermal infiltration can mimic SSc; more common are alopecia, ecchymoses, and nail dystrophy.
Immunological/ inflammatory	Chronic graft versus host disease	Skin changes favor the trunk, hips, and thighs, but can affect the entire body. Associated with pruritis and hypopigmentation.
	Eosinophilic fasciitis	Associated with painful induration of the skin, hypereosinophilia, and hypergammaglobulinemia. Early skin changes described as "peau d'orange"
	Overlap/ undifferentiated autoimmune rheumatic disease	Mixed connective tissue disease (MCTD) is associated with RNP-positivity, and is sometimes classified as a form of scleroderma. Polymyositis-scleroderma overlap syndromes are associated with antibodies to the PM/Scl complex
	Scleredema	Occurs with diabetes, monoclonal gammopathies, and after certain infections (e.g., strep throat). Unlike SSc, occurs without Raynaud's phenomenon and has predilection for the back

(Continued)

Table 13.1 Scleroderma-like syndromes

	Scleromyxedema	Papular waxy induration of the skin along the forehead, neck, and behind the ears. Systemic involvement may mimic scleroderma; neurologic involvement may be fatal
	Nephrogenic fibrosing dermopathy	Rapid induration of the skin and other organs associated with exposure to gadolinium-based contrast used for MRI in patients with renal insufficiency/failure
	Idiopathic pulmonary fibrosis	Patients diagnosed with idiopathic pulmonary fibrosis should be evaluated for the presence of Raynaud's, capillary loop dilatation, and other signs of SSc and other CTD
	POEMS	Polyneuropathy, organomegaly, endocrinopathy, M-protein, and skin changes. Hyperpigmentation is most common but acrocyanosis/ skin thickening are seen.
Acquired	Lipodermato-sclerosis	Hyperpigmentation and induration of the lower extremities associated with chronic venous insufficiency
	Eosinophilic myalgia syndrome and toxic oil syndrome	Acute syndromes caused by exposure to L-tryptophan and aniline-denatured rapeseed oil, respectively. Largely of historical interest.
	Bleomycin exposure	Used as a model to study scleroderma

Table 13.2 The classification of systemic sclerosis

1. "Prescleroderma"	Raynaud's phenomenon, nail fold capillary changes
	Disease-specific antinuclear antibodies:
	centromere (ACA)
	nucleolar (antitopoisomerase-1 (Scl-70))
2. Diffuse cutaneous SSc	Skin changes within 1 year of Raynaud's.
	Proximal and acral (face, arms, hands, feet) skin involvement
	Tendon friction rubs
	Early, significant organ disease:
	interstitial lung disease
	oliguric renal failure ("scleroderma renal crisis")
	myocardial disease
	gastrointestinal disease
	Nailfold capillary dilatation and/or "dropout"
	Scl-70 antibodies in up to 60% of patients
	RNA polymerase III antibodies in 25% of patients
3. Limited cutaneous SSc	Raynaud's phenomenon for many years
	Acral skin involvement
	Late incidence of pulmonary hypertension with or without interstitial lung disease
	Skin calcification and telangiectasia
	Nailfold capillary dilatation and/or "dropout"
	ACA antibodies in 70–80% of patients
4. Scleroderma sine scleroderma	Raynaud's
	No skin involvement
	Presentation with lung fibrosis, renal crisis, cardiac or gastrointestinal disease
	Antinuclear antibodies may be present

- These exposures likely explain only a very small fraction of patients who develop scleroderma or similar conditions.
- There are three main abnormalities in scleroderma.
  - *Raynaud's phenomenon:* A vasculopathy is found that manifests clinically as Raynaud's phenomenon, and pathologically as endothelial cell injury. Vascular injury may be the primary event either by vasomotor instability or microvascular intimal proliferation and vessel obliteration. Intravascular pathology in the form of increased platelet activity, red cell rigidity, and thrombosis may also be a factor.
  - *Inflammation* occurs early in scleroderma, and may no longer be present at the time of diagnosis. Clinically, this active phase of scleroderma is associated with doughy, edematous (not indurated) skin and the presence of tendon friction rubs (which can be felt by placing the hand over the tendon during active or passive range of motion).
  - *Fibrosis* is the hallmark of several diseases, and in SSc it is widespread and nonorgan-specific. Excess deposition of collagen and extracellular matrix protein is found in the skin and internal organs of patients with SSc. Current research focuses on the role of several proteins including endothelin-1 and transforming growth factor-β.

Cutaneous features of scleroderma and their treatment

Scleroderma—localized skin changes (morphea; linear)

- This is distinguished from SSc by:
  - the absence of Raynaud's,
  - the absence of vascular or organ damage
  - the distribution of skin lesions.
- Morphea may be "circumscribed" with just one or two lesions or "generalized." The rash is often itchy, violaceous or erythematous, and progresses to firm "hide-bound" skin with hypo- or hyperpigmentation and subsequent atrophy.
  - The "circumscribed" condition tends to resolve within three to five years and treatment is often unnecessary. The acral parts are spared, the trunk and legs being most often involved.
  - The "generalized" form can be disfiguring, leading to contractures, ulceration, and occasionally malignancy. Generalized morphea may respond to PUVA. Methotrexate may also be effective.
- Guttate morphea is a variant with small 10 mm diameter papules and minimal sclerosis, resembling lichen sclerosus et atrophicus. The lesions usually localize to the neck, shoulders, and anterior chest wall.
- Linear morphea describes a band-like pattern of sclerosis, often in a dermatomal distribution. The sclerotic areas often cross over joints and are associated with soft tissue and bone atrophy, and growth defects. Treatment is similar to generalized morphea as above. Physical therapy and appropriate exercises may help to minimize growth defects in the childhood form.
- *En coup-de-sabre* is linear sclerosis involving the face or scalp and associated with hemiatrophy of the face on the same side. The lesion assumes a depressed appearance reminiscent of a scar from a saber.

Scleroderma/systemic sclerosis (SSc)—diffuse skin changes

- The changes in the skin usually proceed through three phases: early, classic, and late. In the early stage, there may be nonpitting edema of the hands and feet, most marked in the mornings and often associated with Raynaud's. The skin then becomes taut, the epidermis thins, hair growth ceases, and skin creases disappear and the classic changes of scleroderma become more pronounced. The classic changes remain static for many years.
- The late phase may evolve at any time. Truncal and limb skin softens such that it can be difficult to know that a person ever had sclerosis. However, the hand changes rarely resolve and continue to show the ravages of fibrosis and contractures. During this phase of the disease digital pitting scars, loss of finger pad tissue, ulcers, telangiectasia, and calcinosis can occur.

- All patients with SSc will have some involvement of the face and the digits (although this involvement may be mild). SSc never involves the mid-back. Skin thickening limited to the fingers is called *sclerodactyly*.
- *Limited scleroderma* (lcSSc) is associated with skin involvement limited to the hands and face. This form of SSc, previously known as CREST, can lead to pulmonary arterial hypertension in the absence of pulmonary fibrosis.
- *Diffuse scleroderma* (dcSSc) is associated with taut hypo- or hyperpigmented skin involvement proximal to the elbow, knee, or clavicle. In this group there is a preponderance of visceral involvement (such as pulmonary fibrosis and renal crisis) in the first five years of symptoms.
- A practical scheme for assessing dcSSc and lcSSc by dividing the disease into early and late stages is shown in Table 13.3.

Raynaud's phenomenon (Table 13.4)

- The overall prevalence of this phenomenon is between 3–10% of the population worldwide, variation depending on climate, skin color, and racial background in particular. In SSc, Raynaud's is present in approximately 95% of cases.
- Raynaud's is more than just cold fingers, which is a common complaint, and often has nothing to do with autoimmunity or vasospasm.
- A patient with Raynaud's experiences episodic vasospasm, with the following symptoms:
  - pallor of the digits (due to ischemia), followed by
  - cyanosis (due to deoxygenation), and then
  - redness with pain and tingling (due to hyperemia following the return of blood).
- All three phases do not need to be observed to make a diagnosis of Raynaud's. Continuous blueness/cyanosis with pain, however, is not characteristic of Raynaud's.
- Symptoms that might suggest secondary Raynaud's include an onset in men, patients older than 35 years, symptoms all year round, digital ulceration, and asymmetry.
- The antinuclear antibodies discussed earlier (Table 13.2) should be sought, and nailfold capillaroscopy should be performed. Pathological changes seen on capillaroscopy include nailfold capillary dilatation, hemorrhage, and dropout. Both have a high predictive power for detecting those patients likely to develop SSc.
- Nailfold capillaroscopy can be performed by placing a drop of immersion oil on the nailfold, and then examining the area with an ophthalmoscope set at +40 diopters. If immersion oil is not available, clear surgical lubricant may suffice.
- Conservative measures should be directed at keeping the core body temperature warm, which encourages vasodilatation throughout the extremities.

Table 13.3 Characterisitc findings in early and late systemic sclerosis

Diffuse cutaneous features	Early (<3 years from onset of disease)	Late (>3 years from onset of disease)
Constitutional	Fatigue, weight loss	Minimal
Vascular	Raynaud's (often mild)	Severe Raynaud's. Telangiectasia
Cutaneous	Rapid progression involving arms, face, and trunk	Stable or some regression
Musculoskeletal	Arthralgia, myalgia, stiffness	Flexion contractures
Gastrointestinal	Dysphagia and 'heart burn'	More severe dysphagia. Midgut and anorectal disease
Cardiopulmonary	Myocarditis, pericarditis, lung fibrosis	Progression of established disease/Pulm. Hypertension
Renal	Maximum risk of scleroderma renal crisis	Crisis uncommon after 4 years
Limited cutaneous features	**Early (<10 years from onset of disease)**	**Late (>10 years from onset of disease)**
Constitutional	None	Digital ulceration or gangrene
Vascular	Severe Raynaud's. Telangiectasia	Stable, calcinosis
Cutaneous	Mild sclerosis on face	Flexion contractures
Musculoskeletal	Occasional joint stiffness	More severe symptoms common. Midgut and anorectal disease
Gastrointestinal	Dysphagia and heartburn	Slow progressive lung fibrosis. Pulmonary hypertension.
Cardiopulmonary	Rarely involved	Right-sided heart failure
Renal	Rarely involved	Rarely involved

Table 13.4 The treatment of Raynaud's phenomenon

Treatment	Examples	Comments
Nonphar-macological	Hand warmers. Protective clothing	Universally helpful
	Evening primrose oil	Effective in clinical trials
	Fish-oil capsules	
Parenteral vasodilator	Nifedipine or Amlodipine	Hypotension is possible with all of these agents.
	Sildenafil	
	Losartan	
	Topical nitroglycerin	High rate of discontinuation due to side effects
	Prostacyclin	For severe attacks, digital gangrene, and prior to hand surgery
Surgery	Digital sympathectomy. Debridement. Amputation	

Systemic features of the disease, investigation, and treatment

The gastrointestinal tract (Table 13.5)

- The gastrointestinal tract is probably the most commonly involved system in SSc. Over 90% of all patients with lcSSc and dcSSc develop esophageal hypomotility, with >50% of patients with lcSSc having serious disease.
- The cause of gastrointestinal dysfunction in SSc is not entirely clear. Possible contributing factors include neural dysfunction, tissue fibrosis, and muscle atrophy. In the earliest stages of neural dysfunction most patients are asymptomatic.
- Prokinetic drugs such as metoclopramide (5–10 mg po BID-TID) may help some patients with esophageal hypomotility.
- Many patients develop reflux esophagitis. Simple advice such as raising the head of the bed, taking frequent small meals, and avoiding late night snacks, may help. Patients often require high-dose proton-pump inhibitors.
- Small bowel disease with hypomobility can lead to weight loss and malabsorption; small intestinal bacterial overgrowth (SIBO) may exacerbate these symptoms. SIBO can be diagnosed using a lactulose breath test, and treated with two-week courses of broad spectrum antibiotics (such as ciprofloxacin, metronidazole, doxycycline, or amoxicillin), which can be used as needed, on a rotating basis. Ultimately the small bowel may fail, necessitating total parenteral nutrition.
- Atony and hypomotility of the rectum and sigmoid colon may cause constipation and incontinence, best managed with bulking agents, although severe cases may need limited surgery or the use of implantable sacral stimulators.
- Anemia due to vascular lesions in the gastrointestinal mucosa is now widely recognized. The classic appearance in the stomach is now called gastric antrum venous ectasia (GAVE, or watermelon stomach), and these lesions may be treated by argon laser therapy if blood loss is significant, although this is not curative.

Pulmonary disease (Table 13.6)

- Pulmonary disease ranks second to esophageal in frequency of visceral disease. With the improvements in management of renal disease, pulmonary disease is now the major cause of death in SSc.
- The major clinical manifestations are parenchymal lung disease (interstitial lung disease, organizing pneumonia, and traction bronchiectasis) and pulmonary vascular disease (isolated pulmonary hypertension, pulmonary hypertension associated with interstitial lung disease, and pulmonary edema). Far less common conditions include pleurisy, aspiration pneumonia, drug-induced pneumonitis, and spontaneous pneumothorax.
- Interstitial lung disease often develops insidiously and established fibrosis is currently untreatable. Early diagnosis is therefore vital. The Scleroderma Lung Study (SLS) demonstrated that treatment with

Table 13.5 Common gastrointestinal disorders in systemic sclerosis

Site	Disorder	Investigation	Treatment
Mouth	Caries, sicca syndrome	Dental radiographs	Oral hygiene. Artificial saliva
Esophagus	Hypomotility	Barium swallow	Metoclopramide
	Reflux		High-dose proton pump inhibitors
	Strictures	Endoscopy	Dilatation
Stomach	Gastroparesis		Metoclopramide
	Gastric ulcer	Barium swallow. Endoscopy	Proton-pump inhibitor
Small bowel	Hypomotility	Barium follow-through	Metoclopramide
	Malabsorption	Hydrogen breath test	Pancreatic supplements. Low-dose octreotide. Nutritional support, antibiotics
		Jejunal aspiration/biopsy	If serologic evidence of celiac disease is present
		Stool bulking agents	Stool cultures
	Barium enema	Large bowel	Hypomotility
Rectal manometry	Surgery. Neurostimulator	Anus	Incontinence

Table 13.6 Cardiopulmonary disorders in systemic sclerosis

Disease	Frequency	Investigation	Treatment
Lung disease:			
Pulmonary fibrosis	Most common in dcSSc (SCL-70+)	Chest radiograph, lung function tests, high-resolution chest CT scan	Controversial; consider cyclophosphamide
Pleurisy	Uncommon	Chest radiograph	NSAIDs. Low-dose oral prednisolone
Bronchiectasis	Rare	Chest CT scan	Antibiotics. Physiotherapy
Pneumothorax	Rare	Chest radiograph	Chest tube, pleurodesis
Pulmonary hypertension	10–15% overall	Doppler echocardiogram. Catheter studies	Endothelia. 1 receptor antagonists (Bosentan), Prostacyclin PDE5 inhibitors Anticoagulation. Long-term oxygen therapy
Cardiac disease:			
Dysrhythmias and conduction defects	Common, but rarely symptomatic	ECG. 24-h ambulatory cardiac monitor	Dependen: on rhythm—drugs, pacemaker
Pericarditis	10–15% overall	Echocardiogram	As pleurisy, above
Myocarditis	Rare		Prednisone, Cyclophosphamide. Diuretics
Myocardial fibrosis	30–50% of dcSSc		Controversial: consider diuretics, ACE inhibitors

oral cyclophosphamide (up to 2m/kg/day) for 12 months resulted in a 2.5% improvement in forced vital capacity. The ongoing Scleroderma Lung Study II (SLS II) compares cyclophosphamide to mycophenolate mofetil.

- The plain chest radiograph is not a sensitive test for early fibrosis. Lung function tests can be discriminatory. The single-breath diffusion test (DLCO) is abnormal in >70% of early cases and lung volumes are often decreased. In the case of a low DLCO and normal lung volumes, the clinician should think of pulmonary arterial hypertension (PAH); a decline in a previously stable DLCO may be indicative of emerging PAH.
- High-resolution CT scanning now plays a major part in detecting and following interstitial lung disease and should be performed whenever possible.
- Pulmonary fibrosis tends to be associated with dcSSc and Scl-70 antibodies, and isolated PAH with lcSSc and anti-centromere antibodies.
- Recent studies suggest a prevalence of PAH of 12–15% in SSc. Right heart catheterization is the gold standard method of diagnosis, but screening using this method is not practical. Annual echocardiography by experienced practitioners, lung function tests (including DLCO), and clinical assessment are essential to help detect subclinical disease.
- Treatment of PAH associated with SSc includes prostaglandins, and inhibitors of endothelin-1 or phosphodiesterase 5 inhibitors.
- Continuous parenteral epoprostenol, a prostacyclin, improves symptoms and pulmonary artery pressures, but not mortality. Subcutaneous and nebulized prostacyclin are also available.
- Bosentan (62.5–125 mg po BID), an oral endothelin receptor antagonist, improves function and is now an accepted treatment.
- Sildenafil (20 mg po TID)and tadalafil(40 mg po QD) inhibits phosphodiesterase type 5, and enhances relaxation of vascular smooth muscle as well as inhibiting their growth. A recent double-blind placebo-controlled study of patients with idiopathic or connective tissue disease associated pulmonary hypertension found that sildenafil significantly improves 6-minute walk times and mean pulmonary artery pressure.

Cardiac disease

- There are many cardiac manifestations including pericardial effusion, arrhythmias, and myocardial fibrosis. Heart block has been reported, but is rare. Many cases are subclinical and careful monitoring is needed. More epidemiological research is needed in this area.

Renal disease

- Renal disease has been superseded by lung disease as the main cause of death in SSc due to the impact of ACE inhibitors in the treatment of hypertensive renal crisis. It remains however a major, life-threatening complication of SSc.
- Both epithelial and endothelial damage occur before becoming clinically detectable.

- The most characteristic pattern of involvement is scleroderma renal crisis, which generally occurs with dcSSc within the first 5 years of disease onset. In high-risk patients the incidence may be as high as 20%, and associated with microangiopathic hemolytic anemia, encephalopathy, and convulsions. Mortality may reach 10%. Patients with antibodies against RNA-polymerase III are at highest risk for scleroderma renal crisis. RNA-polymerase III antiboides are found in 25–30% of patients presenting with scleroderma renal crisis.
- A more insidious pattern of renal involvement is also reported in which there is a slow decline in glomerular filtration rate accompanied by proteinuria. This is very uncommon, but probably reflects a more benign vascular and fibrotic process.
- Hypertension should be treated with angiotensin-converting enzyme inhibitors (ACE-I) and calcium-channel blockers.
- Dialysis or renal transplant may become necessary. It is important to know that considerable recovery of renal function can be made after an acute crisis and that decisions involving renal transplantation should be withheld for at least 1 year.
- Corticosteroids are known to increase the risk of renal crisis in dcSSc. Doses >15 mg daily should be avoided.
- Other associated risks for hypertensive renal crisis include rapidly progressive skin disease, diffuse cutaneous disease, and the presence of antibodies to RNA polymerase III.
- There is no evidence that prophylactic use of ACE inhibitors reduces the risk of renal crisis.

The management of scleroderma renal crisis as an acute rheumatological emergency is discussed in Chapter 22.

Other organ involvement

Table 13.7 summarizes the involvement of other organs in SSc.

Malignancy

It has been suggested that there is an increased incidence of all malignancies in SSc patients. Potential causes include immunosuppressive drug use, increased incidence of cancers in scar tissue, and oncogene overexpression. There is a close temporal relationship in the onset of cancer and scleroderma among patients with antibodies against RNA polymerase III, implying that malignancy may initiate a scleroderma-specific immune response.

Table 13.7 Other organ involvement associated with systemic sclerosis

Organ	Effect	Frequency
Thyroid gland	Spectrum of autoimmune disease. Hypothyroidism common	20–40%
Liver	Primary biliary cirrhosis	3% of lcSSc*
Nervous system	Trigeminal neuralgia	5%
	Carpal tunnel syndrome	3%
	Sensorimotor neuropathy	
	Autonomic neuropathy	
Genital	Cavernosal artery fibrosis causing impotence	Up to 50%

*Antimitochondrial antibodies found in up to 25% of patients with SSc and anticentromere antibodies found in 10–20% of patients with primary biliary cirrhosis.

Antifibrotic and immunosuppressive therapies for systemic sclerosis

- Apart from the specific therapies alluded to in the sections on skin and systemic disease earlier in this chapter, a number of general systemic therapies are under investigation but none have demonstrated marked benefit.
- Currently, no treatment can induce complete remission of the disease. Some therapies can offer partial relief and control of end-organ damage. The evaluation of treatments is extremely difficult given the complexity, heterogeneity, and episodic nature of the disease, as well as the paucity of patients.
- Both antimetabolite and alkylating immunomodulatory agents have been used, particularly in early dcSSc. The majority of these therapies are currently being evaluated in controlled trials (see Table 13.8).
- D-penicillamine was been widely used in the past but a single randomized controlled trial has shown no benefit.
- Novel potential antifibrotic therapies may develop through understanding more about anti cytokine antibodies that block fibroblast activation (e.g., anti-TGFβ, anti-IL6), or by antagonists/gene translocations that influence pre- and post-translational modification of collagen.
- Halofuginone, a type I collagen synthesis inhibitor, has shown beneficial effects in treating scarring and has been used with mixed effect in bleomycin-induced scleroderma. Further work is needed to assess its use in SSc.
- An open label study of minocycline suggests this agent does not work.
- Studies are currently underway looking at the effect of rituximab and tocilizumab in early skin disease that is mainly inflammatory in nature.
- Autologous stem cell transplant has been performed in severe disease, but has a high mortality rate, and the benefit may not be permanent. Its place in treatment strategies needs further research.
- Until definitive data are available, a reasonable approach is to treat patients with severe, active skin involvement with three to six months of oral cyclophosphamide (2mg/kg/day) followed by longer term therapy with mycophenolate mofetil (up to 1.5 g twice daily). Patients with mild, active skin disease may be treated with mycophenolate mofetil alone.

Table 13.8 Antimetabolite and alkylating immunomodulatory agents being evaluated for use in treatment of SSc

Agent	Comment
Cyclophosphamide	Efficacy from trial data on lung fibrosis. Often given with steroids
Mycophenolate	Improvement in skin disease
Methotrexate	Used by some investigators, but controversial
Antithymocyte globulin	Possible benefit in diffuse disease, high morbidity
Pooled gammaglobulin	Limited data
Plasmapheresis	Equivocal and anecdotal
Cyclosporine	Beneficial on skin sclerosis
	Watch for renal crisis
	Reduce dose if on calcium-channel blockers
Chlorambucil	Anecdotal and control trial failed to show superiority over placebo
Plasmapheresis	Equivocal and anecdotal
Photopheresis	Limited data; mixed results

Summary—the approach to systemic sclerosis

Diffuse cutaneous systemic sclerosis

History and physical examination generally establishes the diagnosis and autoantibody profiles may identify poor prognosis. The extent of visceral disease should be assessed by baseline investigations as follows:

- Basic metabolic profile
- Creatinine clearance and urinary protein (repeat annually)
- Barium swallow/GI endoscopy depending on symptoms
- Lung function tests, including DLCO (annually)
- Electrocardiogram (annually)
- Doppler echocardiography (with estimate of pulmonary artery pressure) (repeat annually)
- Chest radiograph at baseline; if lung function is abnormal, this should be replaced by a high-resolution CT of the chest, repeated annually.
- Given the paucity of patients, it is important to be aware of local or national centers of expertise and patient suitability for clinical trials.

Limited cutaneous systemic sclerosis

By the time of presentation physical signs are usually diagnostic. Investigations are as above and treatment is mostly symptomatic, concentrating on vascular (Raynaud's and pulmonary hypertension) and GI disease, with annual review and appropriate testing.

Prognosis

- SSc has the highest case-specific mortality of any autoimmune rheumatic disease. Estimates of 5 years mortality in scleroderma range from 34–73%. Standardized mortality ratios have been estimated at 3–4 times expected. Logistic regression modeling suggests 3 factors—proteinuria, elevated ESR, and low carbon monoxide diffusion capacity—are >80% accurate at predicting mortality >5 years.
- Patients with renal crisis have been estimated to have a 50% mortality, although the use of ACE inhibitors and renal replacement therapies may have reduced this.
- Anti-topoisomerase and anti-RNA polymerase antibodies have also been associated with SSc-related mortality.
- Advances in the understanding of mechanisms leading to pulmonary hypertension have led to new therapies that, with time, may show significant impact in slowing disease progression.

Scleroderma-like fibrosing disorders

Eosinophilic fasciitis

- This is an uncommon idiopathic condition that is characterized by rapid spread of skin changes over the extremities. Skin initially takes on a "peau d'orange" appearance, which is replaced by induration.
- Like SSc, flexion contractures and Raynaud's phenomenon may be present. Unlike SSc, the epidermis is spared (i.e., superficial wrinkling of the skin is intact) and nailfold capillary microscopy is normal.
- This condition may resolve spontaneously. Otherwise, 70% of cases respond to corticosteroids.
- This condition may be a paraneoplastic phenomenon. It is overrepresented in women and in the hematologic malignancies in this respect. The paraneoplastic condition often fails to respond to steroids and resolves on successful treatment of the underlying malignancy.
- Methotrexate or mycophenolate mofetil may be helpful, but this has not been well studied.

Nephrogenic systemic fibrosis (NSF)

- Also known as nephrogenic fibrosing dermopathy, the current nomenclature reflects the systemic nature of this disease, which can lead to fibrosis in the muscles, myocardium, lungs, kidneys, and testes.
- NSF is characterized by the presence of skin induration, nodular plaques, and flexion contractures in the absence of Raynaud's phenomenon.
- Lesions develop over days to weeks, and initially favor the lower extremities.
- The majority of patients will have end-stage renal disease and a history of exposure to gadolinium-based contrast.
- Histologically, NSF lesions are characterized by collagen bundles surrounded by fibroblast-like epithelioid or stellate cells and mucin deposition, which can extend into the fascia and muscles.
- Response to immunosuppressive agents is disappointing. Early institution of physical therapy to prevent contractures and muscle wasting is important. Pain management may be especially challenging.
- Because of precautions taken by the radiology community, new cases of NSF have become progressively uncommon.

Scleromyxedema

- This is characterized by papular waxy induration of the skin along the forehead (glabella), the neck, and behind the ears.
- Unlike SSc, scleromyxedema may also affect the middle of the back, which is generally spared in scleroderma.
- Scleromyxedema can be associated with esophageal dysmotility and myopathy; case reports have also demonstrated an association with severe neurologic sequelae, including encephalopathy, seizures, coma, and psychosis.
- This condition may respond to intravenous immunoglobulin(0.4 g/kg/day for 5 days).

Scleredema

- Scleredema is a scleroderma-like disorder associated with doughy induration of the skin along the back, neck, face and chest.
- Unlike scleroderma, scleredema typically spares the distal extremities.
- This disorder is generally seen in association with poorly controlled diabetes, monoclonal gammopathy, or following certain infections, such as streptococcal pharyngitis.
- Prognosis depends on the underlying etiology. Scleredema that occurs after infection may resolve spontaneously. Scleredema associated with diabetes may improve with better glucose control.
- For some patients, ultraviolet light therapy (such as UVA-1, PUVA and photopheresis) may be beneficial.

Idiopathic inflammatory myopathies— polymyositis (PM) and dermatomyositis (DM)

Epidemiology and diagnosis

- The idiopathic inflammatory myopathies are characterized by proximal muscle weakness and evidence of autoimmune-mediated muscle breakdown. These disorders include:
  - Polymyositis
  - Dermatomyositis
  - Juvenile dermatomyositis
  - Myositis associated with neoplasia
  - Myositis associated with connective tissue disease
  - Inclusion body myositis
- Polymyositis (PM) and dermatomyositis (DM) are the most common forms of idiopathic inflammatory myopathy, the latter distinguished by the presence of a characteristic rash. Overlap syndromes with other autoimmune rheumatic diseases occur in 15–20% of cases.
- These conditions are rare. PM has an estimated incidence of 2–8 per million. Incidence increases with age and is highest between the ages of 40–65 years. The male to female ratio is 2:1, but is lower in myositis associated with malignancy, and higher during the childbearing years (5:1). A small amount of evidence suggests that the incidence in African-Americans compared to white Caucasians is 3–4:1.
- The uncertainty about etiology makes classification of these conditions difficult. However, a modification of Bohan and Peter's classification (1975) shown in Table 14.1 serves this purpose at present.
- There are a number of secondary causes of myositis and myopathies. These will be discussed later in this chapter.
- The criteria for the diagnosis of PM and DM are shown in Table 14.2.

Table 14.1 Modification of Bohan and Peter's classification of PM and DM

1	Primary idiopathic polymyositis
2	Primary idiopathic dermatomyositis
3	1 or 2 above, with malignancy
4	Juvenile poly(dermato)myositis
5	Overlap syndromes with other autoimmune rheumatic diseases
6	Inclusion-body myositis
7	Rarer myositis:
	granulomatous
	eosinophilic
	focal
	orbital
8	Drug-induced

Table 14.2 Criteria for the diagnosis of poly/dermatomyositis

1	Compatible weakness. Symmetrical proximal muscle weakness developing over weeks or months
2	Elevated serum muscle enzymes, creatine kinase and aldolase
3	Typical electromyographic findings: myopathic potentials (low amplitude, short duration, polyphasic) fibrillation, positive sharp waves, increased insertional activity, complex repetitive discharges
4	Typical muscle biopsy findings
5	Dermatological features of DM: Gottron's papules, involving fingers, elbows, knees, and medial malleoli Heliotrope sign around the eyes Erythematous and/or poikilodermatous rash

Clinical features of PM and DM

Myositis

- Muscle weakness is the main clinical feature in both conditions and is almost universal, tending to develop insidiously over months but occasionally developing with great speed.
- The weakness is usually symmetric and diffuse, involving the proximal muscles of the neck, shoulders, trunk, hips, and thighs; the lower limb muscles tending to be clinically symptomatic first.
- Weakness of the distal muscles is rare but can occur late in the disease. The face and ocular muscles may also be involved.
- Shortness of breath may be a consequence of diaphragmatic and intercostal muscle weakness (as well as other causes that will be discussed later), and should be looked for.
- Myalgias occur in about 50% of cases; they are usually mild and sometimes difficult to distinguish from polymyalgia rheumatica.
- There may be atrophy in chronic disease, more so in PM than DM, and contractures may occur in disease of long duration.
- Often the distinction between an autoimmune rheumatic disease overlapping with PM/DM versus an autoimmune rheumatic disease with myositis as a manifestation can be very difficult. The relative severity of clinical symptoms and the serological picture may be of help.

Cutaneous disease

- The rash of DM commonly precedes the weakness by weeks to months. The rash may parallel the weakness or remain independent, persisting after the myositis resolves. Erythematous or violaceous papules or plaques (Gottron's papules) or macular patches (Gottron's sign) may occur over the metacarpophalangeal and proximal (occasionally distal) interphalangeal joints. Occasionally these lesions may be found on the extensor surfaces of the knees, wrists, elbows, or medial malleoli. The rash is present in up to 80% of cases.
- A macular eruption may involve the upper chest, neck, shoulders, extremities, face, and scalp. This may develop into poikiloderma, hyper- or hypopigmentation with atrophy and telangiectasia. Typical features include the "V" sign at the base of the neck anteriorly, and the "shawl" sign at the back of the neck and across the shoulders.
- The heliotrope rash, found in 30–60% of cases, is a purple/lilac colored suffusion around the eyes, often associated with periorbital edema. It is characteristic but not pathognomic.
- Some patients have typical cutaneous DM but do not develop overt myositis. The term *amyopathic DM* is applied. The same risk of malignancy and systemic complications remains.
- Calcinosis, cutaneous vasculitis, and ulceration, rare in adults, are more common in juvenile DM.

Malignancy

- Studies suggest a modest increase in malignancies within 1–2 years of onset in DM. The malignancy may predate, predate, or postdate the onset of myositis. In the majority of cases, cancer and myositis have an independent course.
- The largest population studies suggest the presence of malignancy to occur in 15% of cases of DM (relative risk in men 2.4, in women 3.4) and 9% of cases of PM (relative risk in men 1.8, and in women1.7). Cancer deaths in studies suggest an increase in DM but not PM, supporting a true association with DM, rather than a study bias due to intensive searching. The highest risk appears to be in men older than 45 years with DM who lack myositis autoantibodies or overlap autoimmune rheumatic disease.
- Tumors frequent in the general population are frequent in PM and DM. There does, however, appear to be an increase in ovarian, breast, lung, stomach, colon, and bladder cancers out of proportion to that of other tumors.
- The extent of investigation is controversial. Thorough physical assessment should always include rectal, pelvic, and breast examination. Specific investigations should include a chest radiograph, urinalysis, prostate-specific antigen in men, fecal occult blood testing, mammography, and cervical smear, and probably pelvic ultrasound and CA 125 levels in women. Further bowel investigations are open to debate and determined by individual patient symptoms. Remember that an elevated ALT may be from muscle and may not indicate liver pathology.
- Malignancy manifesting as paraneoplastic myopathy and its investigation is discussed in Chapter 4.

Systemic manifestations

Table 14.3 shows the systemic manifestations of PM and DM.

Assessment of disease activity and damage

- There is a need to be able to accurately assess disease activity and damage using valid and reliable instruments, as has been developed in systemic lupus erythematosus.
- A disease activity measure might contain the following information:
  - muscle strength measure (e.g., time required to rise from a chair 10 times without using one's arms)
  - patient and physician global disease activity visual analog scale
  - laboratory tests results
  - physical function measures (Health Assessment Questionnaire)
  - patient quality of life measures (e.g., Short Form-36).
- A damage score should contain information on damage to different organs.
- Several activity and damage measures are currently being validated, but no widely-accepted instruments currently exist.

Table 14.3 Systemic manifestations of PM and DM

Organ/system	Features
General	Fatigue, malaise, weight loss
	Fevers—in 40% overall
	Raynaud's phenomenon
Pulmonary	Due to muscle weakness: aspiration pneumonia, respiratory failure (low TLC, VC, high RV)*
	Due to local disease: interstitial fibrosis (20%), pulmonary vasculitis (rare), pulmonary hypertension (rare)
	Due to treatment: hypersensitivity pneumonitis, opportunistic infection
Gastrointestinal	Esophageal dysphagia—in 30%
	Striated muscle dysfunction
	Cricopharyngeal dysfunction
	Low esophageal dysfunction
	Stomach and bowel dysmotility†
Cardiac	Cardiomyopathy—<5%
	Pericardial effusion—up to 20%
	Heart block—rare
	Dysrhythmias—uncommon
Skeletal	Arthropathy
	Deformity, mild erosive arthritis
Renal	Very rare. Possible myoglobinuria

* TLC = total lung capacity; VC = vital capacity; RV = residual volume.

† Intestinal vasculitis, perforation, and pneumatosis cystoides intestinalis, features of juvenile DM, are very rare in the adult.

Investigation of PM and DM

The investigation of potential malignancy in DM has been discussed earlier in this chapter. Specific investigations for PM/DM include the following:

Muscle enzyme levels

- Serum levels of enzymes released from damaged muscle may be helpful both in diagnosis and monitoring of the disease; creatine kinase (CK) is most widely used, although aldolase may be a more sensitive test of muscle turnover.
- There are a number of causes of a high CK level (see Table 14.4), and levels, particularly in DM, may not be increased despite active myositis and may be influenced partly by muscle bulk, i.e., chronic muscle atrophy. The latter is difficult to assess since measures of muscle mass do not necessarily correlate well with degree of inflammation. Tests that measure muscle mass are not currently practical for clinical use.

Muscle biopsy

- All patients should have a muscle biopsy to confirm the diagnosis and to exclude conditions that may resemble inflammatory myositis.
- There is an argument for not doing so in the patient with proximal weakness, elevated enzymes, typical EMG changes, a rash of DM, confirmed myositis-specific autoantibodies, or an overlap autoimmune rheumatic disease and myositis-associated autoantibodies. For most patients, however, it is important to remember that the mimics are more common than the inflammatory myopathies themselves.
- Patients with a clinical diagnosis of PM/DM who do not respond to treatment as expected may benefit from a biopsy in order to confirm a diagnosis.
- A needle biopsy may be adequate in some cases. However, an open biopsy gives the best picture of muscle architecture and is required for certain functional enzyme studies.
  - *Dermatomyositis*: perivascular inflammatory infiltrate (B lymphocytes, CD4 T lymphocytes) with capillaritis
  - *Polymyositis*: intramuscular inflammatory infiltrate (CD8+ T lymphocytes) with muscle fiber degeneration and replacement with fat
  - *Inclusion body myositis*: basophilic intracellular vacuoles ("inclusion bodies")
- Optimal processing and evaluation, minimizing risk of artifact, requires coordination with the pathologist prior to the biopsy taking place.

Table 14.4 The causes of a raised creatine kinase

Cause	Examples
Strenuous prolonged exercise	
Muscle trauma	
Diseases affecting muscle	Myositis
	Metabolic
	Dystrophy
	Myocardial infarction
	Rhabdomyolysis
Drugs	Toxic myopathy
	Induction of myositis
	Inhibition of CK excretion (barbiturates, morphine, diazepam)
Metabolic abnormalities	Hypothyroidism
	Hypokalemia
	Ketoacidosis
	Renal failure
Normal variants	Ethnic group (often higher normal values in the African-American population)
	Increased muscle mass
	Technical artifact

Autoantibodies in myositis

- A high antinuclear antibody (ANA) and myositis-specific autoantibodies (MSA) favor PM/DM over other myopathies. The various associations with autoantibodies are shown in Table 14.5.
- A modest correlation with anti-Jo-1 antibodies is observed but the usefulness of titers as an index of disease activity is not established.
- Other MSA have been identified, but are not widely available.
- Antisynthetase antibodies (such as anti-Jo-1) are associated with interstitial lung disease, arthritis, Raynaud's phenomenon, and "mechanic's hands" (i.e., dry, cracked skin across the digits)
- Anti-SRP antibodies herald an acute-onset, severe illness, often with little evidence of inflammation on biopsy. These patients require aggressive immunosuppression.

Electromyography

- Electromyography (EMG) and nerve conduction studies cannot establish the diagnosis of PM/DM with certainty, but can demonstrate a myopathic process and help to exclude many other neuropathies and certain myopathies (Table 14.6 gives the differential diagnoses of myopathy and Table 14.7 lists drug-induced myopathies in more detail).
- 90% of patients will have abnormal EMG studies.
- Early findings include low-amplitude, short-duration, polyphasic potentials, with early recruitment and full interference patterns (i.e., more fibers are required to achieve a given force). The latter features are in contrast to neuropathies where there is decreased recruitment and interference. With time, reinnervation of denervated fibers leads to high-amplitude, long-duration, polyphasic potentials.
- Other features include spontaneous activity in up to 75% of cases, fibrillations, and repetitive discharges akin to myotonia but of constant amplitude that start and stop abruptly.

Imaging

- Magnetic resonance imaging (MRI), ultrasound, computed tomography, ^{99}Tc and thallium have been used to assess the distribution of disease.
- MRI with T2-weighted images and fat suppression or short tau inversion recovery (STIR) is best at identifying areas of muscle inflammation, atrophy, or fatty infiltration.
- On MRI, active myositis results in the appearance of muscle edema. When evaluating a patient for weakness, MRI may be particularly useful in distinguishing weakness due to active inflammation from weakness due to previous damage or glucocorticoid myopathy (which would not be expected to show muscle edema).
- Because involvement of muscles may be patchy, MRI may also help identify an optimal site for muscle biopsy.

Table 14.5 Antibodies in PM/DM

Antibody class	Antibody subclass	Percentage of PM/DM	Myositis subgroup
Myositis-specific:		In total 30–40	
Anticytoplasmic	Anti-Jo-1	20	Antisynthetase syndrome
	Anti-PL-7/ PL-12/OJ/EJ	<3 each	
	Anti-SRP	4	PM
Antinuclear	Anti-Mi-2	8	DM
	Anti-56 kDa	90	All
Myositis-associated:	Anti-PM-Scl	8	PM/ DM–scleroderma overlap
	Anti-U1-RNP	12	PM/DM overlap syndromes
	Anti-U2/ U5-RNP	<2	PM
	Anti-Ro and Anti-La	5–10	Systemic lupus. Sjögren's syndrome

Table 14.6 The differential diagnosis of myopathy

Agent	Examples
Infectious diseases:	
Viral	Retroviruses
	Picornaviruses
	Adenoviruses
	Influenza
	Hepatitis B and C
Bacterial	Pyomyositis
	Lyme myositis
	Tuberculosis
Protozoa	Toxoplasmosis
	Trypanosomiasis
Parasites	Trichinosis
	Cysticercosis
Fungal	Candida
Idiopathic:	
Inclusion body myositis	
Autoimmune rheumatic disease	
Other disorders	Granulomatous myositis
	Eosinophilic myositis
	Focal/orbital myositis
Other myopathies:	Dystrophies and congenital myopathies
	Enzyme deficiencies and lipid storage disorders
	Carcinomatosis
	Rhabdomyolysis
	Neurological: motor neuron disease, myasthenia gravis, Guillain–Barré syndrome
	Endocrine: hypo/hyperthyroidism, cortisol excess
	Metabolic: hypocalcaemia, hypokalemia
	Malnutrition
	Drugs

Table 14.7 Drug-induced myopathy

Clinical picture	Examples
Drugs implicated in autoimmune myopathy	D-penicillamine
	Cimetidine
	L-tryptophan
	Zidovudine
Myopathy with weakness, myalgia, and high CK	Colchicine
	Hydroxychloroquine
	Lipid-lowering agents
	Cyclosporine
	Vincristine
	Carbimazole, propylthiouracil
	Alcohol
	NSAIDs—rare in aspirin
Rhabdomyolysis picture	Alcohol
	Illicit drugs—cocaine, heroin
	Amphetamines
	Barbiturates
	Statins (particularly high dose)
	Anesthetics—malignant hyperthermia
	Psychotropics—neuroleptic-malignant syndrome

Other tests

- The ESR is elevated in 50% of cases but correlates poorly with disease activity and response to therapy. The CRP is not specific; high levels would suggest a concurrent infection.
- Complement levels in PM/DM are usually normal.
- Proteinuria may be the result of myoglobinuria.
- Serial spirometry for respiratory muscle weakness may be required.

Treatment of PM and DM

- Treatment should be started promptly pending completion of investigations, particularly in acute onset weakness, dysphagia, respiratory insufficiency, and systemic complications.
- Corticosteroids form the cornerstone of therapy, and 90% of patients will have at least a partial response.
- Most patients, however, will also require treatment with a steroid-sparing agent to maintain disease remission and to minimize corticosteroid-exposure.
- There is a lack of randomized placebo-controlled trials for the treatment of PM and DM.
- An exercise program helps improve fatigue and muscle strength. Exercise should be used with caution during periods of disease activity, but there is no evidence that it causes prolonged worsening in muscle enzyme levels or inflammation.

Corticosteroids

- Oral prednisone at 1 mg/kg/day is continued until a decline in CK and/or a substantial improvement in muscle strength is seen. Severe cases (or extraskeletal involvement) may be treated with IV methylprednisolone 1 g/day for 3 days before starting oral prednisone. High doses may be required for months and a bisphosphonate should be considered early as prophylaxis against steroid-induced osteoporosis. Adequate calcium and vitamin D intake should always be maintained.
- Most patients will respond to treatment, but this can be slow and partial. The CK is often seen to change faster than any apparent improvement in strength. Failure to respond may be due to one of several reasons:
  - incorrect diagnosis
  - hereditary myopathy or 'inclusion-body' myositis
  - steroid myopathy
  - permanent loss of strength
  - unresponsive to steroid therapy.
- When the initial goals have been reached, the dose of steroid should be tapered gradually over a 6-month period.

Immunosuppressive agents

- Methotrexate (MTX) and azathioprine (AZA) have demonstrable efficacy in retrospective analysis and, in the case of AZA, a controlled study.
  - MTX 10–25 mg by mouth or 15–50 mg subcutaneously per week
  - AZA 2–3 mg/kg/day
- AZA may be a better option for patients with interstitial lung disease or hepatitis, but may take longer to show effectiveness. Studies have shown a synergistic effect of MTX and AZA where a single drug has failed. The reader is referred to Chapter 5 for discussion on the monitoring of disease-modifying drugs.
- Cyclosporine is a useful therapy in patients where MTX and AZA have been ineffective or not tolerated. It has been used in combination with MTX or IV gammaglobulin.

- Cyclophosphamide has had variable results and is used in resistant cases or in those cases where there is severe extraskeletal involvement such as vasculitis or lung disease.
- Tacrolimus has been used in refractory patients with synthetase syndromes, with improvement in muscle strength, lung function, and cutaneous manifestations. It can be given as an ointment.
- Mycophenolate mofetil (MMF) and chlorambucil are also used.
- There are several reports of improvements in clinical and laboratory measures in patients with refractory PM/DM after receiving infliximab or etanercept. Further work needs to be done in this area.
- In open label studies, rituximab has been used in refractory DM with clinical improvement.
- Monoclonal antibodies against complement component C5 (eculizumab) are also being used in the treatment of DM.

Intravenous gammaglobulin (IVIg)

- IVIg is obtained from healthy donor serum and contains a large antibody pool. There is increasing evidence of the efficacy of this treatment in both PM and DM. High-dose regimens in the form of 2 g/kg/day for 2–5 days each month have been advocated. However, the effectiveness of each treatment is of limited duration (6–8 weeks), tapering and maintenance regimens are empirical and tachyphylaxis may occur. It can be used safely in immunocompromised patients and there are no reports of transmission of infectious diseases. Further studies are needed to refine the place and optimum treatment dose.

Treatment of extramuscular disease in PM/DM

- The rash of DM may respond to the treatment of the myositis. If lesions persist, hydroxychloroquine at 200–400 mg/day or topical tacrolimus may be of benefit. Photosensitivity can respond to sunscreens. Topical steroids are often not successful.
- The treatment of amyopathic DM is controversial. Sunscreens and hydroxychloroquine can be used and in some severe cases steroids or immunosuppressives are justified for the cutaneous disease. If treatment is withheld due to an absence of myositis, the patient should be followed closely, especially in the first 2 years after onset, to avoid delay in treatment should myositis develop.
- Calcinosis, principally a problem in juvenile disease, is difficult to treat.Treatment of the disease may help to prevent calcinosis, but it does not affect established calcinosis. Inflammation may respond to colchicine and surgical resection may help for accessible deposits.
- Physical therapy and passive exercises help prevent contractures, though active exercise is discouraged in the acute period of muscle inflammation.
- Interstitial lung disease is managed as in other autoimmune rheumatic disease, with oral steroids and oral or IV cyclophosphamide.
- Distal esophageal dysmotility does not generally respond to immunosuppression, but measures similar to treatment of reflux may help.

Drug-induced myopathy

- Table 13.7 lists the drugs that commonly cause a myopathy.
- Recently most attention has been given to HMG-CoA reductase inhibitors (statins) used in lipid-reduction therapy. These drugs are widely prescribed; atorvastatin is the most commonly prescribed drug in the US. In large-scale trials, myalgias have been noted in 11% of patients and significant myositis with elevated CK levels in 0.5%. Myalgias and cramp are the most common symptoms reported, and may be exacerbated by the use of other drugs (cyclosporine and fibrates) or other diseases (hypothyroidism). Patients presenting with muscular symptoms should have their muscle enzyme levels checked and the drug stopped or reduced in dose. Some patients will progress to develop a necrotizing myopathy (see below).

Prognosis in PM and DM

- PM and DM are diseases with a high mortality and morbidity. One retrospective study estimated a mortality rate of 22%, mostly due to malignancy and pulmonary disease.
- The use of prolonged immunosuppressive therapy increases the risk of infection, which may be with unusual organisms. Case reports have described atypical mycobacterial infections in patients with long-standing PM/DM.
- A worse prognosis is associated with increasing age, bulbar muscle, and cardiopulmonary involvement.

Inclusion-body myositis (IBM)

- This is a distinct disorder that comprises 20–30% of idiopathic myositis. It usually begins after the age of 50 years and is three times more common in men. The difficulty in distinguishing it from PM and its insidious onset can lead to considerable delay in diagnosis.
- Early in the disease course, there is a significant inflammatory component that may partially respond to glucocorticoids.
- Distal weakness and wasting can be as common as proximal, often involving the lower limbs before the upper, and sparing the face.
- Unlike PM/DM, IBM can present with diminished hand-grip strength, in addition to proximal muscle weakness.
- Dysphagia is a feature in 40% of cases and myalgias in 20%.
- An open biopsy (as opposed to needle biopsy) is essential to diagnose IBM. A needle biopsy may not be sufficient to allow the recognition of important clues that point away from other forms of myositis.
- Patients do not respond to treatment as well as do those with PM. Immunosuppression may lead to reduction in muscle enzyme levels without improvement in strength or function.
- Treatment usually begins with high-dose corticosteroid for 3 months, adding in MTX or AZA if there is clinical improvement. If there is continued decline in strength or function, immunosuppression should be discontinued.
- Weakness will progress in most patients but this is often very slow. Patients may need assistance with daily activities within 10 years and some may be wheelchair bound within 15 years of onset of symptoms.
- Interferon β may be efficacious for the treatment of inclusion-body myositis.

Necrotizing myopathy

- A rapidly progressive, symmetric, necrotizing myopathy has been described as a paraneoplastic phenomenon. Unlike polymyositis, this form of myopathy is associated with prominent muscle necrosis but little or no inflammatory infiltrate. Although the severity of this myopathy does not mirror tumor progression, the cornerstone of therapy is treatment of the underlying malignancy.
- A second form of necrotizing myopathy has been described in patients with antibodies to HMG-CoA reductase, particularly among patients who have been treated with statins. Unlike polymyositis, patients with this form of myopathy often have minimal weakness. This form of myopathy is responsive to immunosuppression, but is prone to relapse.

PM and DM in children

- The primary clinical feature of both juvenile DM (JDM) and PM (JPM) is chronic, progressive, proximal muscle weakness. Fulfillment of the criteria of Bohan and Peter is needed to establish the diagnosis (see Table 14.8). In addition to the rash, 3 of the other 4 criteria need to be met for DM. These criteria need to be revised in children because biopsies and electromyography are now rarely done as they are invasive painful procedures. MR is increasingly used to define inflammatory changes and to guide biopsies if done.
- Incidence values for JDM and JPM range form 2.5–5 per million.
- The childhood peak for the disease is 5–9 years of age and JDM is 10–20 times more common than JPM.
- Children of African or Asian origin may be at increased risk of chronic myositis. In the United States, Caucasian children with DM are reported more frequently, with a male to female ratio of 2:1. In the United Kingdom, Ireland, and China the ratio is in the order of 5:1.
- JDM is a systemic disease, most commonly affecting the gut, lungs, and nervous system. This is thought to be due to vasculitis that is more marked than in adult disease.
- Antinuclear antibodies are seen in 20–70% of cases of JDM/JPM. Myositis-associated antibodies seen in adult disease (Jo-1) are rarely seen in childhood disease.
- The increased frequency of malignancy seen in adults with DM within two years of onset of disease is not seen in childhood DM or PM.
- Several agents have been associated with the onset of juvenile DM, which may also explain some temporal, seasonal, and regional differences in disease onset. The most prominent agents to date have been RNA picornaviruses, group A β-hemolytic streptococci, and *Toxoplasma gondii*. The true pathogenesis of juvenile DM in relation to infectious agents remains unclear.
- HLA associations include B8 and DRB1.
- TNF-α promoter polymorphisms have also been implicated in pathogenesis.
- In general the clinical features of juvenile DM/PM are similar to adult disease. Fever, abdominal pain, dysphagia, dyspnea and peripheral arthritis are seen. Skin ulceration is seen in 20% of patients and can be severe and disabling. Lipodystrophy is a recognized skin finding. Calcinosis is more common in childhood (10–30% of patients) and the outcome of this ranges from spontaneous resolution to chronic deposition and flexion contractures. Calcinosis is difficult to treat and causes long-term morbidity.
- Rapid disease control is important to help prevent damage. IV or oral corticosteroids are first line, followed by MTX.
- JDM in particular benefits from early and aggressive therapy, which may prevent calcinosis and other complications:
  - Methylprednisolone 30 mg/kg/dose (up to a maximum of 2g) twice weekly for one month
  - Prednisone 2 mg/kg/day
  - Intravenous immunoglobulin 2g/kg administered in divided doses over 5 days

Table 14.8 Bohan and Peter's criteria for the diagnosis of juvenile DM/PM

Feature	DM	PM
Characteristic rash	Yes	No
Symmetrical proximal muscle weakness in the absence of other rheumatic/endocrine disease	Yes	Yes
Elevated muscle enzymes	Yes	Yes
Muscle histopathology	Yes	Yes
Electromyographic changes of inflammation	Yes	Yes

- Other treatments that have been used include IV immunoglobulin and cyclosporine A. Cyclophosphamide is used for severe multisystem disease.
- Infliximab and IV bisphosphonates have shown some effect on muscle disease and calcinosis. Rituximab and autologous stem cell transplantation have been used in a small number of cases.
- Early physiotherapy and muscle strengthening is vital, and evidence suggests that this does not affect the inflammatory process.
- Disease activity and damage measures are now being used and validated, as in adult disease.

Primary vasculitides

Introduction

- The vasculitides are a heterogeneous group of relatively uncommon diseases that can arise as primary conditions or secondary to an established disease such as RA (see Chapter 5) or SLE (see Chapter 10).
- The vasculitides are linked by the presence of vascular inflammation, which can lead to one of two common outcomes:
  - *Vessel wall destruction*, leading to aneurysm or rupture
  - *Stenosis*, leading to tissue ischemia and necrosis
- In 1990, the American College of Rheumatology developed a classification system based on vessel size, with the inclusion of a division between primary and secondary vasculitis (see Table 15.1).
- In 1994, the Chapel Hill Consensus Conference (CHCC) developed a standard nomenclature for the primary systemic vasculitides based on clinical and laboratory features, and categorized by vessel size:
  - Large vessel: Aorta and its major branches ("great vessels")
  - Medium vessel: Main visceral arteries (e.g., renal, mesenteric)
  - Small vessel: Capillaries, arterioles, and venules
- In 2012, the second Chapel Hill Consensus Conference recognized two additional categories of vasculitis:
  - Variable vessel vasculitis: Vasculitides that can affect any caliber blood vessel
  - Single organ vasculitis: Vasculitides that are inherently restricted to a single organ (as opposed to a very limited presentation of a systemic vasculitis).
- The 2012 Chapel Hill Consensus Conference also adopted a new nomenclature that de-emphasizes the use of eponyms:
  - Granulomatosis with polyangiitis (GPA) for Wegener's granulomatosis (WG)
  - Eosinophilic granulomatosis with polyangiitis (EGPA) for the Churg-Strauss Syndrome (CSS)
- ANCA (see below) is helpful to define a subset of the small vessel vasculitides that have a predilection for the respiratory tract and kidneys. These "ANCA-associated vasculitides" include granulomatosis with polyangiitis, microscopic polyangiitis, and eosinophilic granulomatosis with polyangiitis.
- This classification system is not perfect:
  - Patients with "large vessel vasculitis" and "small vessel vasculitis" can have disease that affects some medium-sized vessels.
  - Not all patients with "ANCA-associated vasculitis" have detectable levels of ANCA.
- This is still a useful framework for the clinician, however, since categorizing the patient into one of these groups can narrow the differential diagnosis considerably.

Antineutrophil cytoplasmic antibody (ANCA)

- ANCA exist in 2 main forms:
  - Cytoplasmic (C-ANCA): caused by antibodies against proteinase-3 (PR3-ANCA), and is generally associated with granulomatosis with polyangiitis (Wegener's granulomatosis)
  - Perinuclear (P-ANCA): caused by antibodies against myeloperoxidase (MPO-ANCA), and is generally associated with microscopic polyangiitis and eosinophilic granulomatosis with polyangiitis (the Churg-Strauss Syndrome)
- Other ANCA-staining patterns (i.e., noncytoplasmic, nonperinuclear) can occur; moreover, the P-ANCA pattern may be caused by antibodies against antigens other than myeloperoxidase. These are sometimes referred to as "atypical ANCA," and do not predict the presence of vasculitis, although they can be found in Crohn's disease, immune-mediated neutropenia, and other autoimmune diseases.
- Counterintuitively, patients with "ANCA-associated vasculitis" can be ANCA-negative in up to 50% of cases. Therefore, the absence of ANCA does not completely exclude the diagnosis of an ANCA-associated vasculitis.
- Patients with active, untreated disease, however, are more likely to be ANCA-positive.
- The exact role that ANCA may play in the pathogenesis of vasculitis is still incompletely undersootod.

Disease and damage assessment

- To be complete, any description of a chronic disease (such as primary systemic vasculitis) must include both a description of disease activity and a description of disease damage.
- The concept of damage denotes the aspects of disease that are unlikely to reverse with immunosuppression (such as pulmonary fibrosis or renal insufficiency).
- Clinical trials of vasculitis commonly use the **Birmingham Vasculitis Activity Score** (BVAS) and **Vasculitis Damage Index** (VDI) to assess activity and damage, respectively.
- These instruments are most helpful for the assessment of the small- and medium-vessel vasculitides.
- Other clinical indices exist. The French Vasculitis Study Group (FVSG) has developed a prognostic **Five Factor Score** (FFS), which was revised in 2008 to include the following elements:
  - Age > 65,
  - Renal insufficiency (i.e., serum creatinine ≥1.7 mg/dL),
  - Cardiac involvement,
  - Gastrointestinal manifestations
  - ENT manifestations (for patients with granulomatosis with polyangiitis (Wegener's granulomatosis) only).
- Each of the first 4 items is worth 1 point. ENT manifestations in patients with granulomatosis with polyangiitis (Wegener's granulomatosis) are associated with decreased mortality; therefore, if present, 1 point is subtracted from the total score (so the maximum FFS for any given patient is 4, not 5).

Table 15.1 A classification of systemic vasculitis

Dominant vessel	Primary disorders	Secondary disorders
Large arteries	Giant cell arteritis. Takayasu's	Aortitis in ankylosing spondylitis. Syphilitic aortitis
Medium arteries	Classic polyarteritis nodosa. Kawasaki disease	Infection, e.g., hepatitis B. Hairy cell leukemia
ANCA-associated (small/medium vessels)	Granulomatosis with polyangiitis (Wegener's granulomatosis). Eosinophilic granulomatosis with polyangiitis (Churg–Strauss syndrome). Microscopic polyangiitis	Vasculitis secondary to autoimmune disease. Malignancy. Drugs. Infection, e.g., HIV
Small vessels (leukocytoclastic)	Henoch–Schönlein purpura. Essential mixedcryoglobulinemia	Drugs. Malignancy. Infection, e.g., hepatitis B/C
Variable vessel	Behçet's disease, Cogan syndrome	
Single organ	Primary CNS vasculitis, cutaneous angiitis	

- The FFS is associated with the 5-year mortality of patients with ANCA-associated vasculitis and polyarteritis nodosa:
  - FFS=0 is associated with a 5-year mortality of 7.5%.
  - FFS=1 is associated with a 5-year mortality of 20%
  - FFS>1 is associated with a 5-year mortality of 47%

Large-vessel vasculitis

- The "large vessels" include the aorta and its main branches (i.e., the subclavian, axillary, carotid, and brachiocephalic arteries). Primary and secondary forms of large vessel vasculitis are shown in Table 15.2.
- The classic forms of primary large vessel vasculitis are Takayasu's arteritis and giant cell arteritis.
- Because of the overlap in symptoms, polymyalgia rheumatica is often discussed with the large vessel vasculitides, as if it were a *forme fruste* of giant cell arteritis. Recent studies demonstrate, however, that it is probably more appropriate to think of polymyalgia rheumatica as a syndrome comprised of bursitis, tenosynovitis, and synovitis that is frequently associated with giant cell arteritis.
- The clinical manifestations of large-vessel vasculitis can be predicted by the pattern of vessel involvement.
  - Arch aortitis leads to aneurysmal dilatation and aortic regurgitation.
  - Subclavian involvement causes arm claudication and diminished upper extremity pulses on examination.
  - Carotid involvement may lead to visual loss, jaw claudication, and stroke.
  - Involvement of any major blood vessel may cause bruits of physical examination.
- Unfortunately, a large vessel vasculitis may not be suspected until one of the above events has occurred.

Table 15.2 The causes of large-vessel vasculitis

Primary	Takayasu's arteritis
	Giant cell arteritis*
Secondary†	Infection: bacterial, fungal, mycobacterial, spirochetal
	Rheumatoid arthritis
	Seronegative spondyloarthropathy
	Systemic lupus erythematosus
	Sarcoidosis
	Relapsing polychondritis
	Juvenile chronic arthritis

* Giant cell arteritis is discussed in this chapter in the section on polymyalgia rheumatica.

† The secondary forms of large-vessel vasculitis are considerably less common that the primary forms; these are discussed in their respective sections.

Takayasu's arteritis

- Takayasu's arteritis (TA) is a chronic granulomatous arteritis that affects the aorta and the great vessels. The pulmonary arteries can also be involved, although this is relatively uncommon.
- It is most common in Japan, Southeast Asia, India, and Mexico. In the United States, its annual incidence is estimated at 2.6 per million.
- TA tends to affect women (90% of cases), with adolescents and young adults between 20–40 years at greatest risk. Classification criteria distinguish TA from giant cell arteritis (GCA) by age at onset (i.e., TA <40 years, GCA >50 years).
- Importantly, TA is not limited to patients of Asian descent; the majority of patients in the United States are white.
- The hallmark of the disease is arteritic inflammatory infiltrates that cause luminal narrowing or occlusion; clinically, this presents with bruits, claudication, and diminished (or asymmetric) pulses.
  - Lightheadedness, visual disturbance, and strokes can occur. **Subclavian steal** (i.e., dizziness caused by retrograde vertebral artery flow) can be an important cause of neurologic symptoms.
  - **Hypertension** may develop as a consequence of (ostial) renal artery stenosis.
  - **Musculoskeletal symptoms**, including arthralgias and myalgias, are not uncommon.
  - **Cardiovascular complications** are an important cause of morbidity, and include aortic insufficiency, congestive heart failure, systemic hypertension, and ostial involvement of the coronary arteries.
- Traditionally, the diagnosis of TA has depended on angiography to demonstrate the characteristic changes of arterial dilatation, thrombosis, and aneurysm formation.
  - **Conventional angiography** has the added benefit of allowing a comparison between central and peripheral blood pressures; because subclavian stenosis is a common consequence of this disease, a standard brachial (arm cuff) blood pressure reading may underestimate central hypertension.
  - **Magnetic resonance imaging/angiography** (MRI/MRA) has excellent resolution at the level of the large vessels, and may be the technique of choice for some patients. MR can also demonstrate evidence of vessel wall inflammation, which could support a diagnosis of TA.
  - **High-resolution ultrasonography** is sensitive for detecting carotid lesions. Ultrasonography has also been used to identify the presence of temporal arteritis among patients with giant cell arteritis (due to the "hypoechoic halo" that forms around the inflamed artery), although this is not routinely used in the United States due to widespread lack of expertise.
  - **PET scanning** is useful to diagnose the presence of a large vessel vasculitis when more conventional technologies fail to demonstrate luminal abnormalities. That said, it is not clear whether it can be used to monitor response to therapy.

Treatment

- Initial medical treatment is with corticosteroids (prednisone 1 mg/kg/day).
- Most patients should also be treated with methotrexate 20–25 mg po/SQ weekly
- Resistant or severe cases may be treated with a TNF-α inhibitor (e.g., infliximab 5mg/kg IV q 4 weeks) or cyclophosphamide 2mg/kg/day po.
- Hypertension can be difficult to manage, and may require angioplasty or surgery to address renal artery stenosis.
- Surgical management ranges from angioplasty to bypass procedures.
  - These are best performed during the inactive phase of disease.
  - Angioplasty is often a temporizing measure, and lesions tend to restenose over time
  - When intervention is required, surgical bypass is the treatment of choice.
  - Overall operative mortality is 4%, associated mostly with aneurysm rupture.
- The prognosis depends mainly on the presence of hypertension and aortic incompetence. The majority of patients (75%) will have some impairment of daily living, and 50% are permanently disabled.
- Mortality is low, 5- and 10-year survival rates reported as 80% and 90%, respectively.
- TA is not a contraindication to pregnancy. Cytotoxic agents should be stopped and steroids kept to as low a dose as possible. Obstetric decisions can be made on their own merits and not because of coexistence of TA. The main complications are exacerbation of hypertension and congestive cardiac failure. The anesthesiologist should be made aware of the diagnosis, as the patient may require invasive blood pressure monitoring during delivery.

Polymyalgia rheumatica and giant cell arteritis

Polymyalgia rheumatica (PMR)

- The diagnosis of PMR is based essentially on clinical symptoms and signs. The criteria of Jones and Hazleman (1981) are succinct and practical (see Table 15.3).
- In 2012, the American College of Rheumatology and the European League Against Rheumatism proposed new classification criteria for PMR. Using the new criteria, a patient 50 years old (or older) with bilateral shoulder pain may be classified as having PMR in the presence of morning stiffness, new hip symptoms, and elevated acute phase reactants (see Table 15.4).
- There may be apparent muscle weakness on testing, which is due to pain rather than intrinsic muscle disease.
- PMR is rare in patients <50 years old; the mean age of onset is 70. Prevalence among patients older than 50 years is 1 in 133, and women are affected more than men (ratio 2:1). There is also a higher frequency of diagnosis in northern latitudes.
- Parainfluenza, parvovirus B19, *Mycoplasma pneumoniae* and *Chlamydia pneumoniae* infections have been shown to have a temporal relation to incidence peaks of PMR, although other studies have found no relationship.
- HLA DRB1*04 and DRB*01 are associated with disease susceptibility.
- Symptoms may start asymmetrically but soon become bilateral.
- Systemic features of malaise, weight loss, low-grade fever, and depression are common.
- Arthralgias and synovitis may occur. Up to 5% of patients with RA (see Chapter 5) have an initial PMR-like presentation.
- Pathological features of PMR are minor and include synovitis with a CD4+ T-cell infiltrate similar to that seen in giant cell arteritis (GCA) (see text below).
- The lack of specific clinical features, a specific laboratory test, and the presence of several conditions that can present with PMR-like symptoms, makes this a diagnosis of exclusion (see Table 15.5).
- Failure to respond to standard doses of corticosteroids after a few weeks should trigger an aggressive evaluation for occult malignancy.
- PMR and GCA have a close clinical relationship, although the reason for this is not clear. One-half of patients with GCA have symptoms of PMR and up to 20% of patients with PMR have histological or clinical evidence of GCA. The pathogenesis for both conditions is not known.

Giant cell arteritis (GCA) (Table 15.6)

- GCA is a granulomatous arteritis of the aorta and larger vessels, with a predilection for the extracranial branches of the carotid artery. It is the most common form of primary systemic vasculitis in the United States; the annual incidence is estimated at 18 per 100,000.
- Like PMR, the female to male ratio is 2:1

Table 15.3 Criteria for the diagnosis of PMR

1.	Shoulder and pelvic girdle pain which is primarily muscular in the absence of true muscle weakness
2.	Morning stiffness
3.	Duration of at least 2 months (unless treated)
4.	ESR >30 mm/h or CRP >6 mg/ml
5.	Absence of inflammatory arthritis or malignancy
6.	Absence of muscle disease
7.	Prompt and dramatic response to corticosteroids

Jones JG and Hazeleman BL. The prognosis and management of polymyalgia rheumatica. Annals of Rheumatic Diseases, 1981; 40: 1–5. Reprinted with permission of BMJ Publishing Group, Ltd.

Table 15.4 2012 ACR/EULAR Criteria for the Classification of PMR

A score of 4 or more is required to classify a patient as having PMR if the following criteria are met: (1) ≥50 years old; (2) bilateral shoulder aching; (3) elevated ESR/CRP

1.	Morning stiffness duration >45 minutes	2 points
2.	Hip pain or limited range of motion	1 point
3.	Absence of RF or ACPA	2 points
4.	Absence of other joint involvement	1 point

Dasgupta B *et al.* 2012 provisional classification criteria for polymyalgia rheumatica: a European League Against Rheumatism/American College of Rheumatology collaborative initiative. *Ann Rheum Dis* 2012; 71: 484–92.

Table 15.5 Conditions that can mimic polymyalgia rheumatica

1.	Rheumatic disease in the elderly, including rheumatoid arthritis and systemic lupus erythematosus
2.	Inflammatory myopathy
3.	Hypo/hyperthyroidism
4.	Carcinoma, myeloma
5.	Chronic sepsis
6.	Bilateral shoulder capsulitis
7.	Osteoarthritis
8.	Depression
9.	Parkinsonism

- Infectious and genetic associations are also similar to PMR with evidence of disease "clustering."
- GCA is rare among African Americans.
- Severe headache and scalp tenderness localized to the occiput or temporal area are common initial symptoms, and are present in 70% of cases. The temporal artery can be swollen, tender, and pulseless. Scalp necrosis has also been reported.
- Large arteries are affected in 15% of cases, leading to claudication, bruits, absent neck and arm pulses, and thoracic aorta aneurysm and dissection. Asymptomatic large-vessel abnormalities, present on imaging studies, are considerably more common.
- Visual disturbance is usually an early finding. Patients may complain of amaurosis fugax, but visual loss due to retinal ischemia may be irreversible within hours. Diplopia and ptosis may also be seen.
- Fundoscopy may show optic disc pallor, hemorrhages, and exudates. Optic atrophy is a late finding.
- Arteritic anterior ischemic optic neuropathy is the most common ophthalmologic finding, and must be differentiated from nonarteritic anterior ischemic optic neuropathy, an idiopathic cause of painless visual loss that does not respond to steroids.
- Jaw, arm, and tongue claudication are other common sinister features.

Table 15.6 Diagnostic criteria for GCA

Diagnostic scheme	Criteria
Jones and Hazleman (1981)	Positive temporal artery biopsy or cranial artery tenderness
	One or more of: visual disturbance, headache, jaw pain, cerebrovascular insufficiency
	ESR > 30 mm/h or CRP > 6 mg/ml
	Response to corticosteroids
American College of Rheumatology	Three or more of:
	Age at onset >50 years
	New headache
	Temporal artery tenderness or decreased pulsation
	ESR over 50 mm/h
	Abnormal artery biopsies showing necrotizing arteritis with mononuclear infiltrate or granulomatous inflammation usually with multinucleated giant cells

Jones JG and Hazleman BL. The prognosis and management of polymyalgia rheumatica. Annals of Rheumatic Diseases, 1981; 40: 1–5. Reprinted with permission of BMJ Publishing Group, Ltd.

- Malaise, fatigue, weight loss, fever, and anemia are common.
- Tongue claudication and dry cough are less common manifestations.
- The ESR and CRP are characteristically elevated, but can be normal in up to 5% cases.
- Patients suspected of having giant cell arteritis should be evaluated with bilateral temporal artery biopsies, taking segments of 1.5 cm each. Treatment should not be delayed; biopsies may be helpful to confirm the diagnosis up to two weeks after treatment with steroids was initiated.
- Unlike most forms of vasculitis, GCA does not cause fibrinoid necrosis; the presence of fibrinoid necrosis on a temporal artery biopsy should prompt a search for another form of vasculitis, such as granulomatosis with polyangiitis (Wegener's granulomatosis), microscopic polyangiitis, or cryoglobulinemic vasculitis.
- Even following this protocol, temporal artery biopsies may be negative in up to 12% of patients with GCA. A negative temporal artery biopsy does not exclude this diagnosis.
- Doppler ultrasound and (more recently) MR have both been studied as possible substitutes for temporal artery biopsy, although this is not common practice in the United States. Ultrasound in particular is operator-dependent, and it may be difficult to find someone with the appropriate expertise to evaluate a patient for GCA.
- Similarly, PET is useful in showing abnormal metabolic activity in the aorta of many patients with GCA, but this is most useful to establish the initial diagnosis. It has not been validated to follow response to therapy.

Treatment of PMR and GCA

- Both conditions require corticosteroid treatment; however, the amount and duration of treatment required are quite different.
- PMR responds dramatically to low dose corticosteroids (e.g., prednisone 10–20 mg daily) within 24 hours; many patients will report substantial relief within hours after their first dose. After treatment for 2–4 weeks, the prednisone dose may be decreased by 2.5 mg every 2 weeks until the patient reaches a maintenance dose of 10 mg/day. Prednisone may subsequently be tapered in 1 mg increments.
- GCA requires treatment with high-dose steroids (e.g., prednisone 1 mg/kg/day, up to 80 mg daily), and the patient may take a week or longer to experience substantial relief. After treatment for 1 month, prednisone may be gradually tapered over 12 months.
- Some studies have demonstrated the efficacy of MTX as a steroid-sparing agent for both GCA and PMR. A recent meta-analysis of trials in GCA indicates that the use of adjunctive MTX lowers the risk of relapse and cumulative corticosteroid dose, although the benefit is very modest. Although MTX for the treatment of GCA and PMR is not standard, it is worth considering for some patients.

- The treatment of GCA requires a few additional considerations:
  - Patients with visual symptoms associated with GCA should be treated with intravenous pulse methylprednisolone therapy (1 g daily for 3 days) prior to initiating therapy with prednisone
  - Daily low-dose (e.g., 81 mg) aspirin may prevent cranial ischemic events such as stroke and blindness, and should be considered if there is no contraindication.

Polyarteritis nodosa

- Polyarteritis nodosa (PAN) is a necrotizing vasculitis of medium-sized arteries, leading to cutaneous ulcers, kidney infarction, mesenteric angina, and mononeuritis multiplex.
- Mesenteric angina (i.e., abdominal pain 1 hour after eating) may be a late manifestation of splanchnic vasculitis, which may present as diarrhea due to hypoperfusion of the intestines.
- Some cases of PAN have been linked to infection with hepatitis B. Patients with PAN should be screened for viral hepatitis, since these patients may require antiviral therapy in addition to immunosuppression.
- The Chapel Hill Consensus Conference created a distinction between "classic" PAN (i.e., an ANCA-negative, medium-vessel vasculitis associated with renal infarcts) and microscopic polyarteritis nodosa (i.e., an ANCA-positive, medium- and small-vessel vasculitis characterized by glomerulonephritis). This re-classification (and the hepatitis B vaccine) have made PAN increasingly uncommon.
- "Classic" PAN should further be distinguished from cutaneous polyarteritis nodosa, which presents with large, painful ulcerations of the lower extremities in the absence of internal organ involvement, and therefore is associated with a much lower mortality rate.
- The clinical features are shown in Table 14.8.
  - Patients often present with nonspecific features of systemic disease including myalgias, arthralgias, weight loss, and fever.
  - About 50% of cases develop a vasculitic rash, often with "punched out" ulcers in the lower extremities.
  - GI and renal involvement is common; 50% in both cases. Non-specific abdominal pain, gut/gallbladder infarction, and pancreatitis are all features.
  - Renal disease usually appears in the form of renal infarct. Renal impairment is often mild and present in around 20% of cases.
  - Isolated organ involvement is rare, but disease affecting the skin, testes, epididymis, breasts, uterus, appendix, and gallbladder has been reported.

Treatment and prognosis in all the small- and medium-vessel vasculitides is discussed at the end of this section.

Granulomatosis with polyangiitis (Wegener's granulomatosis)

- Granulomatosis with polyangiitis (GPA)is the most prevalent of the so-called ANCA-associated vasculitides (AAV), a group of diagnoses that includes microscopic polyangiitis and eosinophilic granulomatosis with polyangiitis (EGPA; the Churg-Strauss syndrome).
- Renal-limited vasculitis and drug-induced ANCA-associated vasculitis are less-common members of this group.
- GPA is a worldwide disease with a variable incidence of 4–9 per million. GPA is slightly more common in men than women, and most often appears in the fourth and fifth decades (see Table 15.7).
- Classically, GPA is described as a clinical triad, with manifestations affecting the upper respiratory tract, lower respiratory tract, and kidneys. However, patients may present with a wide range of clinical manifestations.
  - Some patients may have an indolent presentation characterized by respiratory tract involvement, such as sinusitis and pulmonary nodules.
  - Others may have a more fulminant presentation, including rapidly progressive glomerulonephritis and pulmonary hemorrhage.
- Different treatment strategies for these manifestations are discussed below.

The clinical features of GPA

Ear, nose, and throat
- Up to 90% of patients have ear, nose, and throat involvement.
- Chronic sinusitis is a common initial presentation for GPA, and many patients will have been treated with several courses of antibiotics before the correct diagnosis is reached.
- Other manifestations include nasal septal perforation, bloody nasal discharge ("crusts"), and nasal bridge collapse due to erosion of underlying cartilage ("saddle nose").
- Patients may also complain of diminished hearing, either due to sensorineural hearing loss or Eustachian tube dysfunction.
- Subglottic stenosis is a classic feature of GPA, and may present with hoarseness and stridor. Subglottic stenosis may worsen even when a patient is otherwise in remission, and responds better to localized therapy (i.e., direct steroid injections) than systemic therapy.
- In the oral cavity and oropharynx inflammation can lead to mucosal ulcers or gingivitis ("strawberry gums")
- It is thought that *Staphylococcus aureus* has a role in disease pathogenesis. Nasal carriage in GPA patients is 3 times that of healthy populations. The exact mechanisms leading to disease are unclear, but trimethoprim/sulfamethoxazole may benefit patients with WG by eliminating *S. aureus* colonization.

Table 15.7 Modified American College of Rheumatology 1990 classification criteria of granulomatosis with polyangiitis (Wegener's)—diagnosis requires 2 or more of the following:

1.	Nasal or oral inflammation: Development of painful or painless oral ulcers or purulent or bloody nasal discharge
2.	Abnormal chest radiograph: The chest radiograph may show nodules, cavities, or infiltrate
3.	Urinary sediment: Microscopic hematuria or red cell casts
4.	Histological changes of granulomatous inflammation on biopsy
5.	PR3-ANCA (C-ANCA) positivity

Pulmonary disease

- 80% of cases have pulmonary disease.
- The classic pulmonary manifestation is cavitary parenchymal lesions, mimicking infection or malignancy.
- The tracheobronchial tree may be locally involved before any signs of generalized disease. Subglottic pseudotumors and/or stenosis cause stridor or dyspnea. Lower bronchial stenosis may cause atelectasis and obstructive pneumonia. Multiple nodules with or without cavitation may be found in the lungs of asymptomatic patients.
- Severe pulmonary disease is associated with alveolar capillaritis, hemorrhage, and hemoptysis, with ground glass infiltrates on computed tomography (CT). The radiograph typically shows an alveolar or mixed alveolar–interstitial pattern; the appearance may mimic pulmonary edema and focal infection.

Renal disease

- Up to 90% of patients with generalized ("severe") GPA have renal involvement.
- Renal involvement can range from milder focal and segmental glomerulonephritis (GN) to fulminant diffuse necrotizing (rapidly progressive) and crescentic GN, which may rapidly lead to end stage renal disease.
- The milder form of the condition is not common, manifesting in the asymptomatic patient as a nephritic picture of microscopic hematuria, active sediment, and mild renal impairment.

Skin disease

- 40% of cases have skin disease.
- Features include palpable purpura due to a leukocytoclastic vasculitis, necrotic papules ("Churg-Strauss nodules"), livedo reticularis, and pyoderma gangrenosum.

Musculoskeletal symptoms
- Musculoskeletal symptoms are observed in 60% of cases.
- Symptoms can range from mild myalgias (in 50% of the cases) and arthralgias to overt arthritis. 20–30% of rheumatic symptoms may be related to a nonerosive and nondeforming polyarthropathy.
- Migratory arthralgias are a classic presentation for WG.

Nervous system
- About one-third of patients with GPA have involvement of the nervous system. Mononeuritis multiplex and distal sensorimotor polyneuropathy are the main lesions. Seizures and cerebritis are much less frequent events.
- Disseminated granulomatous lesions ("pachymeningitis") can spread to the retropharyngeal area and skull base with involvement of cranial nerves I, II, III, VI, VII, and VIII; pachymeningitis can also be associated with diabetes insipidus and meningitis.

Eye disease
- Granulomatous lesions may obstruct the nasolacrimal duct and cause orbital pseudotumor, with optic nerve compression from masses developing in the retrobulbar space. Rarely a purulent sinusitis may spread and cause secondary bacterial orbital infection.
- Manifestations in the generalized stage of GPA include scleritis, episcleritis (red eye), vasculitis of the optic nerve, and occlusion of retinal arteries, in addition to the granulomatous lesions described above.

Investigation of GPA
- Laboratory investigation should include ANCA, CBC with differential, routine chemistries, ESR, CRP, and urinalysis to look for an active sediment.
- Not all patients with GPA will be ANCA-positive; a negative ANCA test does not necessarily exclude this diagnosis.
- When suspicion of kidney disease exists, renal biopsy may be useful to confirm a diagnosis of GPA, and may provide prognostic information as well.
- Sinus biopsies confirm a diagnosis of GPA in only 33% of cases; biopsy often shows nonspecific evidence of inflammation, and is most useful to exclude concomitant infection or malignancy.
- Pulmonary nodules are often asymptomatic; a patient diagnosed with GPA should undergo some form of chest imaging, regardless of symptoms.

Treatment and prognosis of GPA is discussed with the other AAV, below.

Other forms of AAV: microscopic polyangiitis (MPA) and eosinophilic granulomatosis with polyangiitis (EGPA)

Microscopic polyangiitis (MPA)

- MPA is classified as a pulmonary-renal (hemorrhage) syndrome, a group that also includes Goodpasture's disease and systemic lupus erythematosus. GPA and cryoglobulinemic vasculitis may also present as a pulmonary-renal syndrome.
- MPA lacks the granulomatous manifestations characteristic of WG, such as sinus disease, subglottic stenosis, and pulmonary nodules.
- Unlike GPA, MPA is characterized by MPO-ANCA antibodies, which are associated with a P-ANCA staining pattern. Up to 80% of patients with MPA will be ANCA-positive.
- Like PAN, the male:female ratio is 2:1, with the majority of patients being Caucasian. The mean age of presentation is 50 years.
- Most patients with MPA will present with renal involvement in the form of a necrotizing glomerulonephritis, similar to what can be seen with GPA. Unlike most forms of vasculitis, glomerulonephritis from AAV is "pauci-immune" (i.e., there is only minimal immunoglobulin deposition on immunofluorescence stains).
- Pulmonary hemorrhage presents as hemoptysis, and can be surprisingly subtle in some patients. Although classically described as a life-threatening manifestation, younger patients may be minimally symptomatic. Bronchoscopy with bronchoalveolar lavage will demonstrate hemosiderin-laden macrophages. Chronic pulmonary capillaritis may eventually lead to pulmonary fibrosis.
- Other clinical features of the disease are shown in Table 15.8.

Eosinophilic granulomatosis with polyangiitis (EGPA; Churg–Strauss syndrome)

- This condition is often described as a clinical triad of adult-onset asthma, eosinophilia, and vasculitis.
- Typically, the asthma gradually worsens in intensity until the patient requires daily oral steroids for symptom control. Many of these patients will have been treated with a leukotriene inhibitor (although leukotriene inhibitors do not cause the disease).
- Peripheral blood hypereosinophilia is typically mild, and resolves quickly upon treatment with oral corticosteroids.
- Other manifestations of hypereosinophilia include "fleeting" pulmonary infiltrates, myocarditis, and interstitial nephritis; frank glomerulonephritis is much less common in this diagnosis.
- Nerve involvement is a common manifestation of vasculitis among patients with the CSS, and patients should be examined for evidence of a sensory neuropathy or mononeuritis multiplex.

Table 15.8 Clinical features at presentation (as % of cases) in classic polyarteritis nodosa, microscopic polyangiitis, and eosinophilic granulomatosis with polyangiitis (Churg–Strauss syndrome)

Clinical feature	Polyarteritis nodosa	Microscopic polyangiitis	EGPA
Renal impairment	25%	90%	50%
Pulmonary disease	40%	50%	General 50%, asthma 100%
Fever	60%	40%	
Skin vasculitis	40%	50%	50%
Gastrointestinal disease	45%	20%	60%
Cardiovascular disease	15%	20%	45%
Peripheral neuropathy	10%	10%	60%
Ear, nose, and throat	10%	20%	
Ocular disease	10%	20%	

- Classically, it is said that the asthmatic component improves dramatically after the onset of the vasculitis, although this is often not the case.
- Cutaneous granulomas that form along the elbows and fingers are called "Churg-Strauss nodules"; ironically, they appear more commonly in association with GPA.

ANCA-associated vasculitis: treatment and prognosis

The AAV are approached using the same treatment strategy, which consists of a *remission induction* phase and a *remission maintenance* phase.

Remission induction

- In the United States, it is standard to use a modified National Institutes of Health protocol for the treatment of "severe" systemic vasculitis (i.e., vasculitis that threatens life or the function of a vital organ): oral cyclophosphamide (CYC) 2mg/kg/day (1.5 mg/kg/day in the elderly or in patients with renal insufficiency) for 6 months, followed by an antimetabolite steroid sparing agent (MTX, AZA) for 1 year or longer.
- Rituximab 375 mg/m^2 IV weekly for four weeks has been approved by the US Food and Drug Administration for the treatment of granulomatosis with polyangiitis (Wegener's granulomatosis) and microscopic polyangiitis, and may also be effective for the vasculitic manifestations of eosinophilic granulomatosis with polyangiitis

(the Churg-Strauss syndrome). Patients should be premedicated with methylprednisolone 60–125 mg IV prior to each infusion.
- Prednisone 1mg/kg/day (up to 80 mg/day) for the first month is used in conjunction with cyclophosphamide or rituximab. Patients with rapidly progressive disease may benefit from initial treatment with methylprednisolone 1 g IV daily for 3 days.
- Pulse IV CYC (15 mg/kg IV every 2 weeks for 6 weeks, then every 3 weeks for 6 months) is as effective as oral CYC for remission induction, but is associated with a higher risk of relapse.
- Patients with renal failure due to glomerulonephritis or pulmonary hemorrhage may also benefit from plasmapheresis.
- Patients with mild disease may be treated with oral MTX 20–25 mg weekly and prednisone 0.5 mg/kg/day for remission induction.
- Patients receiving CYC should also receive trimethoprim/sulfamethoxazole for prophylaxis against *P. jiroveci* pneumonia (PCP). Patients receiving chronic steroids should receive osteoporosis prophylaxis.

Remission maintenance
- Once remission has been achieved with CYC, a less toxic drug may be used for remission maintenance. MTX and AZA (1.5–2.0 mg/kg/day) are both standard remission-maintenance drugs, but mycophenolate mofetil (2–3 g/day) and leflunomide (20–30 mg/day) may also have a role in the treatment of some patients.
- Patients should receive remission maintenance therapy for at least 1–2 years, or longer in patients with a history of relapsing disease.
- There are limited data supporting the use of rituximab 500 mg every 6 months for remission maintenance. This strategy may be particularly useful for patients who have previously failed other remission-maintenance strategies.

Other treatments
- Among patients with renal failure due to ANCA-associated vasculitis, plasmapheresis improves short-term renal survival, but does not improve long-term renal survival or overall mortality.
- IV immunoglobulin (0.4 g/kg/day for 5 days) may be used for remission induction in patients at high risk of systemic infection.
- Anecdotal reports have shown the benefit of infliximab in combination with methotrexate or cyclophosphamide for treatment of resistant vasculitis, although this is highly controversial in the United States, and has fallen out of favor. Case series demonstrate some efficacy in patients with refractory disease, but in exchange for a high risk of infectious complications
- There is evidence that respiratory tract infections may trigger a relapse of GPA. Trimethoprim-sulfamethoxazole in patients with stable disease on maintenance therapy may decrease respiratory infection, and is also useful for prevention of PCP among patients treated with CYC.

Other vasculitides
- Most other forms of vasculitis are treated by analogy to the ANCA-associated vasculitides, with severe forms being treated with cyclophosphamide and high dose glucocorticoids (e.g., prednisone

1 mg/kg/day), and milder forms treated with methotrexate, azathioprine, or other anti-metabolites, in addition to lower dose glucocorticoids (e.g., prednisone 0.5 mg/kg/day).

- The major exception to this rule is giant cell arteritis, which is typically treated with glucocorticoids alone.
- Treatment of a vasculitis associated with an infectious disease (e.g., hepatitis B-associated PAN, hepatitis C-associated cryoglobulinemic vasculitis) should always include treatment of the underlying pathogen whenever possible.

Prognosis

Prior to the introduction of cyclophosphamide and steroids, mortality associated with generalized AAV approached 100%. Modern immunosuppressive regimens have transformed these diseases into chronic conditions, characterized by cycles of relapse and remission. For many patients, the consequences of treatment (such as steroid-associated complications) may lead to greater morbidity than the underlying disease itself. Mortality due to infection continues to be an important consideration for patients treated for AAV; indeed, patients with "treatment resistant" AAV should be carefully evaluated for the presence of *Nocardia*, *Aspergillus*, and other infections that can mimic some of the manifestations of the AAV.

Small-vessel and single organ vasculitis

The definition of small vessel vasculitis is open to different interpretations. Small vessel disease can be one feature of granulomatosis with polyangiitis (Wegener's granulomatosis), microscopic polyangiitis, and eosinophilic granulomatosis with polyangiitis (the Churg–Strauss syndrome). However, there are a range of clinical and pathological features that define a specific group of small-vessel vasculitides outlined in Table 15.9. Patients who have a small-vessel vasculitis restricted to the skin who do not have evidence of a systemic vasculitis (or another rheumatic diseaes) are now thought of as having a "single organ vasculitis".

Leukocytoclastic vasculitis

- Histologically, leukocytoclastic vasculitis appears as a neutrophilic infiltrate in and around small vessels, with fragmentation of the neutrophils (leukocytoclasis), fibrin deposition, and endothelial cell necrosis. Immune complex deposition appears to be important in pathogenesis.
- Small-vessel vasculitis usually presents in the skin, although the microvasculature of any tissue may be affected, especially joints or kidneys.
- Some forms of cutaneous vasculitis are predominantly lymphocytic, without evidence of neutrophils or leukocytoclasis. However, the division into leukocytoclastic and non-leukocytoclastic (lymphocytic) vasculitis is not absolute. Likewise, the clinical presentation of cutaneous vasculitis can vary considerably.
- The finding of leukocytoclasis should prompt a thorough review of drug treatment (e.g., sulfonamides, penicillin, thiazides), a search for infection (hepatitis B, human immunodeficiency virus, B -hemolytic streptococcus), a screen for autoimmune rheumatic disease, malignancy (in particular myelo- and lymphoproliferative diseases), inflammatory bowel disease, chronic active hepatitis, and cryoglobulinemic vasculitis (see below).

Allergic (hypersensitivity) vasculitis

- Allergic vasculitis is the most common pattern of presentation in adults, both sexes being affected equally.
- Nonblanching hemorrhagic papules (palpable purpura), purpuric macules, plaques, pustules, bullae, and ulcers may occur, classically distributed maximally over the lower leg.
- A low-grade fever, arthralgias, and microscopic hematuria may accompany such presentation.
- Often the condition is self-limiting and identifiable causes should be managed as appropriate. Analgesia may be needed and systemic steroids may be required for acute organ disease, especially progressive renal impairment.
- Dapsone (100 mg po daily), hydroxychloroquine (400 mg po daily), or colchicine (0.6 mg po twice daily) may help decrease the frequency or severity of manifestations in some patients.
- AZA (2 mg/kg/day) may be appropriate for refractory disease, but removal of the offending drug or exposure is the most effective treatment strategy.

Table 15.9 Conditions associated with small-vessel vasculitis

Leukocytoclastic vasculitis	Allergic vasculitis (hypersensitivity angiitis): drugs, infection, inflammation, autoimmune disease, malignancy, Henoch–Schönlein purpura
	Urticarial vasculitis (hypocomplementemic vasculitis)
	Cryoglobulinemic vasculitis
	Hypergammaglobulinemia
	Erythema elevatum diutinum and granuloma faciale
Non-leukocytoclastic vasculitis	Drugs (penicillins, thiazides)
	Nodular vasculitis (see 'panniculitis')
(Lymphocytic vasculitis)	Livedo vasculitis
	Pityriasis lichenoides

Henoch-Schönlein purpura

- This tends to be regarded as a special form of allergic vasculitis. It occurs most often in children but can affect young adults as well.
- IgA is usually detected in skin, gut, or renal biopsies. If suspected, one should request direct immunofluorescence (DIF) in advance, since this requires special processing of the biopsy.
- The classic presentation is with purpura, arthritis (50%), hemorrhagic GI disease (40%), and glomerulonephritis (50%).
- Corticosteroids given early may relieve joint and GI symptoms but there is little evidence that they prevent progression of renal disease or influence overall outcome. If renal function is rapidly deteriorating, pulsed methylprednisolone and/or plasmapheresis may be of benefit.
- Patients who present with a nephritic or nephrotic syndrome have an increased lifetime prevalence of renal complications, including hypertension.
- Although most cases are self-limited, this can (rarely) become a chronic, relapsing disease. Such patients should be evaluated for the presence of a monoclonal IgA antibody, which may herald a pre-malignant lesion, and is often refractory to therapy.

Urticarial vasculitis

- Urticarial lesions with arthralgias are the most common features of this condition, with men outnumbering women 2:1. The typical age of onset is 40–50 years.
- Morphologically, the skin lesions resemble ordinary urticaria and sometimes may be mistaken for erythema multiforme. Unlike ordinary urticaria, the lesions of urticarial vasculitis tend to last for days (not hours) and tend to be burning and painful (not pruritic).
- Patients are generally classified as having **normocomplementemic** or **hypocomplementemic** urticarial vasculitis, with the latter being more frequently associated with systemic complaints.

- Patients with hypocomplementemic urticarial vasculitis tend to develop more systemic features such as renal, GI, and pulmonary disease. Less common manifestations include lymphadenopathy, uveitis, and benign intracranial hypertension. These patients are often ANA positive, and some may evolve into SLE.
- Systemic antihistamines are widely used but tend to be disappointing. Several antihistamines used in combination at higher-than-normal doses may be needed to see a clinical response.
- There are anecdotal reports of success with indomethacin, hydroxychloroquine, colchicine, cyclosporine, and dapsone. AZA (2.0–2.5 mg/kg/day) or sulfasalazine (1g po twice daily) may be particularly effective.
- For the majority of patients, the condition is chronic and benign. The normocomplementemic form of urticarial vasculitis may be self-limited in some patients. For those with end-organ damage, chronic immunosuppression may be necessary.

Cryoglobulinemic vasculitis

- Cryoglobulins are immunoglobulins that precipitate when cold. They are divided into three types: type I (monoclonal), type II (mixed monoclonal and polyclonal), and type III (polyclonal).
- Mixed cryoglobulins are associated with autoimmune rheumatic diseases, infection, and lymphoproliferative disorders. Hepatitis B and C viral infection should always be excluded; the latter in particular is strongly associated with mixed essential cryoglobulinemia.
- Cryoglobulins are commonly present in patients with hepatitis C, and do not mandate immunosuppressive therapy in the asymptomatic patient.
- Mixed essential cryoglobulinemic vasculitis presents with purpuric skin lesions showing a leukocytoclastic vasculitis on biopsy; polyarthralgias (70%), weakness, progressive renal disease (55%), and transaminitis (70%) are common. Women are affected as twice as frequently as men.
- Less common problems include edema, hypertension, leg ulcers, Raynaud's phenomenon, abdominal pain, neuropathy, glomerulonephritis, and pulmonary capillaritis (hemorrhage).
- The prognosis is worse with renal disease; the main causes of death among patients with cryoglobulinemic vasculitis include renal failure and infection.
- Treatment requires management of the underlying cause; immunosuppression by itself is frequently unsatisfactory. Choice of immunosuppression should be dictated by the disease manifestations; the most severe forms may require treatment with cyclophosphamide, pulse steroids, and plasmapheresis. Rituximab may also be effective, particularly for patients with hepatitis C-associated cryoglobulinemic vasculitis who cannot be treated with antiviral agents, but relapse after cessation of therapy is common.

Hypergammaglobulinemic purpura

- This is a rare, benign IgM condition presenting as long-standing leukocytoclastic purpura similar to the cutaneous features of Sjögren's syndrome (see Chapter 12).

- It should not be confused with Waldenström's macroglobulinemia, a monoclonal IgM paraproteinemia associated with lymphoma.

Erythema elevatum diutinum (EED) and granuloma faciale (GF)

- These are rare but distinctive forms of chronic localized leukocytoclastic vasculitis. There is no systemic involvement and the etiology is unknown.
- EED is characterized by slowly enlarging edematous purplish-brown plaques or blisters over the backs of the hands, elbows, or knees. They heal very slowly (months to years) with fibrosis. It may respond to dapsone.
- GF presents as single or multiple pink-brown, well-defined, smooth papules and plaques on the face. They persist for years. It is distinguished histologically from EED by the presence of eosinophils and a normal collagen beneath the epidermis. It may respond to intralesional steroids.

Nonleukocytoclastic (lymphocytic) vasculitis

- The differential diagnosis of nodular forms of cutaneous vasculitis embraces a wide range of disorders, including the panniculitides (see Chapter 18).
- **Erythema induratum** (nodular vasculitis) is regarded as a distinct group characterized by recurrent subcutaneous nodules usually found on the legs of young to middle-aged women. Erythema induratum is more likely to present on the posterior aspect of the legs than is erythema nodosum, which tends to appear on the anterior aspect. Patients are otherwise healthy. Streptococcal infection may be found. The term "Bazin's disease" is sometimes used to describe the nodular vasculitis that can occur in association with tuberculosis. The condition often resolves spontaneously but may take many years. Intralesional triamcinolone or dapsone (100 mg po daily) may help.
- **Livedoid vasculopathy** is characterized histologically by endothelial proliferation and intraluminal thrombosis leading to ischemic damage. Patients typically present with painful ulcerations of the lower extremities. Livedoid vasculopathy has been attributed to elevated levels of plasminogen activator inhibitor-1. Similar lesions can be seen in the antiphospholipid syndrome, so a diagnosis should not be made based on the appearance of the lesions alone. The lesions heal with white atrophic scar ("atrophie blanche"). Pressure stockings, subcutaneous heparin, and assiduous wound care may all help with the resolution of the active lesions.
- **Pityriasis lichenoides** is a uncommon disorder of pink papules which enlarge rapidly and may become hemorrhagic before becoming necrotic and heal with scarring. It is usually self-limiting and may respond to ultraviolet B irradiation.

Kawasaki disease

- This is a febrile, acute vasculitic illness of childhood. It is probably more common than rheumatic fever as the cause for rheumatic heart disease in children <5 years of age and is associated with coronary artery aneurysms, myocarditis and myocardial infarction. Other organs involved include liver, pancreas, and kidney.
- It is seen most often in Japanese Americans with a peak prevalence age of 18 months to 2 years, and is more common in males, ratio 5:1.
- Fever is usually present for >5 days and associated with conjunctivitis, erythema, and edema (skin, lips, and pharyngeal), and lymphadenopathy. Joint inflammation may also occur during the acute phase.
- Myocarditis may appear early but arterial aneurysm formation appears later, its risk of occurring increases after longer periods of being febrile (14–16 days).
- There are no specific blood tests. Acute phase markers are usually high and cultures negative.
- An ECG and echocardiogram may show conduction defects and myocardial inflammation, respectively.
- Treatment should start with IVIG (2 g/kg) administered over 8–12 hours and aspirin (80–100 mg/kg/day, divided into 4 doses). Patients who fail to respond may benefit from re-treatment with IVIG, or pulse methylprednisolone therapy. The role of plasmapheresis and anti-TNF-α therapy is less clear.
- For further information, the reader is referred to the 2004 Scientific Statement from the American Heart Association on the diagnosis and management of Kawasaki's disease.[1]

---

[1] Newburger JW et al. Diagnosis, Treatment, and Long Term Management of Kawaski Disease. *Circulation*, 2004; 110: 2747–71.

Metabolic bone diseases and disorders of collagen

Osteoporosis

- Osteoporosis can be defined as a decrease in bone mass and strength resulting in an increased risk of fracture. Unlike osteomalacia, the ratio of matrix to mineral deposit in bone is normal in osteoporosis.
- The World Health Organization defines osteoporosis on the basis of bone density compared to the mean bone density for a young adult; this is known as a T-score. *Osteopenia* refers to bone mineral density (BMD) that falls 1.0–2.5 standard deviations (SD) below the BMD of a young adult. *Osteoporosis* is used if the BMD falls more than 2.5 SD below the BMD of a young adult.
- The risk of osteoporotic fracture is greater in women than in men; in both sexes, risk of fracture varies with site (see Table 16.1).
- The age-adjusted incidence of hip fractures has been increasing steadily. The Centers for Disease Control and Prevention note that 345,000 hip fractures occur annually in the United States, and the incidence increases with age. The annual incidence of a hip fracture in a 65-year-old woman in the United States is 1.6 per 1,000. Recent estimates places the cost of in-patient and community care at $8 billion.

Pathogenesis and classification (see Table 16.2)

- During childhood and adolescence, growth and modeling lead to an increase in the size, shape, strength, and composition of bone. Growth ceases with the closure of the growth plates (epiphyseal cartilage). However, remodeling and mineral homeostasis continue throughout life with bone resorption and deposition coupled by the interaction between osteoclasts and osteoblasts, respectively.
- Peak bone mass, or maximal bone density, is usually achieved in the third decade. Peak bone mass is determined by both genetic (e.g. vitamin D receptor gene polymorphism, estrogen receptor–cytokine interaction), and environmental factors. Changing lifestyle and behavior patterns have been suggested as a effective ways of increasing peak bone mass.

Table 16.1 Risk of osteoporotic fracture with site

Fracture site	Overall lifetime risk of fracture (%)	
	Men	Women
Hip	6.0	17.5
Vertebral	5.0	15.6
Distal forearm	2.5	16.0
Any of above	13.1	39.7

Table 16.2 Classification of osteoporosis

Major type	Causative factor(s)	Details
Primary (physiological)	Postmenopausal Age-related	
Idiopathic		
Juvenile onset		
Secondary	Endocrine	Hyperparathyroidism
		Hypopituitarism
		Thyrotoxicosis
		Hypogonadism
		Cushing's syndrome
		Insulin-dependentdiabetes
	Drugs	Corticosteroids
		Excess thyroxinereplacement
		Heparin
		Anticonvulsants
		Cyclosporine A
	Hemopoietic	Multiple myeloma
		Lymphoma
		Leukemia
		Mastocytosis
		Gaucher's disease
	Inflammatory diseases	Rheumatoid arthritis
		Ankylosing spondylitis
	Congenital	Osteogenesis imperfecta
	Immobilization	
	Idiopathic hypercalciuria	
	Osteoporosis of pregnancy	

- After the age of 35 (presumably due to declining osteoblast activity), the amount of bone laid down is less than that resorbed during each remodeling cycle sequence. The net effect is an age-related decrease in bone mass. Trabecular and cortical bone mass decline by approximately 6% and 3% per decade, in women and men, respectively.
- Further bone loss occurs at the time of menopause with declining ovarian function and levels of estrogens. Up to 15% of bone mass can be lost over the 5-year period immediately after menopause. A further 15% of bone mass can be lost if vitamin D deficiency coexists.
- The mechanism of age-related bone loss is unknown. Several possibilities exist:
  - Decreased intestinal calcium absorption
  - Decreased synthesis of vitamin D
  - Hyperparathyroidism (caused by the above)
  - Increased osteoblast function
  - Fatty infiltration of the bone marrow, leading to loss of precursor cells and locally generated growth factors.
- Bone mineral density measurement is specific but not sensitive for identifying patients at high risk of fracture. Almost 50% of postmenopausal women over 50 years old who have an osteoporotic fracture do not have osteoporosis based on their T-score. Conversely, treating all patients based on T-score generally overtreats younger women, who may be at low risk of bone fracture despite their T-score.
- To address this shortcoming, the World Health Organization has developed a Fracture Assessment Tool (FRAX) to identify patients at highest risk for osteoporotic fractures. The clinical risk factors identified by FRAX include:
  - Age
  - Sex
  - Prior fragility fracture
  - History of corticosteroid use (≥ 5 mg qd for ≥ 3 months)
  - Parental history of hip fracture
  - Rheumatoid arthritis
  - Secondary osteoporosis (e.g., type 1 diabetes, hypogonadism, premature menopause, chronic malabsorption, longstanding hyperthyroidism)
  - Current smoker
  - Alcohol use of greater than 2 drinks daily
  - Low body mass index.
- The complete FRAX tool is available online at www.shef.ac.uk/FRAX
- Bone mineral density measurement should be considered in any patient with these risk factors, or in any woman older than 65. Because of lack of data, it is difficult to know if older men also benefit from routine screening in the absence of known risk factors for osteoporotic fracture (such as concurrent glucocorticoid use).

Idiopathic osteoporosis

- Idiopathic osteoporosis defines occurrence of the condition in pre-menopausal women or men under the age of 60 years, with no apparent cause. The female: male ratio is 10:1. Most cases are found to have "low bone turnover" with low rates of bone formation. Some cases have "high bone turnover" with hypercalciuria; these cases may respond to antiresorption drugs such as calcitonin and bisphosphonates.

- It is not clear if the majority of patients in this group will benefit from therapy. For most patients with idiopathic osteoporosis, in the absence of other risk factors, the absolute risk of fracture remains low. Anticatabolic (antiresorptive) agents are unlikely to shift the risk of fracture significantly.

Juvenile idiopathic osteoporosis (JIO)

- Juvenile osteoporosis (JIO) is an uncommon disorder that occurs before or at onset of puberty. It affects the sexes equally. The cause is unknown and there are no consistent biochemical abnormalities (see Table 16.3).
- The child presents with pain, nontraumatic fractures around the weight-bearing joints, and collapsed vertebrae. No specific treatment is available and for most, bone mass increases to normal values as puberty progresses; however, in some cases fractures may lead to deformity. Supportive physical therapy should be made available.
- In the same way that height and weight charts are used to assess childhood development, there may be a role for serial bone density measurement in children with known low bone mass, as a surrogate assessment of appropriate development.

Table 16.3 The causes of juvenile idiopathic osteoporosis

Type	Causative factor(s)
Primary	Calcium deficiency
	Idiopathic
	Osteogenesis imperfecta
Secondary	Endocrine (see Table 16.2)
	Intestinal:
	malabsorption
	biliary atresia
	type I glycogen storage disease
	Inborn errors of metabolism—homocystinuria
	Leukemia
	Congenital cyanotic heart disease

Glucocorticoid-induced osteoporosis (GIO)

- GIO is a major concern. Treatment should be offered to all patients taking prednisone for a period likely to be >3 months. The risk is present at doses as low as 2.5 mg daily, although data would suggest it increases considerably for doses > 5mg daily.
- There is conflicting evidence about the effect of inhaled corticosteroid on fracture risk. Patients on maximal doses of inhaled corticosteroids should be assessed for additional risk factors for osteoporosis and may require prophylaxis.
- The pathogenesis of GIO is controversial. Corticosteroids can affect calcium and phosphate metabolism both directly and indirectly in bone, kidney, and the intestine. Possible mechanisms are shown in Table 16.4.

Primary hyperparathyroidism

Primary hyperparathyroidism is a relatively common disorder with an adult prevalence of about 0.2% in the fifth to seventh decades of life. It is three times more common in women than men, due to an increased incidence after the menopause. Mild hyperparathyroidism is often diagnosed after an incidental finding of hypercalcemia on routine blood tests. The management of this condition will be discussed later in this chapter.

Table 16.4 Possible pathogenesis of corticosteroid-induced osteoporosis

Mechanism	Site	Effect
Reduced bone formation	Osteoblasts	Reduced activity
		Reduced recruitment
		Reduced collagen synthesis
		Reduced growth hormone
		Reduced cytokine levels
	Adrenal–testis	Reduced gonadal hormones
Increased bone resorption	Adrenal–testis	Reduced gonadal hormones
	Parathyroid	Increased PTH
	Intestinal	Reduced calcium absorption
		Reduced sensitivity to vitamin D
	Renal	Reduced calcium resorption
	Muscle	Decreased muscle mass

Hypogonadism

- Hypogonadism due to any cause may lead to an increased risk of osteoporotic fracture.
- Causes of amenorrhea include primary ovarian failure, use of estrogen antagonists (e.g., in the management of endometriosis), hyperprolactinemia, anorexia nervosa, and low body mass index (e.g., elite sportswomen).
- Causes of decreased testosterone levels include Klinefelter's syndrome, hypogonadotrophic hypogonadism, hyperprolactinemia, anorexia nervosa, and testicular dysfunction following mumps orchitis.

Hyperthyroidism

Hyperthyroidism leads to osteoporosis as a consequence of high bone turnover, enhanced osteoclast recruitment, and increased bone resorption.

Malignancy

Malignant infiltration and replacement of marrow tissue occurs in multiple myeloma, lymphoma, leukemia, systemic mastocytosis, and diffuse bone metastases. Mechanisms differ, for example:

- Overproduction of osteoclast-activating cytokines (such as IL-1 and TNF) in myeloma.
- Local synthesis of 1,25-hydroxyvitamin D by malignant cells in lymphoma.
- Overproduction of heparin, histamine, and prostaglandins that stimulate osteoclasts in mastocytosis.

Other factors

Potential factors that may cause generalized osteoporosis in inflammatory disorders, such as RA and AS, include the systemic effects of inflammatory products, alterations in sex hormones, altered calcium metabolism, changes in load bearing, and the effect of drugs used in treatment. Immobilization per se leads to a net loss of bone (rates as high as 5% per month in the first 6 months).

Evaluation of osteoporosis and low-trauma fracture

- Low-trauma fracture in those aged 50–75 years should be investigated to exclude the possibility of osteoporosis. The three most common sites of fracture are the wrist, vertebrae, and hip. Many now consider a low-trauma fracture in a person >75 years of age as strongly suggestive of osteoporosis and would treat without measuring bone mass. Assessment and investigation for possible underlying disease is still required.
- Plain radiographs are an insensitive method of assessing bone mass. The high correlation between bone mineral density (BMD) and bone strength and, therefore, bone fragility has led to the development of several techniques for assessing BMD.
- The standard technique for measuring BMD is dual energy X-ray absorptiometry (DEXA). It is quick, has high resolution, precision and accuracy, and can assess the lumbar spine, femoral neck, wrist, and whole body. DEXA gives two readings, the "T" and "Z" scores.

The T score is the individual's bone mineral density compared with the mean bone density achieved at peak bone mass for the same sex (and, more recently, race). The Z score is the individual's bone mineral density compared with the mean bone density for someone of the same age and sex (and, more recently, race). Most analyses and studies have focused on the T score. The score is recorded as a + or − figure above or below the mean. For every one standard deviation (SD) below the mean there is a twofold increase in the risk of fracture, i.e., an individual three SD below the mean has an eightfold risk of fracture compared with a "normal" individual of the same age, bearing in mind also that base-line risk increases with age in the "normal" population.

- Quantitative CT allows volume measurements and can distinguish between cortical and trabecular bone in vertebrae. It is, however, costly and entails a high radiation exposure.
- Ultrasonography is a noninvasive technique that is currently being correlated with DEXA. US can be performed at the heel (calcaneus) and patella. Correlation seems poor and its role in clinical diagnostics remains unclear.
- Since the advent of noninvasive techniques, transiliac bone biopsy is no longer essential unless there is the need to diagnose osteomalacia as the underlying cause. Bone biopsy may be used as a tool in research, in particular for the quantification of rates of bone turnover.
- Routine biochemical and hematological tests are usually normal in osteoporosis. Investigation of the newly diagnosed osteoporotic person should include a screen for malignancy and metabolic bone biochemical abnormalities. This at least would include an ESR, CMP, LFT, serum immunoglobulins, calcium and phosphate. Measurement of the sex hormones should also be considered.
- Biochemical markers of bone turnover are available but their precise clinical role has not been established. These include:
  - bone formation: serum bone alkaline phosphatase, osteocalcin (bone gamma carboxyglutamic acid-containing protein), type 1 procollagen peptides
  - bone resorption: fasting urine calcium and hydroxyproline, urine collagen cross links (deoxy)pyridinoline, serum tartrate-resistant acid phosphatase.
- These markers may be helpful in comparing "high bone turnover" with "low bone turnover" cases in established osteoporosis, and in monitoring the effects of and compliance with treatments.

Management of osteoporosis and low-trauma fractures

Prevention

Bone mass at any one time will be determined by "peak bone mass," rate of bone loss with aging, and, with women, the rate and duration of postmenopausal bone loss. Genetic factors cannot be manipulated but nutritional and environmental factors may. Pharmacological intervention in at-risk individuals is good prevention practice. Currently this would include those in the age group 50–65 with a T score of ≤−3.0, or with a T score ≤−2.5 with other risk factors (especially fragility fracture), and those >65 with a T score of ≤−2.5 regardless of presence of additional risk factors.

Calcium

- Calcium supplementation is sensible in those who have a low-calcium diet (poor in dairy products, green leafy vegetables, nuts, dried fruits, etc.). There is conflicting evidence about whether supplements have any effect on preventing bone loss and, therefore, risk of fracture per se in the young adult.
- Calcium supplementation in prepubertal children enhances the rate of change in bone mineral density but whether this translates into higher peak bone mass is unknown.
- In postmenopausal women, calcium supplements can lead to a reduction in the rate of decline of total-body bone mineral density.
- There is a role for calcium and vitamin D supplementation in the elderly osteoporotic; it can help prevent cortical bone loss and subsequent vertebral fractures.
- At present the use of calcium supplements is recommended for:
  - definite osteoporosis
  - poor calcium diet (< 400 mg intake per day)
  - supplement to any anticatabolic (antiresorptive) treatment in the elderly.

Exercise

There is some evidence to suggest that physical activity decreases the rate of bone loss around the time of menopause, although the level and type of activity remains unclear. The activity must, however, be weight-bearing. There is little impact of exercise in improving bone mass once osteoporotic, though it may aid in preventing further loss.

Hormone replacement

- Estrogen replacement therapy is an effective way of preventing postmenopausal bone loss. The addition of a progestogen allows endometrial shedding and minimizes the risk of hyperplasia and neoplasia. The minimum oral dose of estrogen required is 2 µmg/day, and conjugated estrogen 0.625 mg/day. Gels and transdermal/depot treatments should be started at around 3 mg/day or 50 µg/day, respectively.
- Evidence suggests that the use of HRT increases the risk of deep vein thrombosis, coronary artery disease, breast cancer, and stroke. These agents should therefore be used with caution.

Treating established disease

- Virtually all the treatments listed below have demonstrated in the order of 40–50% reduction in risk of fragility fracture, either vertebral or at the hip in postmenopausal women with established osteoporosis.
- Bisphosphonates are now the most commonly used of all agents available in the treatment of established osteoporosis. They are potent inhibitors of bone resorption (anticatabolic). Cyclical disodium etidronate (400 mg daily for 2 weeks, every 3 months) is approved for use in the Canada and Europe, but not the United States. Alendronate (10 mg daily or 70 mg weekly), risedronate (5 mg daily or 35 mg weekly), ibandronate (2.5 mg daily or 150 mg *monthly*), and zoledronate (5 mg IV *yearly*) are the agents currently available.

- In general, bisphosphates are well-tolerated but should be used with caution in renal impairment and history of esophageal reflux/hiatus hernia. Symptoms of nausea and reflux can be lessened by taking these medications with plenty of water and avoid lying down for at least 30 minutes afterwards. These agents should also be taken on an empty stomach as absorption is poor.
- Recent reports have identified an association between bisphosphonates and jaw osteonecrosis, although this remains very uncommon.
- Long-term bisphosphonate use has also been associated with (rare) atypical fractures of the femoral shaft. Therefore, it is becoming common to stop bisphosphonate use for a year (i.e., a "drug holiday") for every 5 years of continuous use.
- Compliance rates with therapy are variable with reports from the United States of < 30% but reports in the United Kingdom of > 80% at 2–4 years' duration of therapy.
- Calcium supplements should be taken alongside bisphosphonate therapy unless otherwise contraindicated.
- Calcium (800–1000 mg) and vitamin D supplements (400–800 IU) are recommended in the elderly and those whose diet is poor in them.
- HRT may be used as described above. Selective estrogen receptor modulators (SERMs) such as raloxifene may become more popular in the future as alternatives to HRT.
- Calcitonin is useful for its analgesic effect early after osteoporotic fractures. It has only a modest effect on bone mineral density and, therefore, is generally not used as a primary treatment for osteoporosis.
- Strontium ranelate has been shown to both increase osteoblastic bone formation and reduce osteoclastic bone resorption. Given at 2 g daily orally, studies have shown 36–41% reduction in fracture risk (hip and vertebral) against placebo. Strontium may be FDA-approved for this indication in the near future, but is not yet widely available in the United States. Furthermore, strontium, by its incorporation into bone structure, gives false high readings on DEXA scanning, making assessment of change in BMD following therapy difficult to interpret at present.
- Teriparatide (20 mg SQ daily) is a parathyroid hormone analogue and an anabolic agent now available for use in severe osteoporosis. It is available in a pre-filled "pen" (or delivery device), and is given as a subcutaneous injection daily for 1 year. Teriparatide should not be co-administered with bisphosphonates.
- Denosumab (60 mg SQ every 6 months) is a fully human monoclonal antibody that binds RANK ligand, which is necessary for osteoclast maturation. It is approved by the United States Food and Drug Administration for the treatment of postmenopausal women at high risk for fracture, or patients with multiple risk factors who are intolerant of other drugs. It is important to note that this drug may be associated with an increased risk of infection.

- A phase II study of ronacaleret, a calcilytic that works by blocking the calcium-sensing receptors on the parathyroid gland, was stopped due to lack of clinical efficacy.
- Acute back pain due to vertebral collapse is discussed in Chapter 20.

A flow chart for the management of fractures in osteoporosis is provided (see Figure 16.1).

Fig. 16.1 Treatment pathways for postmenopausal women with one or more fragility fracture (based on NICE, UK guidelines 2005).

Osteomalacia and rickets

- Osteomalacia and rickets are characterized by defective mineralization of bone and cartilage and the accumulation of unmineralized bone matrix (osteoid), i.e., there is, unlike osteoporosis, a decline in the ratio of mineralized bone to matrix.
- Rickets is the term used for this defect in growing children before the closure of the epiphyses.
- There are many causes of osteomalacia but essentially they all occur due to either a deficiency or resistance to vitamin D, or a non-PTH related defect in renal handling of phosphate (see Table 16.5).
- Both vitamin D_2 (ergocalciferol) from vegetables in the diet, and D_3 (cholecalciferol) from animal tissues and de novo synthesis in skin, are metabolized in the liver to 25-hydroxyvitamin D and then in the kidney to 1,25-dihydroxyvitamin D_3. The latter affects calcium metabolism by acting on the parathyroid glands (negative-feedback loop on PTH stimulation of renal vitamin D hydroxylases), GI tract (decreased absorption of calcium and phosphate), and bone (both bone resorption and osteoblast activation with bone formation).

Clinical and laboratory findings

- Classical symptoms are bone pain and tenderness, bone deformity (depending on age of onset), and a proximal muscle weakness with a "waddling gait." Muscle enzymes and biopsy are normal. Proximal myopathy is not a feature of X-linked hypophosphatemic rickets.
- The hypocalcemia of osteomalacia is usually silent but some individuals develop parasthesias and tetany. Rarely is it severe enough to cause cardiac dysrhythmia, convulsions, or psychosis.
- Children may be hypotonic and apathetic with growth retardation and delayed walking. On weight-bearing, bones become bowed, and there is irregularity of the metaphyseal–epiphyseal junction, usually at the wrist and costochondral junctions. The latter gives rise to the feature "rachitic rosary." An indentation may also arise along the attachment of the diaphragm to the softened ribs (Harrison's groove). Rapid growth of the softened skull leads to craniotabes, parietal bone flattening, and frontal bossing. Dentition is also delayed and poor.
- Many bony deformities persist despite treatment (unless due to simple dietary deficiency and treated early) and may require surgery, e.g., tibial/fibial osteotomy to correct lower limb alignment.
- The classical radiographic change of osteomalacia is the pseudo fracture (Looser's zone), found most often at the following sites:
  - ribs and clavicles
  - outer border of the scapulae
  - pubic rami
  - femoral neck
  - metatarsals.

They appear as incomplete, radiolucent fracture lines perpendicular to the cortex, with poor callus formation.

- Lab tests indicative of vitamin D deficiency include a low serum calcium and phosphate, elevated serum alkaline phosphatase, low

Table 16.5 The classification of osteomalacia

Abnormal vitamin D metabolism	Reduced availability	Poor diet
		Inadequate exposure to sun
		Malabsorption
	Defective metabolism	Hepatobiliary disease
		Chronic renal failure
		Anticonvulsant drugs
		Vitamin D-dependent rickets type I
		X-linked hypophosphatemia
		Oncogenic hypophosphatemia
	Receptor defects	Vitamin D-dependent rickets type II
Altered phosphate homeostasis	Malabsorption	
	Renal phosphate loss	X-linked hypophosphatemia
		Fanconi syndrome
	Defective mineralization	Aluminum and fluoride toxicity
		Bisphosphonate toxicity
		Hypophosphatasia
		Fibrogenous imperfecta ossium

urinary phosphate and low urinary calcium excretion, low levels of 25-hydroxyvitamin D, and a mild secondary hyperparathyroidism. The latter may cause a mild hyperchloremic acidosis due to renal bicarbonate loss. Severe acidosis suggests a renal tubular defect (see Features and Treatment of Altered Phosphate Homeostasis, later in this chapter).

- Levels of 1,25-dihydroxyvitamin D may be normal and are, therefore, not helpful. If the serum calcium and 25-hydroxyvitamin D levels are normal as well, then the defect is likely to be renal handling of phosphate or end-organ resistance. If doubt remains as to the diagnosis of osteomalacia, a transiliac bone biopsy can be taken.

Features and treatment of abnormal vitamin D metabolism

- Vitamin D deficiency through poor diet intake is rare unless combined with exposure to sunlight. It is a phenomenon seen most often in the housebound elderly, and in immigrant Asian populations.
- Bone pain and muscle weakness respond quickly to replacement therapy, though laboratory and radiological features may take longer to return to normal. Limb deformity can be prevented if simple vitamin D deficiency is treated early. Vitamin D_2 (ergocalciferol) at physiological doses of 200–400 IU/day (5–10 mg) daily can prevent

disease. In severe disease, a loading dose of ergocalciferol 50,000 IU can be administered weekly for 4–8 weeks.

- Intestinal disorders that lead to fat malabsorption can cause vitamin D deficiency, as vitamin D is fat-soluble. Cortical bone loss is usually irreversible in this group. Prevention of further damage is best achieved by annually monitoring levels of serum 25-hydroxyvitamin D and, if levels are low-to-normal or less, replacement with ergocalciferol or calcitriol and calcium. Calcium should be supplemented at doses of 800–1000 mg/day for adults.

- Chronic renal failure and renal osteodystrophy are discussed in the section on parathyroid disease and related disorders later in this chapter. Essentially two problems arise as a consequence of renal failure: (1) a decline in production of 1,25-dihydroxyvitamin D, and (2) poor phosphate excretion and subsequent hyperphosphatemia. The latter worsens hypocalcemia that in turn leads to parathyroid hyperplasia and secondary hyperparathyroidism.

- Type I vitamin D-dependent rickets is a rare autosomal recessive disease. Defective 25-hydroxyvitamin D 1 hydroxylase enzyme activity leads to low levels of 1,25-vitamin D. Children are often affected with rickets before the age of 2 years, and fail to respond to normal levels of vitamin D replacement. Treatment is most effective with physiological doses of calcitriol.

- Type II vitamin D-dependent rickets is a rare receptor defect disorder. About 70% of patients will have alopecia and this is an important prognostic feature when discussing likely outcome of treatment. In patients with normal hair, a remission can be achieved with high doses of vitamin D (as above). In patients with alopecia a tenfold increase in vitamin D dosing is often required and about 50% will not respond.

Features and treatment of altered phosphate homeostasis

- Osteomalacia from phosphate depletion is rare and usually occurs as a consequence of abuse of phosphate-binding antacids over many years. Histologically it appears the same as vitamin D deficiency, although biochemically serum calcium is usually normal and vitamin D is high. Treatment is with phosphate supplements and avoidance of antacids.

- X-linked hypophosphatemic rickets (also known as familial hypophosphatemic rickets) is a disorder of vitamin D resistance. It is important to diagnose early as treatment can prevent deformity. It manifests itself as short stature and rickets in the homozygous men, with variable growth and expression of bone deformity in women. Dental delay occurs but dentition is usually normal. Proximal myopathy is not a feature of this condition. Laboratory tests show a low serum phosphate, normal serum calcium and PTH, and a low/normal 1,25-dihydroxyvitamin D. Urine phosphate excretion is increased in the absence of abnormal acidification, glycosuria, or aminoaciduria. A combination of calcitriol (0.125–1.5 µg/day) and phosphate (25 mg/kg/day in infants, and 1–3 g elemental phosphorus in adults) is the most effective therapy. The induction of hypercalcemia is a risk and the serum calcium should be monitored regularly every

2 weeks for a couple of months on induction of therapy and thereafter approximately every 3 months.
- Renal tubular acidosis (RTA) and Fanconi syndrome may be associated with osteomalacia and rickets. In RTA there is a disorder of bicarbonate handling leading to low plasma bicarbonate, metabolic acidosis, and an inappropriate urine pH. Type I, distal tubular RTA occurs as a result of failure to secrete hydrogen ions (see Table 16.6).
- Type II, proximal RTA is a consequence of bicarbonate wasting. Type II is often associated with Fanconi syndrome. The development of rickets in both forms of RTA is due to hypophosphatemia. The acidosis should be treated and vitamin D supplements given.
- Fanconi syndrome is associated with a number of acquired and inherited disorders. These include multiple myeloma, amyloidosis, heavy metal toxicity and disorders of carbohydrate metabolism. The net effect of the proximal renal tubular defects is glycosuria, aminoaciduria, phosphaturia, and hypophosphatemia. Treatment of the bone disease is with phosphate and calcitriol supplements.
- Oncogenic hypophosphatemic osteomalacia is a phenomenon seen with some tumors (usually mesenchymal). The proposed mechanism is the production of a humoral factor that affects proximal renal tubular handling of phosphate. The bone disease regresses after removal of the tumor. A similar condition occurs in fibrous dysplasia and neurofibromatosis. Treatment involves phosphate and calcitriol supplements.

Table 16.6   Some causes of type I, distal RTA

Hereditary	Primary	
	Renal	Medullary sponge Polycystic kidney
	Fructose intolerance	
	Ehlers-Danlos syndrome	
Acquired	Rheumatic	SLE Sjögren's syndrome Sarcoidosis
	Renal	Obstruction Pyelonephritis Transplantation
	Endocrine	Hyper/hypothyroidism Hyperparathyroidism Hyperprolactinaemia
	Hepatic	Chronic active hepatitis Liver cirrhosis
	Tuberculosis	
	Lithium toxicity	
	Cryoglobulinemia	

Parathyroid disease and related disorders

This section will discuss hypercalcemia in adults and children and its relation to musculoskeletal disorders. Hyper- and hypoparathyroidism, and renal osteodystrophy are considered. For further information on vitamin D and phosphate imbalance the reader is referred to the previous section on osteomalacia and rickets.

Hypercalcemia

- The clinical picture of hypercalcemia can range from the asymptomatic to an acute medical emergency.
- Calcium plasma concentrations are normally balanced between the homeostatic mechanisms operating in the gut, skeleton, kidneys, and extracellular fluids. Hypercalcemia arises most often as a result of excessive loss of calcium from bone but may also occur due to excessive gut absorption. The excessive bone loss combined with a failure of the kidneys to handle high loads of calcium, and a failure of bone to reclaim minerals quickly enough, leads to the imbalance. Accelerated bone loss (osteoclast stimulation) may be driven by several causes including parathyroid hormone (PTH) and cytokines interleukin-1 (IL-1), TNF, and transforming growth factor (TGF). PTH also induces calcium reabsortion from the kidneys.
- The clinical presentation of moderate to severe hypercalcemia includes:
  - joint, bone, muscle pain
  - muscle weakness
  - dehydration and polyuria
  - lethargy
  - fatigue
  - acute confusional state—unconsciousness
  - abdominal pains and vomiting
  - renal colic pains
  - electrocardiogram findings—short QT interval, etc.
- Hyperparathyroidism and malignancy are the most common causes of hypercalcemia, accounting for 90% of all cases. A thorough history and examination is required when considering the cause of serum calcium (see Table 16.7).
- Treatment options depend on the level of serum calcium, the presence of symptoms, renal impairment, and the underlying cause. For example, borderline high serum calcium in an asymptomatic individual with a mildly elevated PTH may simply warrant observation in the absence of renal impairment or vitamin D deficiency. On the other hand an individual with severe hypercalcemia, dehydration, and renal impairment due to a treatable malignancy would require urgent aggressive management.
- Dehydration is very common. Early rehydration is very important and often given for 24–48 h prior to review of serum calcium levels and the instigation of further therapies such as bisphosphonates and loop diuretics (see Table 16.8).

Table 16.7 Some cause of hypercalcemia

Common	Primary hyperparathyroidism	
	Malignancy	Lytic metastases: TNF, IL-1
		Ectopic PTH and TGF-α
		Ectopic 1,25 vitamin D
Uncommon/ rare	Drugs	Thiazide diuretics
		Lithium
		Aminophylline
	Granuloma	Sarcoidosis
		Tuberculosis
		Histoplasmosis
	Endocrine/ metabolic	Thyrotoxicosis
		Pheochromocytoma
		Excess vitamin A or D
		Renal failure
	Immobilization	

Table 16.8 Treatment of hypercalcemia

General principles	Rehydrate with normal saline 4 liters in 24 h if needed
	Correct hypokalemia and hypomagnesemia
	Mild metabolic acidosis need not be treated
Specific treatment	Loop diuretics when hydrated
	Bisphosphonates (pamidronate)
	Calcitonin
	Glucocorticoids (hematologic malignancies and granulomatous diseases)

Hypercalcemia in infancy and childhood

- Chronic hypercalcemia of infancy may not be associated with the more common clinical features mentioned earlier. More often there is a failure to thrive, abdominal pain, and irritability. Acute hypercalcemia is very rare in children.
- Conditions to consider are listed in Table 16.9.

Table 16.9 Conditions that may be responsible for hypercalcemia in infancy and childhood

Williams' syndrome	A spectrum of aortic valve stenosis and facial dysmorphism ("elfin" facies).
	Radioulnar synostosis impedes growth in 25% of cases. There is a deletion of the elastin gene on chromosome 7; pathogenesis otherwise is unknown
Idiopathic infantile hypercalcemia	Similar milder appearance to Williams' syndrome can be seen. There are also features of inguinal hernias, hypertension, strabismus, and kyphosis
Familial hypocalciuric hypercalcemia	See later in this section
Neonatal primary hyperparathyroidism	
Other	Fat necrosis
	Sarcoidosis
	Jansen syndrome (metaphyseal dysplasia)
	Overdosing of milk/vitamin D

Parathyroid disorders

Primary hyperparathyroidism

- Primary hyperparathyroidism (HPT) is a relatively common condition with an incidence of 1 in 1,000. It occurs at all ages though is much more common after the age of 60 with a female to male ratio of 3:1. It is unusual in childhood and should raise the possibility of familial multiple endocrine neoplasia (MEN) type I or type II.
- A single benign adenoma accounts for 80% of cases of primary HPT. Generalized gland hyperplasia accounts for 15–20% of cases. Parathyroid carcinoma is very rare.
- The condition is associated with bone, renal, GI, and neuromuscular complications. Bony problems can be seen on plain radiographs and range from mild subperiosteal bone resorption to full osteitis fibrosa cystica with bone cysts, "brown tumors," bone resorption of the distal phalanges and clavicles, patchy osteosclerosis (classic "rugger (rugby) jersey" spine), and multiple lytic lesions of the skull. These changes may often, however, be nonspecific.
- Renal stones are a common complication. GI manifestations include peptic ulceration and pancreatitis. The myopathy of primary PT is rare and more often a syndrome of fatigue and weakness is seen.
- Primary HPT is diagnosed by assaying PTH levels. The assays are sensitive and able to distinguish between nonparathyroid tumor secreting PTH and parathyroid hormone.

Treatment
- Medical management includes adequate rehydration and avoidance of high calcium intake. Clinical trials with calcimimetic agents (stimulate calcium receptors with consequent inhibition of PTH secretion) and in particular cinacalcet hydrochloride are ongoing and may be effective in primary HPT. At the time of writing, cinacalcet has received FDA approval for the treatment of secondary HPT in patients with chronic kidney disease.
- Some individuals (especially the elderly) have physiological mild elevation of PTH due to vitamin D deficiency with normal calcium levels. Vitamin D should be replaced and the serum calcium and PTH levels monitored after 8–10 weeks.
- Parathyroidectomy should be offered to individuals with moderate-to-high serum calcium and/or symptoms and complications of the condition, the latter regardless of whether serum calcium levels are "borderline" raised or not. US imaging, thallium/technetium scans, MR and CT are all useful ways of establishing the position of an adenoma. However, exploration by an experienced surgeon is equally effective.

Secondary and tertiary hyperparathyroidism
Secondary hyperparathyroidism occurs as a consequence of abnormalities in serum calcium and homeostatic "sensing" of calcium levels. With time, PTH secretion becomes autonomous and the abnormality is then called tertiary hyperparathyroidism. This is most often seen in conditions such as end-organ renal disease and vitamin D resistance. Calcimimetics may have an important role to play in controlling secondary HPT but at present parathyroidectomy is the best treatment option. Vitamin D replacement to lower PTH secretion does not appear to be effective in patients with otherwise normal vitamin D levels.

Familial hypocalciuric hypercalcemia (FHH) or familial benign hypercalcemia (FBH)
- This condition is common but most often asymptomatic. It is inherited as an autosomal dominant with high penetrance. Radiographs, PTH, and renal function are usually normal. Although parathyroid gland hyperplasia occurs, parathyroidectomy is invariably unsuccessful at lowering serum calcium levels.
- The two indications for parathyroidectomy are neonatal severe hyperparathyroidism and adult relapsing pancreatitis. Use of diuretics, estrogens, or phosphate to regulate serum calcium has been unsuccessful. Patients should, therefore, be followed without intervention unless complications arise.
- In pregnancy the three situations to be aware of are:
  - asymptomatic hypercalcemia in the affected offspring of a carrier
  - severe neonatal hypercalcemia in affected offspring of an unaffected mother (intrauterine secondary hyperparathyroidism, which usually resolves spontaneously)
  - hypocalcemia in the unaffected offspring of an affected mother (fetal parathyroid suppression).

Familial hyperparathyroid syndromes

Up to 10% of cases of hyperparathyroidism may have a hereditary syndrome. The most common of these is multiple endocrine neoplasia (MEN). Type I, autosomal dominant and equal in both sexes, is associated with pancreatic and pituitary adenomas, and adrenal hyperplasia. Type IIA, autosomal dominant Sipple's disease, is characterized by pheochromocytomas and medullary carcinoma of the thyroid.

Parathyroid hormone resistant syndromes

- Pseudohypoparathyroidism (PHP) occurs as a result of resistance to PTH by target tissues. The biochemical consequences are hypocalcemia, hyperphosphatemia, and elevated PTH.
- Cyclic AMP (cAMP) mediates many actions of PTH. Administration of bioactive PTH to normal individuals leads to increased urinary excretion of cAMP. The abnormal response to this test in individuals with PHP classifies them either type I—no increase in urine cAMP with bioactive PTH—or type II—normal increase in urine cAMP but abnormal phosphate handling.
- The net effect is features similar to those of hypoparathyroidism of any cause (such as congenital parathyroid absence, or surgical removal).
- Common symptoms include:
  - neuromuscular irritability (due to associated hypocalcaemia)
  - muscle cramps
  - pseudopapilledema
  - extrapyramidal signs
  - mental retardation
  - cataracts
  - coarse hair/alopecia
  - abnormal dentition
  - personality disturbance.
- PHP type Ia (Albright's hereditary osteodystrophy (AHO)) manifests as short stature, round facies, obesity, brachydactyly, and subcutaneous ossification. Albright observed that some individuals have these features without PHP. The term pseudopseudohypoparathyroidism was coined. This group has a normal serum calcium and PTH/cAMP test.
- Cases with PHP type I but who lack features of AHO are classified type Ib. They often have the skeletal abnormalities seen in cases of hypoparathyroidism.
- In type II PHP there is a normal cAMP response but an abnormal phosphate response in the kidney.
- The mainstay of therapy is the maintenance of serum calcium and phosphate levels. The complication of calcium and vitamin D supplements is the increased risk of renal stones due to hypercalciuria. One gram a day of calcium is recommended and products rich in phosphate (e.g., dairy foods) should be avoided. Hydroxyvitamin D supplements are valuable but serum calcium and phosphate levels should be checked weekly for 4–6 weeks up to steady state and then every 3–6 months.

Renal osteodystrophy
- The kidneys regulate calcium/phosphate balance, are a target organ for PTH, and produce 1,25-dihydroxyvitamin D (calcitriol). Renal osteodystrophy is the net effect on bone that occurs due to derangement of calcium homeostasis in chronic renal failure. Renal bone disease is classified as 'high turnover' or 'low turnover' depending on whether serum PTH levels are high or low/normal respectively. Low turnover, adynamic osteodystrophy, is related to excess bone aluminum deposition in dialysis patients and is also seen in diabetes mellitus and corticosteroid therapy and as part of aging.
- Hyperphosphatemia, hypocalcemia, impaired calcitriol production, and skeletal resistance to PTH all contribute to secondary HPT in chronic renal failure. Serum PTH varies too widely in the condition to be useful in assessing treatment. Serum alkaline phosphatase is increased and is a useful marker though it does not distinguish between high and low turnover states.
- The clinical manifestations of renal osteodystrophy are shown in Table 16.10.

Table 16.10 The clinical manifestations of renal osteodystrophy

Clinical feature	Comment
Bone pain	Common
Skeletal deformity	Common. Affects appendicular and axial skeleton
	Children: onset <3 years, rachitic; onset <10 years, bowing of long bones, widened metaphyses, pseudoclubbing, slipped epiphyses
	Adults: lumbar scoliosis, kyphosis, distorted thorax
Growth retardation	
Proximal muscle weakness	
Ectopic calcification	Soft-tissues. Visceral. Vascular—if severe, individuals may develop ischemic necrosis

The management of renal osteodystrophy

- Good dietary control of phosphate can maintain normal calcium levels, but low-phosphate diets are often unacceptable and normal phosphate levels are best achieved with binding agents, e.g., calcium carbonate or calcium acetate.
- Small doses of calcitriol (vitamin D) may help to lower serum PTH levels. Some individuals may be sensitive to calcitriol and serum calcium levels may increase. Most patients require doses of 0.25–0.5 µg daily; children may require higher doses.
- Parathyroidectomy is indicated in persistent symptomatic hypercalcemia, ectopic calcification, and severe bone pain.

Ectopic calcification and ossification

- Ectopic calcification can arise from any one of a number of causes of hypercalcemia or hyperphosphatemia. These include renal failure, hyperparathyroidism, and sarcoidosis. Dystrophic calcification is also a feature of SScl (see Chapter 12), DM (see Chapter 13), and 1° calcinosis.
- Ectopic ossification can be seen posttrauma and following myositis. It is also a feature of several rare conditions including pseudo-hypoparathyroidism and myositis ossificans progressiva. Early signs of muscle ossification are best detected with MR scanning. Later ossification it easily visible on plain radiographs. Treatment is difficult but includes physiotherapy to maintain suppleness and possibly heparins or bisphosphonates to halt bone formation.

Paget's disease of bone

- Paget's disease is a chronic disorder of accelerated bone resorption and formation resulting in deformity in size and shape of bone as well as fragility despite apparent "thickening" of bone.
- The condition is common (about 5% of the population over the age of 55) in the United Kingdom, the United States, Australia, and New Zealand, with a male to female ratio of 3:2. It is uncommon in Asia, and non-White races.
- Very little is known of the molecular basis of Paget's disease. There is evidence to suggest that it may be triggered by exposure to a slow virus. Paramyxovirus antigens found in bone cells, and compatible with measles, respiratory syncytial virus, and canine distemper have all been implicated.
- The clinical features of Paget's disease are shown in Table 16.11.

Diagnosis and treatment

- Serum alkaline phosphatase, a measure of bone formation, is the most useful marker and may be elevated as much as 30 times above normal. Occasionally, in limited Paget's, the enzyme is normal. This should not be a deterrent to treating painful lesions. The differential diagnosis of increased bone alkaline phosphatase includes metastatic bone disease, osteomalacia, hyperparathyroidism, and hyperphosphatasia.
- Urine hydroxyproline excretion is also increased. Hydroxyproline is a breakdown product of collagen and a marker of bone resorption. Other markers of bone turnover are available but most remain experimental and are not needed for the diagnosis and treatment of Paget's disease.
- There is a wide variation in radiographic appearance of the condition but the main features are sclerosis, bone expansion, and coarse, disorganized, trabecular bone.
- Isotope bone scanning is a sensitive investigation for defining the extent of lesions.
- Many rare hereditary dysplastic conditions are associated with bone sclerosis. These include osteopetrosis, Engelmann's disease, and pycnodysostosis. These conditions are beyond the scope of this book.
- Sclerosis is also a feature of many other conditions including metabolic disease (fluorosis, hypervitaminosis D, parathyroid disease, renal osteodystrophy), malignancy (lymphoma, myeloma, skeletal metastases), infection, sarcoidosis, and tuberous sclerosis.
- Thermographic improvement and pain reduction are correlated with effective treatment of Paget's; thermographic observations probably demonstrate a decline in bone and periosseous blood flow after treatment.
- There are several indications for treatment of Paget's disease:
  - pain arising from pagetic sites
  - deforming disease
  - skull disease
  - complications: progressive neurological syndrome, fractures, hypercalcemia, high-output cardiac failure, serum alkaline phosphatase (over twice upper normal).

Table 16.11 Clinical features of Paget's disease of bone

Clinical feature	Details
Pain	Deep, boring pain, possibly correlated to blood flow
Bone expansion and deformity	Hands or feet 10% of cases
	Pelvis 75%
	Lumbar spine 50% of cases
	Femur 35% of cases
	Sacrum 35% of cases
	Skull 35% of cases
	Tibia 30% of cases
	Radius 15% of cases
Fractures	
Heat	
Neurological syndromes	Deafness (sensorineural or conductive)
	Tinnitus
	Headache
	Brainstem/cerebellar compression
	Spinal cord/root compression
	Cranial nerve entrapment
High-output cardiac failure	Rare—occurs when > 40% of the skeleton is involved
Malignant osteosarcoma	Seen in 0.1% of cases, esp. if disease present for > 10 years
Immobilization hypercalcemia	Serum calcium levels are nearly always normal
Gout	
Retinal angioid streaks	

- Pagetic and related osteoarthritic pain may be reduced by simple analgesics but pure Pagetic bone pain responds poorly to this. In most cases now, the choice of treatment falls between bisphosphonates and calcitonin. These drugs are discussed in the Osteoporosis section at the beginning of this chapter.
- Etidronate may be given for 6 months at a dose of 5 mg/kg/day. Vitamin D supplements may minimize the mineralization defects that can occur with even low doses of etidronate. Oral tiludronate 400 mg daily for 3 months has been FDA approved for the treatment of Paget's disease. IV pamidronate may also be used and many in current practice offer a single dose infusion of 30–90 mg (depending on renal function) to symptomatic patients, with follow-up and measurement of

serum alkaline phosphatase after 3 months. Transient flulike symptoms of fever, myalgia, and arthralgia often occur after the first dose of IV pamidronate. Risedronate may also be given at 30 mg daily for one month.

- SQ or IM calcitonin may also be used in Paget's disease. The disadvantages are common symptoms of nausea and diarrhea, relapse on therapy, and expense. Nasal spray calcitonin may be useful but the therapeutic effect is weaker than with bisphosphonates. Typical dosing for salmon calcitonin would be a 10 IU test dose followed by 50–100 IU daily, reducing to 50 IU 2–3 times per week once a symptomatic response is achieved (usually after 4–8 weeks). If there has been no symptomatic response after 3 months, calcitonin therapy should be stopped.
- There is no consensus about whether or when to treat Pagetic joints per se prior to joint replacement.

Miscellaneous diseases of bone

Osteochondritis and osteonecrosis

- The osteochondroses are a heterogeneous group of disorders, defined by their radiological appearances. In a few instances, radiological osteochondritis may be an incidental finding, not associated with symptoms and may represent a normal developmental variant. Usually, however, it is painful, occurs in the growing skeleton between the ages of 3–16 years, and is more frequent in men and in the peripheral skeleton. Some cases are due to infarction (osteonecrosis) of subchondral bone. For others the etiology is unknown.

- Osteonecrosis (synonyms: avascular necrosis, ischemic necrosis, aseptic necrosis) can occur at several sites and is associated with as many eponyms (see Table 16.12). Bone infarction and subsequent pain occurs in susceptible areas because of limited collateral circulation and low perfusion pressure, e.g., in the femoral head. First, bone and adjacent marrow becomes necrotic. Granulation tissue then advances into the dead bone, which is resorbed. Osteoblasts then lay down new osteoid. Advanced osteonecrosis leads to secondary osteoarthritis, severe disability, and eventually the need for joint replacement. In the acute phase, core decompressive surgery may help preserve the joint, although some patients may require total joint replacement.

- Etiological factors for osteonecrosis include trauma, sepsis, radiation, thermal, and electrical injury. Caisson's disease is an obliterative endarteritis of the femoral head caused by expanding nitrogen gas in divers who decompress too quickly. Hematological causes include hemophilia, coagulopathies, and hemoglobinopathies. Endocrine causes include Cushing's syndrome and glucocorticoid use (high dose >60 mg/day over a period of months). There is an increased susceptibility to the condition in several rheumatic conditions including RA (Chapter 5), SLE (Chapter 10), SScl (Chapter 13), and vasculitis (Chapter 15). Finally, a miscellaneous group of associations with osteonecrosis include bisphosphonate therapy, alcohol abuse, organ transplantation, dialysis, HIV infection, pancreatitis, chronic liver disease, hypertriglyceridemia, and pregnancy.

- Osteonecrosis complicates 20% of cases of intracapsular hip fracture.

- Fat embolism may account for some cases, e.g., in alcoholism and Cushing's disease.

- Asymptomatic osteonecrosis in SLE may be as high as 35% (it is symptomatic in 5–10%).

- Osteonecrosis is diagnosed and classified radiologically: (Arlet and Ficat classification): I = normal; II = osteoporosis, cysts, sclerosis giving mottled appearance; III = subchondral bone collapse; IV = abnormal bone contour and joint space loss. Bone scintigraphy, CT, and MR are more sensitive. MR can identify early changes in bone marrow before bone necrosis and has greatest specificity once bone changes occur.

- Legg–Calvé–Perthes' disease is osteonecrosis of the femoral epiphysis and occurs in children from 3 to 8 years old, and affects boys more than girls (ratio 4:1). It is bilateral in 10–20% of cases. Symptoms

Table 16.12 The osteochondroses

Skeletal area		Disease eponym	Mechanism
Upper limb	Basal phalanges	Thiemann	Trauma
	Second metacarpal head	Mauclaire	Trauma
	Lunate	Kienbock	Osteonecrosis
	Carpal navicular	Prieser	Trauma
	Humeral capitellum	Panner	Trauma/osteonecrosis
Lower limb	Second metatarsal base	Freiberg	Osteonecrosis
	Fifth metatarsal base	Iselin	Trauma
	Tarsal navicular	Köhler	?Trauma/normal variant
	Talus	Diaz	Trauma-related
	Calcaneal	Sever	Traction apophysitis*
	Apophysis of tibial tubercle	Osgood–Schlatter	Traction apophysitis*
	Proximal tibia	Blount	–
	Inferior patella pole	Sinding–Larsen-Johansson	Traction apophysitis*
	Femoral epiphysis	Legg–Calvé–Perthes	Osteonecrosis
Axial skeleton	Vertebral epiphysis	Scheuermann	Repeated trauma

*Due to repetitive overloading of tendons, usually from sports.

    include an insidious onset of limp and pain in the groin or referred to the knee/thigh which is relieved by rest. Limitation of hip internal rotation and abduction (due to adductor spasm) is typical. Leg length inequality suggests bone collapse. There may be spontaneous resolution, especially in younger patients, in whom conservative management is indicated.

- Osgood–Schlatter's disease is probably due to repetitive trauma at the site of patellar tendon insertion into the tibial tubercle, typically in athletic adolescents, especially young men aged 14–16 years. Pain on exercise usually eases with rest. The diagnosis is made clinically and on demonstrating an enlarged fragmented tibial tubercle on a lateral view radiograph. Bilateral knee views helps to distinguish normal from abnormal.

- Scheuermann's disease, though not consistently defined, is thought to be a vertebral epiphyseal osteochondritis that occurs in adolescence. Although it can be an incidental radiographic finding, it is also associated with diffuse spinal pain that is more likely to be present if the osteochondritis is thoracolumbar (25%) rather than thoracic (75%) and the child is an athlete or very active. It can present with painless dorsal kyphosis with compensatory lumbar lordosis and lateral spine radiographs show irregularity of vertebral end-plates, anterior vertebral wedging, and kyphosis.
- Sinding–Larsen–Johansson's disease occurs as a consequence of over-loading of the patella at its secondary center of ossification producing a traction apophysitis at the patella lower pole. Though not exclusive to the group, it is a typical sports-related injury in adolescent athletes who jump, e.g., high-jump, basketball. Treatment is with simple analgesia or NSAIDs, and rest.
- Köhler's disease is osteonecrosis of the tarsal navicular. Changes may represent a developmental variation in ossification and it presents with a painful limp. Weight bearing is more comfortable on the outside of the foot and the navicular is tender.
- Freiberg's disease, osteonecrosis of the metatarsal (usually the second) head following trauma, is most common in adolescent women. Pain is localized and worse on weight bearing, and swelling may be detectable.

Osteochondritis dissecans

- This is usually a solitary lesion of the medial femoral condyle. A fragment of articular cartilage and subchondral bone becomes demarcated and may form an intra-articular loose body. The cause is unknown but may be due to abnormal ossification or trauma. Similar features may occasionally be seen at the elbow, hip, and talus.
- The condition is seen most often in male adolescents. Symptoms are mainly acute onset pain, an effusion, and limited movement of the joint.
- Plain radiographs will show a well-circumscribed, sclerotic lesion.
- In young patients before skeletal maturity there is a good chance of healing. After the epiphyses have closed, however, there is more risk of a loose body and secondary osteoarthritis. Arthroscopy can assist in assessing the degree of damage and removing loose bodies. Surgery ranges from drilling the lesion *in situ* to encourage healing, to bone osteochondral allografts.

Osteoid osteoma

- This is a benign osteoid-forming tumor that can be an elusive cause of bone pain, radiculopathy, or arthritis in children and adults. It is uncommon and accounts for 10% of benign bone neoplasia. It is 2–3 times more common in men than women and the incidence is highest in the second and third decades of life. More than two-thirds of lesions occur in long bones and especially the femur and tibia.
- Pain is the primary symptom and may be referred.
- The typical lesion is seen on plain radiography as an isolated, well-defined area of sclerosis with a radiolucent nidus often containing

speckles of calcium. Isotope bone scanning is a sensitive method of isolating a lesion and CT is valuable for localizing the nidus before surgical resection.
- Most individuals will respond, in part, to aspirin or NSAIDs. Provided the nidus is completely resected, surgery is curative.

Fibrous dysplasia

- This condition manifests as sporadic isolated or multifocal fibrous bone cysts and occurs most often in the second to third decade of life in isolated (mono-ostotic) disease, and before the age of 10 years in multifocal (polyostotic) disease.
- McCune-Albright syndrome is a triad of fibrous dysplasia, hyper-pigmented "*café-au-lait*" patches, and endocrine abnormalities.
- Laboratory tests are usually normal.
- There is no specific treatment. Some lesions regress. Fractures heal in the normal way. Girls with McCune–Albright-associated precocious puberty may respond to the aromatase inhibitor testolactone.

Molecular abnormalities of collagen and fibrillin

- Collagen and fibrillin are major connective tissue proteins with important mechanical functions. This section will deal briefly with osteogenesis imperfecta, Ehlers-Danlos syndrome, and Marfan syndrome.
- There are a number of types of collagen and a number of gene mutations leading to subtypes of collagen diseases. In this respect we will focus only on common aspects of these uncommon conditions, although the reader should be aware that joint hypermobility syndrome (akin to Ehlers-Danlos hypermobility type) is probably far more common than most clinicians realize, and therefore, it is underdiagnosed.

Osteogenesis imperfecta (OI)

- OI (also known as brittle bone disease) is a spectrum of conditions ranging from stillbirth to asymptomatic signs. The pathogenesis centers around abnormalities of type I collagen that is found not only in bone but also ligaments, teeth, sclerae, and skin.
- Ligament laxity, joint hypermobility, easy bruising, and poor dentition are common features. The differences between the four types of OI are shown in Table 16.13.
- Generalized osteopenia, deformity, and fractures are common bone and radiographic findings. The differential diagnosis in children includes juvenile osteoporosis, Cushing's disease, and homocystinuria.
- There is no effective medical therapy for OI. Patients may need surgery in late childhood/adulthood for deformities, and good dental hygiene.
- Children may present with multiple injuries that lead the clinician to consider child-abuse as a source for these—absolute care must be taken in ensuring neither OI or another collagen disorder is present before considering further action.

Marfan syndrome

- Marfan syndrome is characterized by long extremities (span/height ratio >1.03), long fingers and feet (arachnodactyly) with a hand/height ratio >11% and hand/foot ratio >15%, tall stature (with upper segment/lower segment ratio <0.89), pectus deformity of the chest wall (increasing risk of chest infections), high-arched palate, mandibular hypoplasia, lens dislocations and myopia, and joint laxity.
- There is a predisposition to mitral valve prolapse and acute aortic root rupture. All patients should have an echocardiogram and thoracic CT/MR to assess the aortic valve and arch.
- Beta-blockade has long been used to decrease the rate of aortic dilatation and improve long-term survival. However, there are little data to support this approach.

- In mouse models, losartan has been demonstrated to be an effective therapy through transforming growth factor-β antagonism, and may be an important advance in the treatment of this disease.
- It is an autosomal dominant condition with complete penetrance and prevalence of 1 in 25,000.

Table 16.13 Clinical and biochemical abnormalities in OI

Type	Clinical features	Inheritance	Defect
I	Normal bone growth. Normal dentition. Hearing loss in 50%. Blue sclera	Autosomal dominant	Decreased production of type I procollagen
II	Lethal. Stillbirths	Autosomal dominant. Autosomal recessive (rare)	Rearrangement of collagen IA/2A genes
III	Often deformed growth at birth and worsens. Poor dentition common. Hearing loss common. May have blue sclera	Autosomal dominant or recessive	Mutations in alpha-1 and alpha-2 collagen chains
IV	Often bone deformity and short stature. Poor dentition common. Hearing loss uncommon. Normal sclera.	Autosomal dominant	Mutations in the alpha-2 chains

- A subgroup similar to Marfan syndrome but without vascular fragility exists. The condition is called congenital contractural arachnodactyly.
- Numerous gene mutations have been found for both conditions, both linked to abnormalities of the protein fibrillin type I and II.
- The main aim of follow-up and assessment of these individuals is the early detection and referral of cardiac valve and aortic disease. Musculoskeletal symptoms should be managed in much the same way as outlined in the section below on joint hypermobility syndrome.

Ehlers–Danlos syndrome

- This is a clinically heterogeneous condition characterized by skin fragility, ligament laxity, short stature, spinal deformity, vascular fragility, and (rarely) retinal detachment. ⚠Retinal detachment and a history of early onset OA should lead the clinician to consider the

diagnosis of Stickler's syndrome, which is often associated with a defect in the collagen 2A1 (COL2A1) gene.
- There are at least nine genetic subtypes of Ehlers–Danlos syndrome (EDS), of which at least five have defined biochemical abnormalities. The classification, genetic abnormalities and clinical features of EDS are shown in Table 16.14. Various inheritance patterns are found dependent on the subtype of EDS. Hypermobility type EDS is the most common of these conditions and probably synonymous with JHS (see text below).
- Clinicians should be very sure they have confidently excluded vascular (type IV) EDS as this is associated with significant mortality.
- Therapy for these conditions centers on graded exercise and joint and skin protection. Some individuals require joint splints. Spinal deformity may need bracing or surgery and retinal disease requires ophthalmic expertise.
- Vascular rupture is a major concern in vascular type (type IV). This may occur even in the absence of documented aneurysms. This risk should always be taken into account during surgery or pregnancy, indeed as should tissue fragility in general for all subtypes.
- Tissue vulnerability should always be at the forefront of planning any surgical intervention.
- Patients are often also resistant to local anesthetics—the cause unclear. Failing to recognize this phenomenon can lead the clinician to inadvertently accuse the patient of being "sensitive" or anxious without realizing that they truly do not get a full effect from the anesthetic.
- Difficulties may arise during pregnancy—patients may get additional joint pain from increased body weight, early rupture of membranes and premature birth, cervical incompetence and spontaneous abortion, excessive tissue trauma during delivery, and musculoskeletal complications in the post-natal period due to lifting and caring for the newborn.
- The diagnosis is primarily clinical. Genetic testing can be done by looking for abnormalities of collagen types I, III, and V, although these tests may not be widely available. A skin biopsy is required.

Benign joint hypermobility syndrome (BJHS)
- Joint hypermobility can be associated with a multisystem clinical picture and may be associated with diffuse chronic pain and fatigue.
- Hypermobility is usually considered present if a person satisfies four or more maneuvers in the nine-point Beighton hypermobility score (see Table 16.15).
- BJHS is excluded in the presence of Marfan syndrome or Ehlers–Danlos syndrome (excluding hypermobility (Type III)). It may be synonymous with EDS hypermobility type.
- The revised (Brighton 1998) criteria for BJHS are shown in Table 16.16. BJHS is diagnosed in the presence of two major, one major and two minor, or four minor criteria. Two minor criteria will suffice where there is an unequivocally affected first-degree relative. The criteria serve to demonstrate the range of clinical findings in the condition.

Table 16.14 Clinical features and genetics of EDS

Type	Inheritance	Genetic defect	Common Clinical picture
Classical (type I and II)	AD	Abnormal pro-alpha 1 and 2 encoded by COL5A1 and A2 gene	Hyper-lax skin. Profound bruising and scarring
Hypermobility (Type III)	AD	Not known. ? Tenascin X insufficiency	See BJHS, Table 16.16
Vascular (Type IV)	AD	Abnormal pro-alpha 1 encoded by COL3A1 gene	Characteristic facies—wide spaced eyes, lobeless ears. Vascular rupture
Kyphoscoliosis (Type VI)	AR	Deficiency of lysyl hydroxylase	Severe hypotonia. Scoliosis. Scleral fragility
Atherochalasia (Type VII subtype)	AD	Abnormal pro-alpha 1 and 2 encoded by COL1A1 and A2	Severe dislocations. Skin laxity. Bruising. Hypotonia
Dermatospraxis (Type VII subtype)	AR	Deficiency of procollagen 1 peptidase	Severe, sagging skin. Bruising. Hernias
Rare forms:			
X-linked (Type V)	X-linked	?	Milder version of Classical type
Periodontal (Type VIII)	AD	?	Classical with gum fragility
Type X	?AR	?	Milder version of classical type with platelet aggregation

AD-autosomal dominant; AR-autosomal recessive

Treatment of hypermobility syndrome

- Although hypermobility diminishes with age, the symptoms tend to continue and may worsen.
- It is important to remember that older patients may have been previously more mobile and that the Beighton score may not be an appropriate measure. A history of joint laxity should be sought.
- Hypermobility extends beyond the joints highlighted in the Beighton scale. The clinician should look at the fingers, shoulders, neck, hips, patellofemoral joint, and skin laxity.
- Analgesics are often unhelpful for chronic pain but have their place for the treatment of acute symptoms. Pain and fatigue cause significant morbidity.
- Joint stabilizing exercises with particular reference to core stability, posture and proprioception are beneficial, as may be advice on avoiding overuse injuries and practical ways of managing day-to-day activities. A global approach to joint stability and function, as opposed to just treating regional symptoms, is effective.
- Pain management should be considered in chronic pain cases. This might include for example, cognitive behavioral therapy and the process is similar to that used in fibromyalgia (see Chapter 18).
- The role of serotonergic/noradrenergic agents in these patients is unclear. In part there may be effective control of depression, however, there may also be direct analgesic properties to these agents.
- Neuroleptic agents for neuropathic pain have not been studied in this group of patients. However, gabapentin or pregabalin and other similar agents may have a role.

Table 16.15 Beighton hypermobility rating

	Subject has the ability to:	Right	Left
1.	Passively dorsiflex the fifth metacarpophalangeal joint to ≥90°	1	1
2.	Oppose the thumb to the volar aspect of the ipsilateral Forearm	1	1
3.	Hyperextend the elbow ≥ 10°	1	1
4.	Hyperextend the knee ≥ 10°	1	1
5.	Place hands flat on the floor without bending the knees	1	
Possible total score		9	

Table 16.16 The Brighton (1998) criteria for benign joint hypermobility syndrome

Major criteria	A Beighton score of 4 out of 9 or greater (current or historical)
	Arthralgias for > 3 months in four or more joints
Minor criteria	A Beighton score of 1, 2, or 3 out of 9
	Arthralgias in one to three joints or back pain, either for longer than 3 months, spondylosis/spondylolisthesis
	Dislocation/subluxation in > one joint, or one joint on > one occasion
	Soft tissue rheumatism in three or more sites
	Marfanoid habitus
	Abnormal skin: striae, hyperextensibility, papyraceous scars
	Eye signs: drooping eyelids, myopia,
	Varicose veins, hernias, uterine/rectal prolapse

Rare chondrodysplasias and storage disorders

There are >150 distinctive chondrodysplasias representing autosomal dominant, recessive, and X-linked patterns of inheritance. The first identified mutations were found in the collagen 2A1 gene, and are associated with premature osteoarthrosis. Such conditions include achondrogenesis, Kniest syndrome, spondyloepiphyseal dysplasia, and the Stickler syndrome. Clinical features in the latter three conditions include premature joint destruction, joint/bone deformity, short stature, and progressive myopia (with or without retinal detachment). Stickler syndrome patients are also prone to hernias and cardiac valvular and conduction disorders.

Storage diseases associated with progressive skeletal dysplasia include:
- Mucopolysaccharidoses, e.g., Hurler, Hunter, Scheie
- Mucolipidoses
- Sphingolipidoses
- Gaucher's disease
- Fabry's disease.

The detail and complexities of these conditions is beyond the scope of this book.

Infection and rheumatic disease

Introduction

Infectious agents have been linked directly and indirectly (through organism-specific and autoimmune responses) to a number of acute and chronic inflammatory rheumatic diseases. This chapter will introduce some examples of inflammatory mechanisms (see Table 17.1) and infectious agents (see Table 17.2) linked to rheumatic disease, and then discuss septic arthritis, osteomyelitis, Lyme disease, and rheumatic fever.

Table 17.1 Pathogenesis of rheumatic disease associated with infection

Inflammatory process	Basic process	Example	Susceptibility
Local infection at musculoskeletal sites	Infection. Tissue inflammation and direct damage	Pyogenic septic arthritis	Structural damage to joint replacement Diabetes, complement and immunoglobulin deficiencies
Pathogen and pathogen-specific immune response	Infection and organism-specific immune response. Immune response to intact organismor fragments, probable immune complex-mediated tissue injury	Syndromes associated with viral hepatitis, e.g., Sjögren's syndrome	Not generally established
Pathogens, immuneresponse, and autoimmunity	i. Cross-reactive immune response ii. Infection inferred but not established autoreactivity	Rheumatic fever Rheumatoid arthritis Juvenile idiopathic arthritis Systemic lupus erythematosus	Certain MHC class I and II genes Receptor genes MHC class I and II genes T-cell receptor genes

Table 17.2 Selected pathogens associated with arthritis

Class	Examples	Disorder
Bacteria	*Staphylococcus and Streptococcus*	Non-gonococcal arthritis
		Septic monoarthritis
		Osteomyelitis
	Neisseria spp	Gonococcal arthritis
	Brucella	Septic monoarthritis
		Spondylarthropathy
	Chlamydia	Reactive (formerly, Reiter's)
Mycobacteria	*M. tuberculosis*	Osteomyelitis
		Spinal disease
		Monoarthropathy
Atypical mycobacteria	*M. avium* complex *M. malmoense*	Septic arthritis in immunosuppressed patients
Spirochete	*Borrelia burgdorferi*	Lyme disease
Viruses	Parvovirus B19	Fifth disease
	Rubella	Polyarthropathy
	Hepatitis B	Polyarteritis nodosa
	Hepatitis C	Cryoglobulinemia
		Sjögren's syndrome
	HIV	Polyarthralgia and myopathy
		Vasculitis
		Sicca syndrome
Protozoa	Toxoplasma	Polyarthritis
	Giardia	Oligoarthritis
		Small-vessel vasculitis
	Trypanosoma	Myopathy
Helminths	Toxocara	All cause myositis and arthritis
	Dracunculus	
	Schistosoma	
Fungi	Histoplasma	Can cause monoarthropathy
	Cryptococcus	

Pyogenic nongonococcal and gonococcal arthritides

- Septic arthritis caused by a pyogenic bacterium is a medical emergency. Incidence in the general population is 2–10 per 100,000, rising to 30–70 per 100,000 in those with autoimmune rheumatic disease or prosthetic joint replacements.
- Most cases are due to hematogenous seeding during transient bacteremia, but septic arthritis can also be caused by direct penetration through the skin or by local spread from a contiguous infected site.
- Joints damaged by chronic arthritis (e.g., RA, OA) and prosthetic joints are at increased risk of infection. Immunodeficiency states and diabetes are added risk factors.
- Transient synovitis, particularly of the hip, is not uncommon in children, and generally occurs after upper respiratory tract infection. The presence of three of the following favors the diagnosis of septic arthritis: an elevated serum white blood cell count, inability to bear weight, recent history of fever, and elevated erythrocyte sedimentation rate.
- The most common pathogens are *Staphylococcus aureus*, *Streptococcus* spp and *Neisseria gonorrhoeae* in adults. Prior to the development of the vaccine, *Haemophilus influenzae* was a common cause of septic arthritis. The clinical features and natural history of gonococcal and nongonococcal arthritis are sufficiently distinct to discuss them separately (see Table 17.3).
- Unusual organisms may be involved in patients with a current history of IV drug abuse, or those who are immunosuppressed.
- Salmonella may cause septic arthritis among patients with sickle cell disease.

Management of pyogenic joint infection

Three principles determine outcome: prompt diagnosis, immediate institution of appropriate antibiotics, and adequate drainage of joint.

- Specific tests for infection should include joint aspiration, Gram stain, and culture of synovial fluid; blood cultures, and (if relevant) skin/rash swabs and oral and urethral swabs.
- Surgical drainage and washout or daily arthrocentesis may be required for nongonococcal septic arthritis.
- Plain radiographs in early disease are unhelpful, since they show only soft tissue swelling. In later untreated disease, joint space narrowing and erosion will be seen. Ultrasound may show a joint effusion.
- An affected joint should be rested and nonweight-bearing until the inflammation and pain have subsided enough to allow passive mobilization. Mobilization should be encouraged as soon as possible.
- Empiric therapy with a third-generation cephalosporin should be started while waiting for culture data. Consider vancomycin in areas where community acquired MRSA is prevalent. *Pseudomonas* spp. should be suspected in intravenous drug users.

Table 17.3 Clinical features of gonococcal and nongonococcal arthritis

Gonococcal arthritis	Nongonococcal arthritis

Causative agents:
  Neisseria gonorrhoeae
  Neisseria meningitidis
	Causative agents:
	  Staphylococcus aureus (50% of cases)
	  Staphylococcus epidermis (15% of cases)
	  Streptococcus pyogenes/pneumoniae (20% of cases)
	  Gram-negative bacteria (10% of cases)
	  anaerobes (5% of cases)

Most often in young, healthy adults	Most often in the elderly, or underlying joint or medical condition
Women > men	Men > women
Hip disease uncommon	Hip disease common (20% of cases)
Migratory polyarthritis common	Polyarthritis uncommon
	Monoarthritis very common
Rash, skin blisters/pustules, tenosynovitis common	Extra-articular manifestations common

Synovial fluid analysis:
 	
  Gram's stain is positive in 25%
  Culture positive, 50%
  Lactate normal
	Synovial fluid analysis:
	
	  Gram's stain is positive in 60%
	  Culture positive, 90%
	  Lactate raised

Rapid response to therapy	Often slow response, may require surgery
Full recovery in most cases	10% mortality; one-third residual damage

- Duration of therapy should be based on the organism and response to therapy. One general approach is to treat with IV antibiotics for 7 to 14 days (until the swelling subsides and blood cultures are negative), followed by another 2–4 weeks of an appropriate oral antibiotic.
- There are no studies comparing long and short courses of antibiotics.
- Septic arthritis involving a prosthetic joint should be treated in a stepwise fashion. First, the prosthetic should be removed and replaced with an antibiotic-impregnated spacer; the patient should receive intravenous antibiotics for six weeks. Two to four weeks after antibiotics are finished, the joint should be aspirated; if there continues to be evidence of infection, intravenous antibiotics should be administered for another six weeks. When the aspirate shows no evidence of infection, the joint can be replaced, using antibiotic-impregnated cement.

- Under no circumstances should a joint be injected with corticosteroid if intra-articular infection is suspected, or if there is superficial infection over the skin covering a joint, e.g., cellulitis/psoriasis. Likewise, there is no benefit from intra-articular antibiotics; indeed, these drugs may cause a chemical synovitis.

Management of septic bursitis

- The two most common sites of bursal infection are the olecranon and prepatellar bursae. These are usually managed with serial aspiration and oral antibiotics. Those who do not respond will need IV antibiotics and surgical incision and drainage.
- Osteomyelitis is a potential complication of chronic infected bursitis.

Mycobacterium tuberculosis

- Until 1985, the United States and Europe saw a decline in the number of tuberculosis (TB) cases. The appearance of acquired immune deficiency syndrome halted that trend. More recently, the recurrence of TB has become an important complication of new disease modifying antirheumatic therapies.
- It is estimated that one-third of the world's population is infected with TB. In industrialized countries <5% of cases of TB develop infection of bone or joints.
- Tuberculosis of bone is usually a low grade and slow progressive infection associated with a variable degree of local and systemic symptoms such as fatigue, weight loss, or night sweats. The onset is insidious and usually mono-articular or mono-osseous. Predisposing factors include pre-existing arthritis, alcoholism, prolonged use of corticosteroids, and immunosuppression.
- TB can affect any part of the musculoskeletal system. The spine is a common site, whether within a vertebral body, disc, or a paravertebral abscess. Spinal-cord compression due to vertebral destruction and/ or soft tissue swelling due to an abscess is a serious complication and must be treated emergently, with review by a neurosurgeon. Spinal stabilization procedures carry a good prognosis in preventing neurological sequelae. Monoarticular disease is seen most often in the weight-bearing joints of the hip, knee, ankle or sacroiliac joint, in that order. The wrist and shoulder are less commonly affected. Osteomyelitis may affect any long bone and is associated with either solitary or multifocal cysts.
- The diagnosis of TB is made by identifying acid-fast bacilli from a lesion or by histopathological changes in excised tissue. Occasionally, a high level of clinical suspicion, in the absence of other identified pathology, will lead the physician to treat empirically. Standard anti-TB regimens should be used for treatment and surveillance for 1 year after the end of treatment is recommended. Surgical intervention may be necessary; this may take the form for example of tissue biopsy, debridement of necrotic tissue, or stabilization of a joint or long bone.
- Because of the association between TNF-α inhibitors and disseminated tuberculosis, the identification of latent TB has become increasingly important. This is accomplished using a tuberculin skin test (PPD). Induration of greater than 5 mm should be considered positive in patients who are immunosuppressed. This is true whether or not the patient has received the BCG vaccine in the past.
- Two blood-based interferon-gamma release assays have been approved by the FDA for the diagnosis of Mycobacterium tuberculosis infection, including latent disease. This is the test of choice in patients who have a history of BCG vaccination, or are unlikely to return to have their tuberculin skin test read.

Atypical mycobacterial infection
- Patients with autoimmune rheumatic diseases on immunosuppressant medication are at risk of developing atypical infections.
- These infections are usually chronic in nature and can mimic an inflammatory flare of rheumatic disease, which can make diagnosis difficult. *M. malmoense* has been described causing tensoynovitis and septic arthritis of the knee. *M. avium* complex and *M. chelonae* osteoarticular infections have also been described.
- Atypical infections should be considered in patients with autoimmune rheumatic disease who present with musculoskeletal symptoms that do not respond to conservative treatment.

Osteomyelitis

- This term is used to describe any infection involving bone or marrow.
- A number of general, local, and systemic factors need to be taken into account when managing osteomyelitis (see Table 17.4).
- *Staphylococcus aureus* is the most common cause of osteomyelitis, but in the immunosuppressed host, it is also important to consider tuberculosis, pseudomonas, and salmonella.

Diagnostic procedures

- No single laboratory test is reliable enough to be used routinely for the diagnosis of osteomyelitis. An elevated white cell count and ESR may not be seen despite infection. Imaging plays an important part in establishing the diagnosis. Whether a particular imaging technique is successful at picking up osteomyelitis depends partly on the stage of the infective process.
- Once the pathogen has reached bone, a suppurative reaction and marrow edema occurs. This can be seen using MR imaging. The next stage, vascular congestion, ischemia, thrombosis, and soft tissue swelling, is readily detected by CT. After 2–3 weeks, bone reactions including new periosteal bone formation and decalcification can be seen on plain films.
- Plain films should always be taken if the clinical setting is appropriate, even in assumed early disease, as they may be highly informative.
- Vertebral osteomyelitis is often seen early on plain films. Erosion of the vertebral body or disc, and paravertebral abscesses and vertebral collapse, are common complications.
- Isotope bone scanning may be helpful in localizing an area of abnormality. ^{99}Tcm-labeled scans are, however, not specific, and the negative predictive value is often greater than the positive predictive value in this scenario. ^{67}Ga- or ^{111}Indium-labeled leukocyte scans may be helpful in localizing infection.

Treatment

- Initial treatment in the acute phase is the same as that for septic monoarthritis (see above). In general, antibiotics are needed for 6 weeks, although chronic infection may require long-term (in excess of 3 months) treatment. In addition to the common IV antibiotics discussed above, an anti-staphylococcal penicillin (such as oxacillin or nafcillin) should be considered. Clindamycin and fluoroquinlones are also used to treat osteomyelitis.
- Surgery is required early in the acute phase especially if there is necrotic tissue, an abscess, or spinal involvement. Chronic osteomyelitis implies that dead bone is present and this will require surgical debridement.
- Hyperbaric oxygen has also been used successfully in the treatment of air embolism, osteonecrosis, myonecrosis, and burn patients with infection.

Table 17.4 Factors relevant to the management of osteomyelitis

Factors	Examples
General	Age: neonates tend to harbor S. aureus, enterobacteriaceae, and β-hemolytic streptococci. In children > 4 years, H. influenzae is common, and in adults S. aureus
	Bone: long bones (especially lower limb) are more susceptible than short bones. Pelvic and cranial bones are infrequently involved
Local	Chronic lymphedema
	Venous stasis
	Arterial disease with poor flow
	Scars
	Sensory neuropathy
	Prosthetic material
Systemic	Malnutrition
	Renal and liver failure
	Immunodeficiency
	Diabetes
	Malignancy
	Extremes of age
	Chronic hypoxia
	Parenteral drug use

Lyme disease

- Lyme disease is a tick-borne infection caused by the spirochete *Borrelia burgdorferi*.
- Cases of Lyme disease have been reported from most states in the United States as well as throughout Europe, the former USSR, China, and Japan.
- The highest incidence is in children under the age of 15 years and middle-aged adults, with seasonal variation, being most common in the summer months of June and July.
- The tick vector, *Ixodes*, is found on rodents mainly and in wooded, brush, or grassy areas. A history of potential exposure in an endemic country within the last 30 days is an important fact to establish in considering the diagnosis. A clear history of a tick bite is not necessary to make this diagnosis.
- The diagnosis is approached clinically, partly based on epidemiological history as well as on classical clinical features (see Table 17.5), and confirmed with laboratory tests.

Laboratory tests

- Confirmation of Lyme disease may be by:
  - isolation of the spirochete from tissue or body fluid
  - detection of diagnostic levels of IgM or IgG antibodies in the serum or CSF
  - detection of changes in antibody levels between acute phase and convalescent paired sera.
- False-positive results occur in other infections such as syphilis and treponema, as well as in RA and SLE. Western blotting is available as a confirming test, distinguishing between true seroreactivity and false positivity.
- Serologies may be negative in early in the disease course, when erythema migrans is present. Note that erythema migrans is sometimes called the "bull's eye rash", although it does not always take on this appearance.

Treatment

Treatment of Lyme disease is summarized in Table 17.6.

Table 17.5 The clinical features of Lyme disease

System affected	Symptoms
Skin	Erythema migrans (EM). Begins as a red macule/papule expanding over days or weeks to a large round lesion often with partial central clearing. The lesion should measure 5 cm or more. There may be smaller secondary lesions*
	An expanding lesion is often accompanied by general symptoms: fever, fatigue, arthralgias, myalgias, headache
	Months later a chronic lesion, acrodermatitis chronicum atrophicans (ACA), can appear (violaceous infiltrated plaques or nodules)
Musculoskeletal system	Recurrent, brief attacks of joint swelling in one or a few joints (may become chronic—60% of untreated cases weeks to years after infection).
	A post-Lyme syndrome of fatigue, arthralgias, and myalgias has been reported. Ongoing infection has been difficult to prove, and this may represent a fibromyalgia/chronic pain syndrome.
Nervous system	Lymphocytic meningitis
	Cranial neuritis (especially facial nerve palsy)
	Radiculoneuropathy (differential Guillain–Barré)
	Encephalomyelitis
Cardiovascular	Acute second- or third-degree atrioventricular conduction defects often associated with myocarditis. Resolve in days to weeks
	Carditis—rare and remits spontaneously

* A similar lesion occurring within hours of a tick bite is usually a hypersensitivity reaction and does not qualify as EM.

Table 17.6 The treatment of Lyme disease

Clinical feature	Treatment
Skin disease	Doxycycline 100 mg twice daily for 3 weeks or Cefuroxime 500 mg twice daily for 3 weeks
Septic arthritis	As for skin disease except may require treatment for up to 30 days
Neurologic disease: Meningitis, Cranial nerve palsy	IV Ceftriaxone 2 g daily or Penicillin G 3–4 million units every 4 hours or cefotaxime 2 g every 8 hours
Carditis	As for neurologic disease, above. Both meningitis and carditis should be treated with 2–3 weeks of parenteral antibiotics

Rheumatic fever

- Rheumatic fever is a delayed, nonsuppurative sequel to a pharyngeal infection with Lancefield group A β-hemolytic streptococci.
- There is a latent period of 2–3 weeks before the appearance of an illness. A symptomatic pharyngitis is seen in 60% cases; migratory arthritis (typically of the large joints), myocarditis and valvulitis, and central nervous system disease (chorea) are all associated with this diagnosis.
- While the infection is often self-limiting, chronic and progressive damage to cardiac valves occur leading to cardiac decompensation and death.
- The use of penicillin within 10 days after a *S. pyogenes* infection decreases the risk of rheumatic heart disease significantly.
- Although there has been a dramatic decline in the United States and Europe, the disease still occurs in these areas, and is common in developing countries. There are an estimated 10–20 million cases per year in these areas, with an annual incidence of 100–200 per 100,000.
- Associations have been described with HLA DR2, 3, and 4.

The clinical features may be summarized in the revised Jones criteria (see Table 17.7).

Clinical manifestations and treatment of rheumatic fever

Arthritis

- Joint involvement is more common and often more severe inteenagers and young adults. It tends to start in the large joints of the lower limbs and migrate. Arthropathy tends to occur early and the pain can be severe in the absence of objective signs of inflammation. It lasts 2–3 weeks and is self-limiting.
- NSAIDs are the main treatment for the condition.
- Where one draws the line between the phenomenon of post-streptococcal reactive arthritis (seen in the absence of carditis) and rheumatic fever is difficult. Most patients will fulfill the Jones criteria and, therefore, should be considered as having rheumatic fever.

Cardiac disease

- Rheumatic heart disease is the most severe outcome of acute rheumatic fever. It remains the major cause of acquired valvular heart disease in the world. The mitral valve (stenosis) is involved more frequently than the aortic valve. When left unchecked, cardiomegaly and cardiac failure secondary to valvular disease develops.
- Carditis may also occur and is associated with cardiomyopathy and conduction defects including second- or third-degree heart block.

Chorea

- Sydenham's chorea (St. Vitus dance) is a neurological disorder consisting of abrupt, purposeless movements, muscle weakness, and emotional disturbance. The hands and face are usually the most obviously affected parts. The movements are not present during sleep

Table 17.7 The revised Jones criteria for the diagnosis of acute rheumatic fever (diagnosis requires 2 major, or 1 major and 2 minor criteria)

Major manifestations	Carditis
	Polyarthritis
	Chorea
	Erythema marginatum
	Subcutaneous nodules
Minor manifestations	Fever
	Arthralgia
	Previous rheumatic fever or rheumatic heart disease
Laboratory tests	Raised ESR or CRP
	Normochromic normocytic anemia
	Prolonged PR interval on ECG
Supporting evidence	Raised ASO titer*
	Positive throat cultures for group A streptococci
	Recent scarlet fever

* ASO = antistreptolysin O antibodies (titers peak at about 4 weeks, which is about 2 weeks into the clinical onset of rheumatic fever; they fall off rapidly over the following 2–3 months).

but do occur at rest, and may be more marked on one side of the body.
- Chorea may be the sole feature suggesting rheumatic fever (beyond observing new cardiac murmurs) and may occur weeks to months after onset of an arthropathy.

Skin
- The subcutaneous nodules of rheumatic fever are firm and painless. They are located over bony surfaces or near tendons, and are present for 2–4 weeks only, and more often in patients with carditis.
- Erythema marginatum is an evanescent, nonpurpuric rash, usually affecting the trunk and proximal part of the limbs, but sparing the face. Because the rash often appears to make a ring, it is also called erythema annulare. The lesions come and go in a matter of hours and heat may make them appear, or become worse. Again, it is more common in association with carditis. They resolve spontaneously.
- Erythema nodosum is rare.

Diagnosis
- There is no diagnostic investigation.
- Raised inflammatory markers are seen, often with a mild anemia.

- Serial rises in antistreptolysin O titers may be seen if measured every 14 days.
- Chest radiograph and ECG to look for conduction defects/cardiomegaly.

Treatment of rheumatic fever

- The mainstay of treatment is an anti-inflammatory agent, usually aspirin.
- If carditis is present, steroids should be started (2 mg/kg/day oral prednisone for 1–2 weeks followed by steroid taper over 2 weeks).
- Penicillin should be taken for 10 days, even in the absence of ongoing pharyngitis.
- Chorea can be treated with haloperidol 1–2 mg/kg/day, often given with prednisone, although there is little evidence that this gives added benefit.
- Recurrence is most common within the first 2 years; however, recurrence rates seem to be low, and the risk of recurrence declines with age at first attack.
- Prophylaxis in those who have had rheumatic fever should probably continue for life, though some clinicians would recommend up to 10 years with antibiotic therapy to cover any dental or invasive procedure. Prophylaxis can be given either as oral penicillin V, 250,000 units twice daily, or as penicillin G, 1.2 million units IM once every 3–4 weeks. Erythromycin at 250 mg daily may be used if there is an allergy to penicillins.

Miscellaneous conditions

Behçet's disease

- Behçet's disease is a systemic inflammatory disorder of unknown etiology. It is most common in the Mediterranean basin, the Middle East, and Asia.
- The usual onset of the syndrome is in the third or fourth decade.
- Onset is rare in children, and after the age of 45 years.
- The male: female ratio is approximately equal, but the syndrome tends to run a more severe course in men and the young.
- Based on registries, the prevalence is about 1 in 300,000 in Northern Europe, 1 in 10,000 in Japan, and 40 in 10,000 in Turkey.
- The syndrome is classically associated with HLA B5—its presence associated with greater disease severity. However, there are geographical variations. Patients from Mediterranean countries and Japan show this association with B5, but patients in the United States do not. In patients of Israeli origin, there is an association with HLA B51.
- The full-blown syndrome might be easy to identify, but there are conditions that mimic the incomplete picture, including reactive arthritis, inflammatory bowel disease, and major aphthous ulcers.
- There are no laboratory findings specific to the condition. The ESR and CRP are often only moderately raised.

Clinical features and their management

Skin and mucosa involvement (see Table 18.1)

- Oral aphthous ulcers are always present, and may precede other features by several years. Idiopathic oral aphthous ulcers are common, and by themselves do not imply the presence of Behçet's. The ulcers associated with Behçet's are indistinguishable from ordinary ulcers, but tend to be multiple, more frequent, and may heal with scarring.
- Genital ulceration in men is most prominent over the scrotum (90%). Urethritis is not seen unless there is a meatal ulcer. In women, the labia are commonly affected. Cervical ulcers are rare.
- Skin lesions may be nodular (resembling erythema nodosum), acneiform, or vasculitic.
- The pathergy reaction, a hyperreactivity of the skin to a needle prick, is peculiar to this syndrome and pyoderma gangrenosum. After skin puncture with a needle, a papule or pustule forms in 24–48 h. The reaction is seldom found in patients from Northern Europe or the United States, but is positive in 60% and 70% of patients from Japan and Turkey, respectively.
- Mild oral and genital ulceration may respond to oral colchicine 0.6 mg po bid. More severe disease may require AZA 2.5 mg/kg/day. Nonsteroidal anti-inflammatory drugs can help control pain.

Eye disease

- This is a serious complication and a negative prognostic factor. Eye disease is more common in men and patients <25 years of age.
- Disease is bilateral in 90% of cases and is usually a chronic relapsing panuveitis. The presence of a hypopyon (cells in the anterior chamber)

Table 18.1 The clinical findings in Behçet's disease

Lesion	Prevalence (%)
Aphthous ulcers	97–100
Genital ulcers	80–90
Skin lesions	80
Eye lesions	50
Arthritis	40–50
Thrombophlebitis	25
Neurological disease	1–15
Gastrointestinal disease	0–25

is almost always associated with severe retinal vasculitis, after which there is almost always some structural damage despite treatment. The extent of this damage determines the course of eye disease in Behçet's syndrome.
- Topical steroids and mydriatics with close supervision may be sufficient in mild disease, but severe disease requires the addition of AZA 2.5 mg/kg/day or anti-TNF-α therapy to the topical regimen.

Musculoskeletal system involvement
- Joint involvement is seen in about 50% of patients.
- It is usually mono- or oligoarticular, but can be symmetric, mimicking RA.
- Chronic synovitis is rare, nonerosive, and nondeforming.
- In general, knees, ankles, wrists, and elbows are involved (in descending order of frequency).
- Back pain is rare.
- Pain may respond to NSAIDs. Inflammatory disease often requires the introduction of methotrexate 20–25 mg PO/SQ weekly.

Cardiovascular and pulmonary involvement
- Endocarditis, myocarditis, pericarditis, coronary vasculitis, and ventricular aneurysms can all occur but are rare.
- Venous involvement is one of the main features of Behçet's syndrome. Thrombophlebitis occurs in 25% of all patients. Limb venous thrombosis is often observed. Occlusion of the suprahepatic veins—Budd–Chiari syndrome—carries a high mortality.
- Pulmonary embolism is rare despite high rates of thrombophlebitis. It might be explained by the difference in architecture of thromboses seen in Behçet's syndrome versus normal (e.g., postoperative) thromboses. The former tends to adhere throughout its length to the vein wall; the latter tends to have a long, nonadherent and potentially embolic tail.
- Arterial lesions can occur anywhere. Aneurysms may develop and rupture. This is frequently fatal.

- The pulmonary pathology of Behçet's disease is related to arterial vasculitis. Aneurysms, thromboses, and infarcts may be found.
- Aspirin and NSAIDs can be used to relieve the symptoms of phlebitis. Aneurysms and arterial occlusion require cytotoxic therapy with cyclophosphamide 2.5 mg/kg/day and prednisone 1 mg/kg/day; surgery may also be indicated. There remains debate about whether to use heparin or oral anticoagulants for the thrombophlebitis, although most physicians will choose to treat with anticoagulation in addition to immunosuppression.

Neurological involvement
- Prospective surveys suggest a prevalence rate of 5% for neurological disease in the condition.
- Pyramidal signs are the most common, followed by cerebellar and sensory symptoms and signs. The most common site is the brainstem. Meningeal irritation and dementia may also occur. As is the case with eye disease, central nervous involvement is often more severe in men.
- In contrast to other vasculitides, peripheral neuropathy is unusual.
- CNS disease should be treated with IV methylprednisolone, and cyclophosphamide should be considered.

Gastrointestinal involvement
- While seen in up to one-third of patients in Japan, gastrointestinal disease is rare in patients from the Mediterranean basin.
- The basic pathology is mucosal ulceration, seen most often in the ileum and cecum. The course is one of relapse and remission, with a distinct tendency to perforate.
- Ulceration may respond to prednisone 0.5–1 mg/kg/day, sulfasalazine 2–3 g/day, or infliximab. Surgical evaluation may be necessary to manage severe sequelae.

Renal involvement
- This is seen much less than might be expected in a systemic vasculitis. There are occasional reports of glomerulonephritis. Amyloidosis usually presents with nephrotic syndrome.
- About 5% of men develop epididymitis. Treatment focuses on symptom control.

Treatment of Behçet's disease
- Colchicine 0.6 mg po bid should be used to treat orogenital ulceration; dapsone (25–100 mg PO daily), thalidomide, and anti-TNF-α therapy all have demonstrated efficacy.
- Azathioprine 2.5 mg/kg/day should be considered for the treatment of the systemic manifestations of Behçet's. Methotrexate 20–25 mg/week may also be effective, particularly for articular symptoms. Arteritis and other life-threatening manifestations should be treated with cyclophosphamide 2.5 mg/kg/day.
- Infliximab (e.g., 5 mg/kg IV every 4 weeks) or rituximab (e.g., 375 mg/m^2 IV weekly for 4 weeks) may be effective for treating ocular manifestations of Behçet's that do not respond to topical therapy.
- Warfarin should be used in the usual way for thrombotic episodes. If thrombosis occurs in the setting of disease flare, immunosuppression may be required as well.

Sarcoidosis

- Sarcoidosis is a multisystem disease of unknown etiology, characterized by the presence of multiple, noncaseating granulomas in involved tissue.
- It occurs worldwide, but the prevalence, clinical features, and outcome varies. It is seen more often in developed versus underdeveloped, Western versus Eastern, and in Northern versus Southern European countries. Sweden and Denmark have prevalence rates of 60 per 100,000: the United Kingdom 20 per 100,000. In the United States, sarcoidosis is 10–15 times more prevalent in the African American population than in Caucasians; African Americans may also present with a more severe form of this disease. There is also an increased incidence of sarcoidosis in families. Recent studies have suggested a link between HLA B8, DR3, and acute sarcoidosis with arthritis.
- Acute sarcoidosis presents with rapid onset fever, erythema nodosum, and hilar lymphadenopathy. This condition has a high rate of remission and a good prognosis; the chest radiograph clears within 1 year in 60% of cases.
- Chronic sarcoidosis is less common and has a subtle, insidious, progressive, and highly variable clinical course (see Table 18.2).
- Sarcoidosis is rare in childhood, and usually indolent. If arthritis occurs, it is usually before 5 years of age and associated with eye and cutaneous disease.

Musculoskeletal manifestations of sarcoid

Joints

- Distinctive patterns of arthropathy are seen in both acute and chronic sarcoidosis. In acute disease, transient arthralgias may precede the emergence of other symptoms. Sarcoid arthritis is usually symmetric and persists for 1–4 months on average, and occurs in association with erythema nodosum (EN). Effusions are common at the knees and ankles. After recovery, acute sarcoidosis only occasionally recurs.
- Chronic arthritis is uncommon in sarcoidosis; when it does occur, it usually appears in the form of monoarthritis or involvement of the spine. Again, knees and ankles appear to be most often involved with inflammatory disease, characterized by acute exacerbation with synovial thickening and effusions. Unlike acute sarcoidosis, a history of EN is unusual. Chronic polyarthritis is also more frequent in women than men. It may cause joint deformity and destruction.

Bones

- Bone involvement occurs in 5% of all patients with sarcoidosis. Bone cysts are seen most often in the hands and feet and are most frequently seen in patients with persistent disease and/or lupus pernio (i.e., erythematous induration of the skin across the face). Cysts are often asymptomatic and found by chance on plain radiographs. Clinically they can present in the fingers and toes with "sausage-like" swollen digits.

Table 18.2 Clinical manifestations in chronic sarcoidosis

Organ/system	Clinical features
Lung	Parenchymal disease in > 90% of cases
Skin	Lupus pernio, plaques, and nodules
Ocular	Uveitis, conjunctivitis, sicca
Lymphatics	Lymphadenopathy, splenomegaly
Bone marrow	Infiltration
Hepatic	Failure, granuloma, portal hypertension
Renal	Nephrocalcinosis, granuloma, glomerular disease
Cardiac	Arteritis, cardiomyopathy, conduction abnormalities
Nervous system	Central and peripheral neuropathy. intracerebral lesions. Meningitis. Seizures
Granulomata	Endocrine and reproductive organs. Gastrointestinal tract. Salivary/lacrimal glands. Nose, tonsils, and larynx

- Other radiological features include thickening of cortical bone, acrosclerosis, and joint destruction.
- Occasionally lytic lesions appear in vertebral bodies, leading to back pain and crush fractures. Lytic lesions may also be seen in the skull bones and long bones.

Muscles

- Often asymptomatic, in the early stages of acute sarcoidosis granulomatous muscle involvement is common (50–80%). It may present as proximal pain, tenderness, and weakness. Involvement may be focal with a granulomatous mass or diffuse and symmetrical myopathy, the latter leading to progressive weakness and atrophy.
- Electromyography looks similar to that of polymyositis.

Diagnosis and treatment of sarcoidosis

- A patient with a new diagnosis of sarcoidosis should receive an electrocardiogram, pulmonary function tests, computed tomography of the chest, and slit-lamp examination, in addition to a thorough physical examination and symptom-driven evaluation.
- The red blood cell count is usually normal. Leukopenia can be seen in up to one-third of cases, and eosinophilia in one-quarter. Thrombocytopenia is a relatively common problem.
- The ESR may be elevated in the acute phase, particularly if EN is present.
- Reports of hypercalcemia vary widely from 2–60%. The level tends to fluctuate and the reasons for such wide variation remain unclear.
- Liver function tests may be abnormal.
- One-third of patients have significant proteinuria.

- Epithelial cells found in the granuloma produce angiotensin-converting enzyme (ACE). Serial measurements of this enzyme may be useful in monitoring the course of the disease, although it is not a reliable screening test for establishing the diagnosis.
- As sarcoidosis can resemble other diseases such as lymphoma and tuberculosis, the diagnosis should be confirmed by histology. Peripheral tissues such as skin or salivary glands may be helpful. Transbronchial lung biopsy is widely used and highly sensitive and specific.
- Acute, transient disease may resolve spontaneously, and require only supportive care.
- More severe disease may require treatment with corticosteroids, either alone or in combination with methotrexate.
- Addition of hydroxychloroquine may also help the skin and joint manifestations of sarcoid. Infliximab may be useful to treat refractory forms of this disease, including lupus pernio.
- Most patients with chronic disease will require steroid therapy, but the decision to treat is more often related to systemic involvement than to articular disease.
- No therapy is required for asymptomatic osseous, cystic bone disease, or asymptomatic muscle disease. The place for steroids in chronic sarcoid myopathy remains uncertain.

Miscellaneous skin conditions associated with arthritis

Panniculitis

Panniculitis refers to inflammation within the subcutaneous fat. It is a dynamic inflammatory process involving neutrophils, leukocytes, and histiocytes that causes fibrosis, and, sometimes, granulomatous change.

There are four categories of panniculitis, based on histopathology:

- Septal panniculitis
- Lobular panniculitis
- Mixed type septal and lobular
- Panniculitis with vasculitis.

Septal panniculitis

This includes erythema nodosum (EN) and Vilanova disease (subacute nodular migratory panniculitis). EN is a common, acute, and self-limiting condition found typically over the anterior tibial surface. It usually heals within 4–6 weeks without scarring, though a rare form can cause ulceration and a migratory form can occur for several years (more often in women around 45 years old). The causes and associations of EN are shown in Table 18.3.

Lobular panniculitis

Listed below are a number of conditions that cause lobular panniculitis.

- *Weber–Christian disease*: a relapsing, febrile, nodular nonsuppurative syndrome. There may be multiple recurrent nodules plus fever; arthralgias, myalgias, and abdominal pain are common. Any area of the body containing fat can become involved, e.g., mesentery, heart, lung, liver, kidney. There is a 10–15% mortality. Investigations may show:
  - typical histological features on biopsy
  - elevated ESR
  - anemia
  - leukopenia or leukocytosis

Many clinicians believe that Weber-Christian disease does not exist as an independent entity, and that this one term has been mistakenly used to represent several diseases with similar presentations. Therefore, at minimum, it should be considered a diagnosis of exclusion; prior to making this diagnosis, it is important to rule out other causes of panniculitis, including:

- *Lipogranulomatosis*: this group of conditions tends to occur in children. Multiple lesions, often on the extremities, resolve with subcutaneous atrophy.
- *Poststeroid use*: the pathogenesis of this rare condition is not understood. It seems to be limited to children, occurs on withdrawal of corticosteroids, and may clear up on steroid readministration.
- α1-*antitrypsin deficiency*: may respond to doxycycline.
- *Acute pancreatitis*.

Table 18.3 Etiological causes of EN

Cause	Examples
Infection	Streptococcal
	TB/leprosy
	Yersinia/Salmonella
	Histoplasmosis
	Blastomycosis
	Psittacosis
Drugs	Penicillin
	Sulfonamides
Pregnancy Diseases	Sarcoidosis
	Inflammatory bowel disease
	Collagen vascular disease (SLE, scleroderma, dermatomyositis)
	Malignancy (rare)
	Sweet's syndrome

- *Calcifying panniculitis* is a feature of chronic renal failure. It is not the same as metastatic calcification. The prognosis is poor even with good calcium-phosphate balance. Parathyroidectomy may help.
- *Lipodermatosclerosis*: this condition may be a result of venous insufficiency and thrombophlebitis. It should be treated with compression stockings. Intralesional corticosteroids or low-dose aspirin may also help.
- *Lupus profundus* is a rare manifestation of chronic cutaneous SLE, occurring in <3% of cases of SLE. The lesions are usually tender and may ulcerate and calcify. The lesions commonly occur on the face, upper arms, and buttocks, and may underlie an area of discoid lupus. The lesions do not seem to follow the course of the systemic disease. It may respond to steroids.
- *Factitious*: self-inflicted injuries may mimic the appearance of a panniculitis.

Panniculitis with vasculitis

This is seen in small-vessel and medium-vessel vasculitis. The reader is referred to Chapter 14.

Treatments include:
- Treatment of the underlying disease or agent
- NSAIDs
- Bed rest and limb elevation
- Antimalarials
- Steroids

- Dapsone
- Colchicine
- Azathioprine
- Cyclosporine.

Neutrophilic dermatoses

The neutrophilic dermatoses are a group of noninfectious disorders characterized by the presence of an angiocentric, primary neutrophilic inflammatory cell infiltrate. The disorders can be divided into those that cause vessel wall destruction (vasculitis) and those that do not. Table 18.4 lists the causes of noninfectious neutrophilic dermatoses. The majority of diseases are discussed in detail in their own chapters in this book. This section will discuss Sweet's syndrome, and pyoderma gangrenosum.

Sweet's syndrome

- This condition is rare and occurs more often in women than men (ratio 3.7:1), between the ages of 30 and 70 years. It has occasionally been reported in children. The pathogenesis is unknown.
- The characteristic features are myalgias, fever, arthralgias, and painful erythematous plaques (or occasionally nodules resembling erythema nodosum). Untreated, the lesions resolve over 6–8 weeks but new lesions will continue to appear. The condition is usually an acute, steroid-responsive, self-limiting disorder. If longer-term treatment is required, steroid dosage may be reduced by the addition of an NSAID, dapsone, colchicine, or possibly methotrexate.
- A secondary cause for the condition should be sought (see Table 18.5).

Pyoderma gangrenosum

- This is an uncommon, ulcerative, cutaneous condition associated with several systemic diseases (see Table 18.6).
- The lesion is characterized by an erythematous, violaceous border overhanging a central area of ulceration and necrosis. The lesions start as discrete pustules, most often on the legs, and are often extremely painful, healing with scars.
- There is no specific treatment. An underlying disease should be sought. Treatments include topical sodium cromoglycate or 5-amino salicylic acid, oral sulfonamides, dapsone, and corticosteroids.
- It is important to exclude potential mimics. Chronic infections, hypercoagulable states (such as the antiphospholipid antibody syndrome) and some forms of vasculitis can all lead to lesions that resemble pyoderma gangrenosum.

Multicentric reticulohistiocytosis

- This is a rare systemic disease, primarily a disorder of adults in their fifth decade. It is recognized clinically by the combination of papular and nodular skin lesions and a severe destructive polyarthritis.
- The disorder is distinct from the solitary nodule lesion of the reticulocytoma in that the latter is not associated with systemic disease. Multicentric reticulohistiocytosis may involve any organ system.

Table 18.4 Noninfectious neutrophilic dermatoses

Group	Examples
Nonangiocentric	Psoriasis
	Reactive arthritis
	Acne fulminans
Angiocentric and vessel destruction	Leukocytoclastic vasculitis
	Polyarteritis nodosa
Angiocentric, no vessel destruction	Sweet's syndrome
	Pyoderma gangrenosum
	Bowel-associated dermatosis–arthritis
	Behçet's disease
	Rheumatoid arthritis
	Ulcerative colitis
	Familial Mediterranean fever

Table 18.5 The associations with Sweet's syndrome

Associations	Examples
Hematological malignancy	Leukemia
	Lymphoma
	Myelodysplastic disorders
Solid tumors	Breast
	Gastric
	Genitourinary
	Colon
Infectious diseases	HIV
	Hepatitis
	Tuberculosis
	Salmonella
Inflammatory bowel disease	Ulcerative colitis
	Crohn's disease
Rheumatic diseases	Rheumatoid arthritis
	Systemic lupus erythematosus
	Sjögren's syndrome
	Behçet's disease

Table 18.6 Diseases associated with pyoderma gangrenosum

Association	Examples
Rheumatic diseases	Seronegative spondyloarthropathy
	Rheumatoid arthritis
	Osteoarthritis
	Psoriatic arthritis
	Systemic lupus erythematosus
	Granulomatosis with polyangiitis (Wegener's)
	Sarcoidosis
	Takayasu's arteritis
Hematological diseases	Leukemia
	Myelofibrosis
	Gammaglobulinemia
	Polycythemia vera
Gastrointestinal diseases	Inflammatory bowel disease
	Chronic active hepatitis
	Primary biliary cirrhosis
Other	Solid tumors
	Diabetes mellitus
	C7 complement deficiency

- The arthritis may mimic a RA pattern. Often the distal interphalangeal joints are involved and the destruction may give a picture similar to arthritis mutilans.
- The skin lesions occur in approximately 90% of cases. Histologically, the infiltrate consists of multicentric giant cells and histiocytes from the monocyte-macrophage lineage. The lesions are usually numerous, nonpruritic, skin colored (or yellow/brown), and range in size from millimeters to several centimeters in diameter. They occur most often on the dorsum of the hands and on the face (at the nose, corner of the mouth, and ears). Extensive facial involvement may lead to a "leonine" facies.
- About 25% of cases have xanthelasma.
- One-third of cases have constitutional symptoms/signs such as weight loss or fever.
- Approximately 25% of cases have been reported to have malignant (mostly solid tumor) disease. The investigation of the condition, therefore, requires a thorough screen for rheumatic and malignant disease.
- There are no specific laboratory markers. Histology is helpful. Biopsies may be taken from skin or inflamed synovium.

- The differential diagnosis includes:
  - rheumatoid or psoriatic arthritis
  - sarcoid dactylitis
  - xanthoma
  - histiocytosis X—a disorder of children
  - histiocytoma or tendon sheath giant-cell tumor—usually solitary.
- As a rule, the condition waxes and wanes, and spontaneous remissions can occur.
- Multicentric reticulohistiocytosis has been associated with numerous forms of malignancy, and a new diagnosis should prompt a thorough investigation.
- Patients with multicentric reticulohistiocytosis may quickly develop a disabling arthritis, and should be treated aggressively. For patients with mild disease, methotrexate may be sufficient, but some patients may require treatment with cyclophosphamide to prevent progressive damage.

Chronic regional pain syndrome

This syndrome is characterized by variable dysfunction of the musculoskel-etal, skin, neurological, and vascular systems. It may occur in a variety of situations with a number of clinical manifestations varying around central core features. As such, several terms have evolved, describing the same phenomenon:

- Reflex sympathetic dystrophy
- Sudeck's atrophy
- Shoulder–hand syndrome
- Transient osteoporosis
- Regional migratory osteoporosis
- Posttrauma painful osteoporosis

Complex regional pain syndrome (CRPS) has two types; type 1 is symp-toms in the absence of nerve injury, and type 2 ("causalgia") is symptoms in the presence of nerve injury.

Epidemiology

- CRPS is a common disorder. It affects both sexes equally and occurs at any age in all races and geographical regions. Typically the syndrome involves the distal part of a limb, e.g. forearm or foot.
- The early clinical features of the condition include:
  - pain
  - soft tissue swelling (may be synovitis if over a joint)
  - reticular/livedo rash
  - warmth over affected part occasionally there may be localized
  - sweating and piloerection.
- The pain has several particular characteristics and is often described as burning. The features include:
  - allodynia—an otherwise innocuous stimulus produces pain
  - hyperalgesia—increased pain perception to a given stimulus
  - hyperpathia—delayed overreaction, often after repetitive cutaneous stimulus.

The net effect is abnormal tenderness to even minor stimuli.

- Trauma (whether accident, burn, surgery, etc.) is the most common triggering event. The event may have even seemed trivial or minor at the time.
- Several neurological conditions may act as triggers, including, for example, hemiplegia and meningitis. Peripheral nerve root injury may also lead to the syndrome.
- Pregnancy, tumors, and prolonged immobilization have also been linked as possible triggering factors. However, 25% of cases have no clear trigger.
- It is important to try and identify psychosocial stresses.
- The signs and symptoms of pain, swelling, etc. (see above), are traditionally placed as stage I of the condition. In most cases the symptoms persist and fluctuate, though they may just gradually resolve. Stage II is a period of dystrophic change. This tends to occur several months after onset of the disorder. The affected region becomes

cool, pale, and often cyanosed in color with abnormal sensation (dysesthesia). There is a decrease in hair and nail growth, osteopenia develops, and eventually atrophy (stage III) of skin and subcutaneous tissue occurs; at this point the condition becomes difficult to treat and reverse. Most cases tend not to progress beyond stage I or, at most, early stage II.

Investigations

- Laboratory values, including acute phase reactants and metabolic profiles, are normal. However, there may be evidence of bone demineralization, with elevated 24-hour urine hydroxyproline excretion.
- Although essentially a clinical diagnosis, CRPS does have some radiological and nuclear medicine imaging characteristics. No technique is diagnostic. Plain radiographs, DEXA, and MR may show features of osteoporosis.
- Thermography can demonstrate changes in cutaneous temperature.
- Perhaps of most value, and high specificity, is the triple-phase technetium scintigraphy study, showing three phases of abnormal early regional blood flow, blood pool, and late bone uptake respectively.

Management

- Success in treatment of this condition probably hinges on focusing on the whole individual and not the regional symptoms, and making an early and accurate diagnosis. Attention to anxiety, psychosocial stressors, pain behavior, and sleep disturbance is important. The patient often requires repeated reassurance and counseling. The aim should be to resume premorbid levels of activity if possible. In this respect, early intervention with physical therapy and hydrotherapy should be considered.
- Tricyclic antidepressants can help correct sleep disturbance and increase the pain threshold.
- TENS may help pain control and allow entry into a physical activity program.
- In severe cases, regional sympathetic or ganglion blocks can control pain sufficiently to start more vigorous physical therapy or exercise programs.
- Some clinicians have also had success with corticosteroids and with pamidronate. There are no controlled trials of this or any other therapy mentioned above.

Relapsing polychondritis

- This is an uncommon multisystem disorder of unknown etiology, characterized by episodic and sometimes progressive inflammation of cartilage leading to destruction and fibrosis.
- Common sites of involvement include the ear, nose, larynx, joints, heart, and eyes (cornea and sclera) (see Table 18.7).
- Similar patterns of disease may be seen in granulomatosis with polyangiitis (Wegener's); also, some patients with relapsing polychondritis are ANCA+.
- The disease predominantly affects Caucasians in the fourth to fifth decades of life.
- Approximately 30% of cases have an underlying systemic rheumatic or autoimmune disease such as RA, systemic lupus, Sjögren's syndrome, thyroiditis, or ulcerative colitis.
- Patients exposed to levamisole-contaminated cocaine are sometimes mistakenly diagnosed with relapsing polychondriitis, due to the appearance of purpuric lesions on the outer ear. Levamisole, however, is not associated with auricular inflammation.
- There are no specific laboratory tests. The diagnosis is made on clinical grounds.

Treatment of relapsing polychondritis

- There are no controlled trials and the condition is rare. Intervention is based on anecdotal experience.
- Mild symptoms may be controlled with NSAIDs alone. Dapsone may also be of value. Corticosteroids (high doses, 1 mg/kg daily) may control systemic disease, particularly respiratory complications. Persistent or severe cases may be treated with azathioprine, methotrexate, or cyclophosphamide.
- Patients should be assessed for tracheal involvement (e.g., stridor or evidence of extra-thoracic obstruction on pulmonary function tests). Some cases may require temporary or permanent tracheostomy if laryngeal involvement is severe.

Table 18.7 Extent of organ involvement in relapsing polychondritis

Organ	Clinical feature	Prevalence (%)
External ear		95
Arthritis	Nondeforming and nonerosive	85
Nose		48
Eye	Episcleritis, uveitis, retinal vasculitis	57
Respiratory tract	Dysphonia, dyspnea, stridor	67
Internal ear		53
Skin	Erythema nodosum vasculitis, Behçet- like ulceration	38
Kidney	Glomerulonephritis (poor prognosis)	8
Heart	Pericarditis, aortic valve incompetence, heart block	8
Blood vessels	Aneurysms	12

Trentham DE, Le CH. Relapsing polychondritis. *Ann Intern Med* 1998; 129: 114–122.

Miscellaneous disorders of synovium

Pigmented villonodular synovitis (PVNS)

- The term PVNS is used for a group of conditions that are characterized by the proliferation of synovial cells and supporting tissues of the joint, tendons, and bursa.
- The condition is rare (estimated 2 cases per million).
- As the name implies, there is a villous and nodular proliferation. This is nonmalignant and associated with iron and fat deposition. Repeated small hemorrhages and lipid deposits stain the synovium red-brown and yellow, respectively.
- The cause of the condition remains unknown though some studies have proposed a link with chronic repetitive trauma or hemarthroses.
- Experimental models and clinical experience with patients with bleeding disorders have not, however, reproduced the condition.
- The classic presentation is with a monoarthritis. Any age may be affected though it tends to occur more often in both sexes in the third or fourth decade. The knee is the most commonly affected joint and "diffuse" disease is more aggressive and more likely to recur.
- Insidious onset of pain and swelling in the absence of trauma, with a serosanguinous synovial fluid aspirate and a characteristic synovial biopsy are the basis for a diagnosis of PVNS. There are some important conditions to consider in the differential diagnosis:
  - malignant synovioma
  - synovial hemangioma
  - synovial chondromatosis
  - tuberculous arthritis
  - amyloidosis
  - hemophilia.
- Imaging may be helpful. Plain radiographs are often normal, but it may show soft tissue swelling that can be radiodense with hemosiderin deposition. Calcification, however, is not a feature of PVNS and would suggest a malignant lesion or perhaps chondromatosis (see below).
- Erosions and subchondral cysts (also on nonweight-bearing surfaces) can be seen. Loss of joint space can occur late in the condition. Typically, this is not associated with juxta-articular osteoporosis or osteophyte formation. MRI can be highly suggestive of PVNS if there is sufficient hemosiderin and fat deposition in the lesion.

Treatment of PVNS

- Localized forms of PVNS are treated by marginal excision of the lesion.
- The prognosis is good.
- Diffuse forms of PVNS tend to be progressive and recurrent. Treatment techniques have included synovectomy, radiation therapy, arthrodesis, and arthroplasty. No one technique has particularly good results; however, there is only limited experience and little long-term follow-up.
- The most commonly reported treatment is surgical synovectomy.

Synovial chondromatosis

- This condition is characterized by chondrometaplasia of the subsynovial connective tissues. The joint is filled with a thickened white/blue nodular synovium.
- The cause is unknown, the disorder uncommon, and the process nonmalignant. It tends to occur more often in middle-aged men and has never been reported in prepubertal childhood.
- Clinically the condition resembles PVNS (above) but tends to be slowly progressive and sometimes self-limiting with regression. Plain radiographs may show punctate calcification outlining the joint margin.
- The diagnosis should be confirmed on synovial biopsy. In rare cases there may be transformation to a chondrosarcoma.
- Treatment is surgical and usually managed with arthroscopy, removing loose bodies and/or the synovial membrane.

Amyloidosis

- A number of disorders and clinical settings are associated with the extracellular deposition of amyloid, a proteinaceous, fibrillar material. The low solubility of amyloid and its relative resistance to proteolytic enzymes contributes to the irreversible and often progressive course of amyloidosis.
- Despite morphological similarities (including the formation of a beta pleated sheet), amyloid is a heterogeneous group of proteins. All types of amyloid fibrils have a carbohydrate moiety in the form of glycosaminoglycans and proteoglycans. Most forms of amyloid also contain the extrafibrillar protein, amyloid-P (protein AP).
- The different amyloid proteins are often related to distinct clinical forms of amyloidosis. At present, at least 17 proteins have been characterized. The detail of these proteins is beyond the scope of this book. However, two types are important as manifestations of a response to chronic systemic inflammation; amyloid-L (AL) and amyloid-A (AA).
- Protein AL consists of monoclonal immunoglobulin light chains and is seen in idiopathic and myeloma-associated amyloidosis. The clinical features of AL and AA are shown in Table 18.8.
- Protein AA (derived from serum amyloid A (SSA), an acute phase apolipoprotein), is associated with conditions such as secondary reactive amyloidosis and FMF (see Table 18.9).
- The mechanisms by which the various precursor proteins are converted to insoluble amyloid fibrils, the reasons for the predilection of certain proteins for particular organs and tissues, and the reasons why not all cases of a particular chronic inflammatory disorder develop amyloid are not clear. The most studied mechanisms are those associated with the reactive AA type amyloidosis.
- Clinically, amyloidosis may be associated with nephrotic syndrome, cardiomyopathy, hepatomegaly, peripheral neuropathy, malabsorption, and orthostatic hypotension.
- Reactive AA amyloidosis is mainly associated with long-standing infectious or noninfectious inflammation, and less frequently with cancer. In the context of rheumatic disorders AA amyloidosis is mainly seen in:
  - Adult RA
  - JIA
  - AS
- There are several rheumatic conditions that are rarely associated with AA amyloidosis. In these conditions there is a relatively low level of the acute-phase protein SAA. These conditions include:
  - SLE
  - systemic sclerosis
  - Sjögren's syndrome

Table 18.8 The clinical features of AL and AA amyloidosis

	Organ/condition	Comment
AL amyloidosis	Heart	Death occurs in 50% of cases from: restrictive cardiomyopathy, congestive heart failure, conduction disturbances
	Lungs	90% develop cough and dyspnea
	Skin	40% of cases: papules, nodules, tumors
	Neuropathy	10% of cases get carpal tunnel syndrome
	Macroglossia	
	Vasculopathy	
	Amyloid arthropathy	
	Autonomic disturbance	
Common to AL and AA	Weakness	
	Fatigue	
	Weight loss	
	Renal	Nephrotic syndrome/renal failure—major cause of death in AA*, cause of death in one-third of AL patients
	Gastrointestinal tract	Malabsorption, obstruction, diarrhea, hepatosplenomegaly*

*In AA amyloid the spleen, liver, and kidneys are often involved first.

Diagnostic procedures
- The diagnosis of amyloidosis is made by tissue biopsy (usually abdominal subcutaneous fat), and alkaline Congo red stain showing the amyloid deposits as apple green/yellow under the polarizing microscope.
- The strong calcium-dependent affinity of protein AP for amyloid fibrils is also used diagnostically in radiolabeled serum amyloid protein (SAP) scintigraphy. This technique may localize amyloid and could be of value in assessing degrees of response to treatment.
- Other laboratory tests include DNA analysis to detect the genetic variants of proteins known to make up the hereditary amyloidoses.

Treatment of amyloidosis
- The condition is progressive and there is no cure. Marked heterogeneity of the hereditary amyloidoses makes counseling difficult as well. The processes by which the disorder may be controlled include liver transplantation for lysosomal amyloidosis and bone marrow transplantation.
- For patients with AL amyloidosis, treatment with melphalan and prednisone prolongs survival.
- In the rheumatic diseases, cytotoxic drugs such as cyclophosphamide (often in combination with corticosteroids) have improved the prognosis in RA and JIA patients.

Familial Mediterranean fever
- This condition has been in the literature since the early 1900s and was more recently characterized in the 1960s.
- Most cases (80%) present before the age of 20 and it is very rare to present with a first attack after the age of 40.
- Abnormalities of the gene coding for the protein pyrin (on chromosome 16) have been identified and constitute the only test specific for the diagnosis of FMF. FMF is an autosomal recessive disorder. It most frequently affects people of eastern Mediterranean descent, especially Armenians, Arabs, and Sephardic and Ashkenazi Jews.
- The most common symptoms of abdominal pain and pleurisy are related to serositis, present in up to 95% of cases. 75% of cases develop an arthritis that may be erosive and is most often isolated to a single joint. A rash with dermal neutrophil infiltration (rather than a vasculitis) is common and looks not unlike erysipelas.
- Amyloidosis can occur in up to 40% of cases and does not appear to be associated with severity or frequency of attacks of FMF. Patients may develop renal failure, proteinuria, or malabsorption.
- Treatment includes NSAIDs for pain and continuous colchicine 0.6 mg po bid-tid. Up to 65% of cases can achieve complete remission with this regimen. A further 30% can achieve partial remission. All remaining cases should stay on daily colchicine to help prevent amyloidosis. Concern over long-term use of prophylactic colchicine in FMF has not been borne out and the benefits of controlling the condition outweighing any potential complication. It is, however, recommended

that amniocentesis be a routine part of antenatal treatment to exclude colchicine-related chromosomal aberrations.

- Newer agents such as anakinra, etanercept, and infliximab may play a role in the management of patients who are refractory to colchicine.

Tumor necrosis factor-associated periodic syndrome (TRAPs)

- This term covers a group of conditions similar to FMF but occurring in non-Mediterranean areas and associated with mutations in the TNF receptor superfamily type 1A.
- The onset is in the second decade and presents with rash, fever, abdominal pain, disabling arthralgias, and myalgias.
- 20% of patients develop amyloid AA.
- Colchicine is not efficacious. Corticosteroids may reduce the length and severity of attacks. Etanercept has been used successfully in some patients.
- Anakinra, an IL-1 receptor antagonist, is now the treatment of choice for these disorders.

Table 18.9 The clinical features of Familial Mediterranean fever

Clinical feature	Comments
Short attacks of high fever (39–40°C)	Repeated and unpredictable
Painful inflammation	Abdomen—90% of cases (may develop adhesions)
	Chest—45% of cases. Often febrile pleurisy
	Joints—most often monoarthropathy, especially the knee with acute onset pain and swelling with resolution over 1–4 weeks. Aseptic necrosis
	Skin—erysipelas-like erythema, often below the knee to the dorsum of the foot
	Other—orchitis, mild splenomegaly
AA amyloidosis	Renal—early, terminal renal failure Cardiac, hepatic, GI—see Table 18.8
Autosomal-recessive inheritance	Virtual ethnic restriction: Sephardi Jews, Ashkenazi Jews, Armenians, Anatolian Turks, Arabs

Fibromyalgia and chronic widespread pain

- Chronic widespread pain (CWP) is a common finding present in 5–10% of the general population. In the absence of diffuse degenerative or inflammatory rheumatic disease the two most common conditions found in association with CWP are fibromyalgia (FM) and joint hypermobility syndrome (JHS) (see Chapter 16).
- CWP affects women more than men with a ratio of 1.5:1, and is defined as pain for >6 months in two or more sites both above and below the pelvis.
- Treatment of CWP is similar to that for FM and JHS.
- Fibromyalgia is a subtype of CWP that is characterized by fatigue, somatic, and cognitive symptoms (see Table 18.10 and Chapter 2).
- American College of Rheumatology Classification Criteria (1990) require tenderness on pressure in at least 11 of 18 specified areas ("tender points") and the presence of widespread pain, but research indicates that in clinical practice, the tender point count often is performed incorrectly, or not at all.
- Using the classification criteria for FM (see Table 18.10), prevalence rates range from 0.5–4% with a female: male ratio of 10:1.
- American College of Rheumatology Diagnostic Criteria (2010) establish a diagnosis of fibromyalgia based on a combination of two factors: a Widespread Pain Index (WPI) and a Symptom Severity scale (SS).
- These criteria define fibromyalgia as WPI ≥7 and SS ≥5, or WPI 3–6 and SS ≥9 (Table 18.11).
- These diagnostic criteria correctly classify 88.1% of cases classified by the ACR Classification Criteria, and are better able to capture patients who no longer have tender points because they have responded to treatment.
- FM cases tend to aggregate within families.
- FM is also found in up to 25% of patients with RA (see Chapter 5), AS (see Chapter 8), and SLE (see Chapter 10). It is also commonly found in the hypermobility syndrome (see Chapter 16) and overlaps symptomatically with this condition and chronic fatigue syndrome in many ways. Care must be taken to avoid misdiagnosing CWP/FM as the only cause for pain when there is autoimmune rheumatic disease present.
- FM is a controversial condition and its existence as a distinct entity remains uncertain. Its etiology is multifactorial, with neurological, psychological, and behavioral factors important in its development.
- Psychological stresses may precede the onset of FM and CWP.
- Both FM and CWP are often associated with other somatic symptoms such as chronic fatigue, irritable bowel syndrome, multiple chemical sensitivities, and headache syndromes. Other causes of fatigue should always be excluded e.g., hypothyroidism, hypoadrenalism, and anemia.

- Alterations in hypothalamic–pituitary axis function in response to stress have been explored, but no differences between FM and controls have been found.
- Both CWP and FM are associated with alterations in peripheral and central pain processing. Painful stimuli are detected at lower levels in affected patients. Allodynia (pain in response to nonpainful stimuli) found in these conditions is thought to be due to central sensitization and an "amplification" phenomenon.
- CSF levels of noradrenaline and serotonin metabolites are decreased in FM. These transmitters are involved in descending spinal cord pain inhibitory pathways, and the observed reduction may be responsible in part for central sensitization.

Treatment

- It is of paramount importance to consider carefully the way in which an explanation is given as to the nature of the condition. Many patients have suffered disappointment and blows to self-esteem and confidence. It may take some time and may be best approached over several visits. Many will be seeking a physical cause for the pain and may misinterpret discussion about pain amplification and its treatment as labeling their condition as psychological. The label "psychological" is in itself also legitimate medically, but to the layperson it often stirs ideas of "crazy," "all in the head," or "malingerer."

Table 18.10 ACR 1990 criteria for diagnosis of fibromyalgia (FM)

History of widespread pain:

Pain is considered when all of the following are present: Pain in the left and right side of the body, pain above and below the waist, axial skeletal pain, pain present for 3 months

The diagnosis is made when there is pain in at least 11/18 tender point sites on digital palpation with 4 kg pressure*. There are 9 tender point sites, which are present bilaterally:

1.	Occiput: at the suboccipital muscle insertions
2.	Low cervical: at the anterior aspects of the intertransverse spaces at C5–C7
3.	Trapezius: at the midpoint of the upper border
4.	Supraspinatus: at origins above scapula spine near medial border
5.	2nd rib: at 2nd costochondral junction
6.	Lateral humeral epicondyles: 2 cm distal from epicondyles
7.	Gluteal: in upper outer quadrants
8.	Greater trochanter: posterior to trochanter
9.	Knees: at medial fat pad proximal to joint line

Fibromyalgia said to be present when both criteria are satisfied. FM is not excluded by the presence of another disorder.

- It is important to assess the effect of symptoms on the patient's life, and to develop a good rapport so that psychosocial issues can be discussed. Chronic fatigue can be very disabling.
- The emphasis in the explanation should be reassurance that there is no serious underlying inflammatory/systemic condition or damage to the joints and muscles. Reassure that other conditions are absent and that no further investigations are needed.
- Although exercise may cause a short-term increase in pain, a prolonged exercise program has been shown to be beneficial. Low impact activities such as Tai Chi and pilates may be especially helpful.
- Pacing of activities is also important, avoiding patterns of periods of overactivity when feeling well, followed by periods of inactivity due to pain and fatigue afterwards. Pacing is one key component of Cognitive Behavioral Therapy, a chronic pain program that, alongside aerobic rehabilitation, may be of significant benefit to patients with FM, CWP, and JHS. This multidisciplinary approach (psychologists, physical therapists, occupational therapists, doctors) has been tried with some success but remains incompletely studied.
- Education of family and partners is invariably helpful and often essential.
- NSAIDs and corticosteroids are not effective as the pain is not due to inflammation or tissue damage, and may cause increased morbidity due to side effects. Narcotics should be avoided. Many patients will have tried analgesics with little effect. This in itself can fuel anxiety about the cause and severity of their underlying condition as well as frustration and lack of confidence in their doctor.
- Tricyclic antidepressants such as amitriptyline (10–50 mg qhs) are often helpful in improving quality of sleep, decreasing morning stiffness and alleviating pain. Patients should be warned of side-effects such as dry mouth and that they may take 3–4 weeks to take effect. Patients are often also wary of being given an antidepressant. An explanation that it is being used as an analgesic is important to improve adherence. Amitriptyline is one of a group of drugs that increase 5-hydroxytryptamine.
- Amitriptyline may be combined with tramadol successfully.
- The efficacy of selective serotonin reuptake inhibitors (SSRI) is controversial. The use of fluoxetine, sertraline, or citalopram improves mood, but are less effective than tricyclics in treating pain, fatigue and sleep disturbance.
- Venlafaxine (serotonin and noradrenaline reuptake inhibitor) in high doses is effective in treating multiple symptoms in FM. Low dose treatment is generally ineffective.
- Sedative hypnotics may be used to improve sleep.
- Both CWP/FM are conditions with relapses and remissions. Most patients will have ongoing symptoms. Patients with appropriate coping strategies, improvements in psychosocial stressors, and good social support networks are more likely to have a better outcome.

Table 18.11 ACR diagnostic criteria for diagnosis of fibromyalgia (FM)

Diagnostic criteria require the presence of the following:

1. WPI ≥7 and SS ≥5, or WPI 3–6 and SS ≥9

2. Symptoms must be present for at least 3 months

3. An alternate diagnosis is not present.

Widespread Pain Index (0–19 points): the total number of areas in which the patient has had pain over the past week. Areas counted include the chest, abdomen, upper back, lower back, neck, and bilateral shoulder girdle, upper arm, lower arm, hip, upper leg, lower leg, and jaw.

Symptoms Severity scale score (0–12 points): the sum of the severity of three symptoms (fatigue, waking unrefreshed, cognitive symptoms) and severity of somatic symptoms in general, when each is rated on a scale from 0 to 3:

  0 points: no problem/symptoms

  1 point: mild problems/few symptoms

  2 points: moderate problems/symptoms

  3 points: severe problems/many symptoms

Wolfe F et al. The American College of Rheumatology Preliminary Diagnostic Criteria for Fibromyalgia and Measurement of Symptom Severity. *Arthritis Care and Research* 2010; 62(5): 600–610.

Common upper limb musculoskeletal lesions

*For a detailed view on the differential diagnosis of the entire range
of upper limb lesions, see Chapter 2*

Shoulder (subacromial) impingement syndrome

Shoulder impingement syndrome is caused by compression of the rotator cuff by the acromion. This results in shoulder pain, particularly when the patient reaches overhead, or rolls over the shoulder at night. Weakness and loss of range of motion at the shoulder are also commonly reported. For diagnostic work-up and steroid injection of the shoulder, see Chapter 2.

- Shoulder impingement syndrome is the most common cause of shoulder pain in adults.
- Pain is often referred to the upper arm.
- The causes include acute rotator cuff tendonitis (which may be calcific), subacromial bursitis, rotator cuff tear with cuff instability and impingement, and glenohumeral instability owing to a number of different lesions (e.g., labral tear, synovitis due to crystalline arthritis).
- Inferior acromial osteophytes/AC joint OA can accompany any subacromial lesion, and are risk factors for recurrent rotator cuff disease.
- Long-term rotator cuff disease can lead to 'cuff arthropathy', with OA of the glenohumeral joint and significant chronic morbidity.
- In children or young adults with shoulder impingement syndrome, consideration of an underlying glenohumeral (instability) lesion is mandatory.

Steps important in making a diagnosis

- Exclude alternate causes of shoulder pain, including rotator cuff tear, adhesive capsulitis, and referred pain from the neck or abdomen (e.g., cholecystitis with pain referred to the shoulder).
- Elicit evidence of shoulder impingement by testing passive range of motion at the shoulder while applying 5–10 lb of pressure down on the acromion (see Table 19.1).
- An AP X-ray can show specific changes (see Plate 2) that identify underlying glenohumeral or bony pathology. Plain radiographs are also useful for identifying calcific tendonitis. Consider requesting an AP view with 30° external rotation at the arm, an outlet Y view, and an axillary view.
- MR may be necessary to rule out subtle glenohumeral pathology. MR characterizes sites of cuff inflammation and is more sensitive than US in identifying cuff tears.

Conservative management of cuff/SA bursal inflammation (see Figure 19.1)

- Avoid overhead arm activities.
- Trial a full-dose regular NSAID for 2 weeks.
- If the rotator cuff is intact, consider steroid injection (e.g., triamcinolone acetonide 40 mg; see Plate 13) and local anesthetic injection (e.g., 5 ml 1% lidocaine). Approach laterally or posteriorly.
- Consider physical therapy 1–2 weeks later if the cuff muscles are weak.
- Consider a second injection after 6 weeks.

Table 19.1 The range of disorders presenting with a subacromial impingement pattern of pain. Clinical testing, though it can be elaborate, has been shown repeatedly in studies not to be as specific as the original literature appeared to suggest.

Condition	Diagnosis made by
Supraspinatus/cuff tendonitis	MR or US
Subacromial bursitis (e.g. trauma, RA, gout, CPPD)	US/MR
Rotator cuff tear (partial or full)	MR
Long head of biceps tendonitis	Clinical, US/MR
OA ACJ (impingement of osteophytes on cuff)	Clinical, X-rays, MR
Glenohumeral instability due to labral trauma (e.g., SLAP lesion), arthritis GH joint	MR
Enthesitis (e.g. deltoid origin at acromion) in SPAs	Clinical, US
Lesion at suprascapular notch (e.g., cyst, tophus)	MR

* Use 20–40 mg triaminolone acetonide (e.g., Kenolog) or methylprednisolone acetate.

Fig. 19.1 Pragmatic algorithm for managing subacromial impingement pain.

Adhesive capsulitis (AC)

Pain and diminished active and passive range of motion (in the absence of an intrinsic joint disorder) is highly suggestive of AC. The etiology is unknown, but it involves capsular and coracohumeral ligament contractures. The condition is more common in women than men (typically affecting women age 40–60 years), and is four times more common in diabetics. AC occurs bilaterally in 15% of patients. Recurrence is unusual. If left alone, pain usually resolves within 2 years, but the patient may be left with long-term restriction of shoulder movement.

Making the diagnosis

- Do not confuse AC with shoulder impingement syndrome. With impingement, passive range of motion remains intact, and is less painful than active movements. With AC, both passive and active ranges of motion are equally impaired.
- Clues to the diagnosis from examination include marked restriction of external rotation; also, with abduction, the scapula moves very early—normally it doesn't move until 30° of abduction has been completed.
- If the presentation is delayed (e.g., >6 months), a secondary impingement syndrome may have evolved as some range of motion begins to return.

Principles of management

- Rule out associated conditions: diabetes, hypothyroidism, lung carcinoma, myocardial infarction, stroke, and protease inhibitor use for HIV infection.
- Control pain during the initial painful–stiff phase of the condition. Consider NSAIDs, intra-articular steroid injections (e.g. 40 mg triamcinolone acetonide + 5–10 ml 1% lidocaine), suprascapular nerve block, or a short course of prednisone (starting with 30 mg/d) for 3 weeks.[1]
- Mobilize with physical therapy early, but be aware this may be limited by poor pain control.
- Consider surgery if conservative management fails after 6 months. Surgical procedures focus on releasing contracted/fibrotic tissue of the anteroinferior capsular structures. Procedures associated with good results include arthroscopic or open release with manipulation under anesthesia (MUA) or arthroscopic release alone. The latter may be combined with steroid injections.

---

[1] Buchbinder R, Hoving JL, Green S et al. Short course prednisolone for adhesive capsulitis: a randomised, double blind, placebo controlled trial. *Ann Rheum Dis* 2004; **63**:1460–9.

Lateral epicondylitis (tennis elbow)

This condition is common, affecting 1–3% of the adult population, typically in the age group 40–60 years. The dominant arm is most affected. It is rare in elite tennis players, but up to 40% of social players get it at some time. About 90% of all patients seen in clinical practice do not get this from playing tennis!

It is thought to be due to cumulative trauma overuse disorder from mechanical overloading. If chronic, it can lead to tendon degeneration and osseous changes. Poor prognosis is associated with manual work, high level physical strain at work, and high baseline pain and distress.

Diagnostic procedures

- The main differential diagnoses are: elbow joint lesions, referred neck pain and enthesopathics (e.g., DISI or enthesitis linked to spondyloarthropathies—see Chapter 8).
- Pain is elicited by resisted force in pronation (e.g., handshakes, turning doorknobs, carrying bags).
- There is tenderness at the lateral humeral condyle with pain elicited by resisted finger and wrist extension. Pain often extends down the extensor side of the forearm.
- Enthesopathies, tendon tears, and joint lesions may be diagnosed by an experienced musculoskeletal ultrasonographer.
- MR may miss mild epicondylitis/enthesitis and appearances are not specific. MR is more useful for ruling out tendon tears and joint lesions. Do not use MR of the elbow to discriminate elbow lesions from referred neck pain.

Principles of management

- During the acute phase, lateral epicondylitis should be treated with activity restriction, pain control, and immobilization.
- Injection around the epicondyle with triamcinolone should be considered if conservative therapy is insufficient.
- Isometric grip exercises may also help with recovery.
- Surgery is rarely indicated, and should be considered only in patients with persistent symptoms despite several months of therapy (see Figure 19.2).

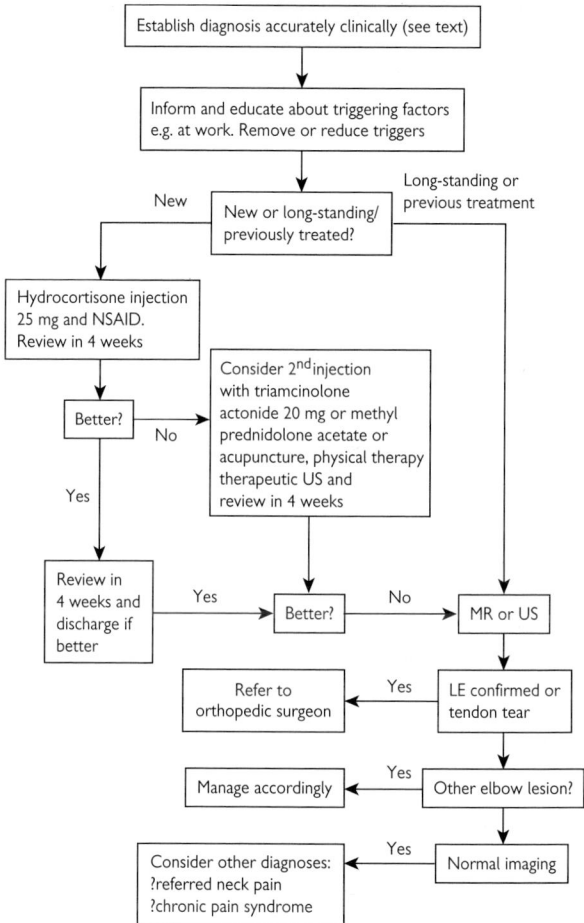

Fig. 19.2 Pragmatic algorithm for managing lateral epicondylitis (LE).

Back pain

Conditions causing acute or subacute back pain in adults

Acute mechanical back pain

- Most cases in a primary care setting are due to lumbar muscle strain or sprain; this presents with diffuse pain in the lower back to buttocks, and resolves spontaneously. If pain is related to posture or movement, especially of the thoracic cage, and local tenderness is felt at the lumbosacral junction, then the pain is highly likely to be musculoskeletal.
- The clinician should be aware of "red flags" that may mandate more thorough investigation, such as cauda equina syndrome, saddle anesthesia, leg weakness, bilateral sciatica, and bladder dysfunction (see Table 20.1).
- Herniated discs account for 4% of lower back pain. Disc herniation presents with leg pain radiating past the knee, and is most common in patients between 20 and 50 years old.
- Degenerative causes of back pain, including degenerative disc disease, facet joint hypertrophy and spinal stenosis, are more common in older patients (see Facet Hypertrophy/Facet Joint Syndromes, later in this chapter).
- The immediate management is adequate and regular analgesia (not "as needed"), advising only minimal bed rest, encouraging mobilization and normalization of activities.
- Short courses of muscle relaxants such as cyclobenzaparine (10 mg po qhs, up to tid) should be considered; these agents decrease muscle spasm and aid sleep.
- The clinician should explore patient fears and, when appropriate, reassure that serious illness is unlikely, tests are not usually needed, severe pain is often short-lived but milder pain may be present for longer, and that recurrences are common.
- Radiographs are likely to be unhelpful for planning management in most cases and radiologists often advise against getting them. MR of the lumbar spine, for example, frequently demonstrates abnormal findings in asymptomatic patients; the relationship between such findings and clinical symptoms is not always clear.
- A rehabilitation approach should be considered (see Table 20.2). The strength of evidence for therapies is variable. Adherence may be a problem with rehabilitation programs but adherence may be augmented by providing patient education literature.
- A study by the U.S. Preventative Services Task Force (USPSTF) concluded that there was insufficient evidence to recommend the use of exercise to prevent back pain, although this may still be worth considering.

Table 20.1 Warning signs for sinister pathology in back pain

⚠ **Red-flag signs:**

1. First pain age <20 or >55 years	6. Immunosuppression/steroids
2. Pain at rest	7. Malaise/weight loss
3. Trauma	8. Osteoporosis
4. Progressive neurologic deficit	9. Intravenous drug use
5. History of cancer	10. Failure to improve in 6 weeks

Table 20.2 Therapies used in facilitating rehabilitation after acute mechanical low back pain

Manipulation	Either done by an osteopath, chiropractor, or physical therapist. Some controversy about the size of benefit due to poor methodological studies. Avoid using in cases of intractable back pain (see Chronic back pain).
McKenzie exercises	Passive extension exercises designed to improve pain and stiffness associated with disc and anterior spinal structure pathology. May aggravate pain from posterior spine structures, e.g., facet joints, spinous processes.
Hydrotherapy or balneotherapy	Poorly studied but warmth can ease movement and augment land-based exercises. Might be considered after initial painful phase to regain normal movements and mobility. Obviously will only suit a few patients and resources may be limited.
Graded activity programs	Useful for patients who require guidance and would be unable to gain optimally from home exercise regime. A plan for rehabilitation with milestones is useful for some patients.
Behavioral programs	Focuses on psychological aspects of pain, involves moderate supervision and planned withdrawal of treatment. Differs from some other approaches in that the therapist takes on the "control" of the back pain. Limited resources may restrict provision of this approach. Choice of patients for program important, although data are limited.

Back pain and nerve root lesions (see also Chapter 2)
- Root compression occurs most often because of acute or subacute disc prolapse or foraminal stenosis. The peak incidence is age 30–50 years. About 70% resolve within 3 months and 90% within 6 months.
- Root compression should be suspected if acute or subacute back pain is associated with segmental nerve or sciatic leg pain.
- Acute sciatic pain (affecting the outer and posterior leg) is often sharp or burning in nature, and most frequently arises from acute disc prolapse of either L4/5 or L5/S1 (>90% cases). Sciatica is characterized by leg pain projecting past the knee, which may be more severe than the associated back pain.
- A patient with a herniated disc may present with complaints of sciatica; evidence of disc herniation may be elicited through physical examination by straight leg raise or crossed straight leg raise (i.e., elevation of unaffected leg). These tests are positive if pain is felt in the buttock or back at a leg angle of 30°–60°. Pain elicited at a leg angle <10° is consistent with musculoskeletal back pain.
- A neurologic examination is essential: L5 root lesions give decreased strength of the foot and great toe dorsiflexion, standing on heel, and decreased ankle reflex and sensation over great toe. S1 root lesions give decreased strength in plantar foot flexion, difficulty weight-bearing on toes, and decreased ankle reflex and sensation on the sole or outer part of foot.

Principles of management
- In general, 30–60% of patients recover in 1 week.
- NSAIDs, acetaminophen, and muscle relaxants should be considered first. Some patients will require narcotics for pain control. Bed rest should be limited; prolonged bed rest leads to worse outcomes.
- An epidural steroid injection can improve pain in the short term, but its impact on long-term outcomes is less clear. A meta-analysis showed that 1 in 7 patients who receive a steroid epidural experience >75% improvement in pain in the short term and 1 in 13 get >50% symptom improvement in the long term.
- Physical therapy and supervised rehabilitation using lumbar extensor exercise regimes may be of benefit.
- MR can characterize lesions, but 25% of asymptomatic people have frank disc protrusions; thus MR gives poor specificity. MR should be used only to confirm a diagnosis.
- The absolute indications for surgery (see Table 20.3) are cauda equina, progressive muscle weakness, and neuropathy causing functional disability.

Facet hypertrophy/facet joint (FJ) syndromes
- FJ OA of the lumbar spine is common in middle-aged/elderly adults, can be part of inflammatory generalized OA, and is associated with spondylolytic spondylolisthesis (i.e., forward slippage of a vertebra, usually L5, in relationship to the vertebrae below).
- Psoriatic arthritis (see Chapter 8) can also affect FJs and is under-recognized as a cause of low back pain.
- CPPD arthritis (see Chapter 16) may also affect FJs.

Table 20.3 Surgical approaches for lumbar disc prolapse

Discectomy	Essential for discs causing cauda equina syndrome and progressive neurological deficits. Excluding aforementioned indications, compared to conservative therapy, in a RCT 66% vs. 33% patients were satisfied following surgery at 1 year, 66% vs. 51% were satisfied at 4 years; thus benefit of surgery in the long term is small. Adverse events with surgery include: mortality (<0.2%), dural tears (4%), permanent nerve root injuries (<1%). 70% success rate in short term. Risk of failure from surgery relates to hysteria or hypochondriasis scores on MMPI* and presence of litigation claims.
Microdiscectomy	Smaller surgical field results in earlier mobilization and less postoperative disability. Outcomes similar to those of conventional discectomy.
Percutaneous discectomy	Suctioning of central disc material causing disc decompression and relieving nerve root pressure. Associated with low complication rate and rapid rehabilitation. Non-RCT data suggest similar efficacy to discectomy.
Chemonucleolysis	Injection of proteolytic enzyme into disc. RCTs suggest standard discectomy is superior. Rare but devastating neurological complications and risk of anaphylaxis (0.3%).
Laser lumbar discectomy	Vaporizing of part of disc by laser introduced through a needle probe. Efficacy possible similar to discectomy. No RCT data.
Prosthetic intervertebral disc replacement	Also indicated for degenerative disc disease, post-laminectomy syndrome and nonspecific persistent low back pain. Artificial discs consist of 2 endplates separated by pliable inner core. Anterior approach needed. Good results reported in open series for pooled patient groups. Complication rate may be high (up to 45%).

*MMPI = Minnesota Multiphasic Personality Inventory.

- Typical symptoms include pain on hyperextension or rotation of the lower back; pain is referred to the upper buttocks, is worse while standing still, and eased by forward lumbar flexion.
- Facet hypertrophy itself cannot be felt, but FJ syndrome is accompanied by muscle spasm and superficial soft-tissue tenderness.
- Arthritic FJs may be seen on oblique spinal radiographs; however, imaging in general cannot reliably identify symptomatic FJ joints. Facet joint injection with anesthetic may confirm the diagnosis if this results in significant pain relief.

Management options for FJ syndromes
- Patients can be treated according to principles applied for all patients with acute mechanical back pain except that extensor exercises are contraindicated because they will aggravate symptoms.

- Short courses of analgesics and/or NSAIDs as for OA (see Chapter 6).
- Generally advise minimal bed rest.
- Steroid injection of FJs is a frequently used treatment modality, although studies have failed to demonstrate benefit over placebo injection.
- Radio frequency denervation of medial branches of dorsal rami supplying FJs can help, but the procedure should only be considered if local anesthetic block works first.

Spinal stenosis

- The diagnosis is frequently missed in the elderly.
- It presents mainly with achy, stiff pains in the legs increasing on walking and eases if the patient stops walking, sits, or leans forward (neurogenic claudication or pseudoclaudication).
- Pain, numbness/tingling, and weakness are the most common symptoms. Neurological leg signs can be accentuated after exercise.
- The diagnosis is made using MR imaging the L-spine.
- Nonsurgical management (including pain control and physical therapy) is often adequate.
- Emergent decompressive laminectomy is required if the patient develops rapidly progressive neurologic symptoms, bladder dysfunction, or cauda equina syndrome.

Nontraumatic vertebral collapse: evaluation

- This is usually due to osteoporosis, collapse into an abnormal vertebra (e.g., vertebral hemangioma), or secondary to malignancy or infection.
- The history should, therefore, focus around identifying risk factors for these conditions. Postmenopausal status or hypogonadism, previous fracture history, steroid use, and alcoholism may all contribute to osteoporosis. Weight loss or B-type symptoms may indicate the presence of malignancy or infection.
- Kyphosis and loss of height can occur after vertebral collapse; a full examination should be performed to evaluate for the possibility of cord compression or malignancy.
- Investigate with AP and lateral spinal X-rays, MR, bone biochemistry (intact PTH), morning LH and free testosterone, 25-OH vitamin D, TFTs, serum/urine electrophoresis, and urine calcium.
- MR is good at discriminating infection and tumors from osteoporosis, but biopsy for histology and culture is essential if tumor or infection has not been ruled out by MR.

Nontraumatic vertebral collapse: treatment

- The patient should be placed on bed rest and monitored for evolving neurological deficits.
- Pain control often requires long acting narcotics, with short acting narcotics for breakthrough pain.
- Calcitonin 100–200 IU sq bid or 200 IU qd by nasal spray has an analgesic effect and reduces bone turnover in osteoporosis. Acetaminophen and NSAIDs alone are unlikely to be sufficient.
- Osteoporosis should be treated aggressively, at minimum with calcium and vitamin D supplements. Teriparatide is the only widely-available anabolic therapy for osteoporosis in the United States. The use of

bisphosphonates in women of childbearing years is controversial due to their long half-lives and unknown impact on the fetus.
- Discuss any pathological malignancy-related fracture with a radiation oncologist.
- If conservative measures fail to relieve pain consider vertebroplasty or balloon kyphoplasty.

Postsurgical back pain
- There are numerous causes and no single entity (see Table 20.4).
- Imaging with gadolinium-enhanced MR may be helpful to delineate inflammatory tissue around the surgical site.
- Persistent pain after surgery may be associated with adverse psychological and social factors and outstanding litigation or insurance claims.
- Nerve root blocks, epidurals, and spinal stimulators may be used.

Sterile discitis
- This is inflammation of the intervertebral disc often associated with annulus enthesitis at the vertebral endplates and vertebral osteitis.
- The causes include disc degeneration, CPPD disease (probably), AS (Romanus lesions) and other SpAs including SAPHO.
- The lesion should be identified with MR and treatment should include bed rest and aggressive analgesia. In RCTs, steroid disc injections have been shown to be little help overall. IV bisphosphonates (e.g., pamidronate 60–90 mg) has anecdotally been shown to help AS and SAPHO discitis in particular.

Table 20.4 Implicated causes of post-surgical back pain

Recurrent disease	E.g., further disc protrusion and radicular features. If re-operation not appropriate consider nerve root block, steroid epidural, etc.
Operation for wrong lesion	MR appearances can highlight lesions, which may not be relevant to clinical features. More than 1 or 2 lesions can co-exist. Detailed clinical assessment prior to imaging is essential.
Misdiagnosis originally	Many rheumatologists will be familiar with cases of failed surgery undertaken for a structural lesion but where inflammatory disease, typically SpA-related disease, was present and causes ongoing symptoms.
Adverse rehabilitation conditions	Resolution of symptoms and regaining functional capacity if slow has been associated with significant psychological and social factors. Poor result of surgery also associated with an outstanding insurance claim or litigation.
Arachnoiditis	Thought to be a direct effect of surgery. Dural tissue becomes inflamed. In nerve root/disc surgery often associated with sensory root symptoms for some months afterwards. Diagnosis with Gd-enhanced MR. Where associated with sensory radicular symptoms, may respond to steroid root block, epidural. If radicular symptoms, chronic and disabling, consider spinal cord (implanted) stimulator.

Management of chronic back pain

Chronic back pain requires a special approach, with an emphasis on psychological and social management. Patients are likely to have set beliefs about their problem, the ability of healthcare systems to help them, and are more likely to have developed coping strategies than patients with acute or subacute back pain. However, those with chronic back pain who continually seek further and different healthcare options are likely to have less successful coping strategies.

Initial approach to the care of patients with chronic low back pain (see Table 20.5)

- Be confident there is no undiagnosed condition affecting back pain and that no new neurological lesions have evolved. If examination raises concern, use MR to rule out lesions.
- Establish empathy and trust, taking time to get information about the patient's:
  - social situation
  - health and illness beliefs
  - intrafamily dynamics
  - true role and perception of their role at work
  - view on conventional and complementary therapies
  - view on what does and doesn't work and on their specific view of exercise therapy.
- With the information just outlined, you will be able to plan a more individually tailored approach to management.
- Plan the management approach with the patient and establish short- to midterm goals, including whether, and what type of, supervision is required (e.g., graded program of exercise) and how often a review is needed.
- Consider domains of therapy under the following headings:
  - physical therapy
  - work/life commitments
  - psychological and social support
  - painkillers and medications
  - education (insight and coping strategies)
- Plan to review progress at regular intervals.
- Evaluate patients carefully at baseline if considering long-term opiate use. There may be an increased risk of dependency if the patient currently or previously abused drugs, if there's a high level of psychological distress, if short-acting opiates are used, or if drugs are prescribed as needed.
- Although many strategies, especially those that combine techniques, can be costly, these costs to healthcare are likely to be offset by the saving in lost wages.

Table 20.5 Management options for chronic low back pain

Exercises	RCT evidence supports use. Greater evidence of effect when combined with behavioral methods. Aerobic exercises augment effect of "back school." Should be essential part of outpatient physical retraining program. Less evidence on how much should be supervised, by whom, and how often.
Manipulation	Trials show efficacy on pain in the long term.
Transcutaneous electric nerve stimulation (TENS)	Disappointing results from 2/3 RCTs in patients with chronic back pain but efficacy for other specific diagnoses unknown.
Posture training	May be more appropriate than corset use and easy to combine training with supervised exercise therapy.
Oral medications	NSAIDs best reserved for acute-on-chronic pain exacerbations. Low-dose tricyclics (e.g., amitriptyline, nortryptiline) are useful particularly if chronic neuropathic pain present. Try to avoid long-term opiate drugs.
	Chronic opiate use for chronic low back pain has not been extensively studied. A mental health evaluation before long-term prescribing is essential to avoid triggering dependency (see text); short courses initially for a trial period are sensible. Best supervised by specialist with experience in pain management.
Back school	Regular program carrying an educational component. Programs vary from one to many sessions. May be more effective in occupational setting. Long-term changes in behavior not extensively studied. Noncompliance and relapse are problems.
Psychologically oriented rehab programs	Intensive courses often run by psychologists and "hands-off" physical therapists can help (highly) selected patients. Focus on learning to cope with pain and control the effects of pain on functioning and psyche. Not suitable for many patients. Courses are few and far between. Cost-effectiveness of courses not proved.
Complementary therapies	Increasingly used (see Chapter 21). By consensus, chiropractic has been shown to be helpful for chronic low back pain. Acupuncture has yet to be proved successful in robust studies. Poor evidence base otherwise.
Intrathecal opiates	Conflicting results from (only) noncontrolled studies. Generally, results show overall short-term improvements regarding pain perception but not function. Best reserved for patients where all else has failed.
Spinal cord stimulator (SCS)	A number of good studies show that SCS is effective for neuropathic including radicular pain. Technique is relatively safe. Careful patient selection is important. Studies show 50% reduction in pain long term.

Management of back pain in children and adolescents

Children with spinal problems present with deformity, back pain, limping, systemic features, neurological features, or a combination of effects. Back pain in children is common—up to 30%. It is rare in the young <10 years. If severe enough to warrant hospital admission there is frequently an underlying cause. Age determines likelihood of cause, with infection and tumors being more common in young children compared with adolescents (see Table 20.6).

The principles behind history and examination in children are discussed in Chapter 2.

Nonspecific low back pain

- The annual incidence is 10–22% in schoolchildren.
- Adolescent back pain is linked with familial clustering, physical inactivity, sports injuries, and psychosocial factors.
- Most children have self-limiting symptoms.
- Management should focus on an explanation of the short natural history, reassurance, addressing predisposing factors (see above) that remain a trigger for recurrence and increasing general health/exercise to improve muscle strength.

Idiopathic scoliosis

- This is often vertebral malalignment in the coronal plane associated with spinal rotation accentuated on spinal flexion.
- It occurs in up to 3% of schoolchildren.
- Most (70%) are asymptomatic. Progression is more likely in the presence of pain or thoracic curve convex to the left—conditions that should be investigated for more serious underlying spinal pathology.
- Progressive scoliosis (see Figure 20.1) requires bracing or surgery. Usually curves of 25–45° are braced and those >45° are best considered for surgery.

Congenital (CS) and neuromuscular (NMS) scoliosis

- CS is associated with genitourinary malformations (20%) and, rarely, congenital heart disease. CS is associated with spinal dysraphism (20%), myelodysplasia, and Klippel-Feil syndrome.
- NMS is associated with cerebral palsy, muscular dystrophy, spinomuscular atrophy, and myelodysplasia.
- To avoid rapid progression and increased long-term morbidity and disability, refer for prompt correction of progressive curves. Orthotic treatment is an adjunct to, not a substitute for, surgery.

Table 20.6 Causes of back pain in children

Developmental
Painful scoliosis
Spondylolysis and spondylolisthesis
Scheuermann disease
Infection
Discitis
Vertebral osteomyelitis
Spinal epidural abscess
Inflammation
Juvenile arthritis
Osteoporosis
Mechanical
Herniated disk
Muscle strain
Fractures
Neoplasms
Benign (osteoid osteomas, osteoblastoma, aneurysmal bone cyst)
Malignant (leukemia, lymphoma, sarcoma)
Visceral
Pyelonephritis, appendicitis, retroperitoneal abscess

Scheuermann's osteochondritis

- This is perhaps the most common cause of spinal deformity and back pain in children and adolescents (3–5% of all adolescents, usually 13–17 years). The etiology is unknown.
- If severe, it can lead to kyphosis and then frequently becomes symptomatic. Compensatory lumbar lordosis evolves.
- The typical radiographic pattern is one of wedge deformities (<10°) of contiguous thoracic vertebrae with irregular vertebral end-plates.

Management of symptomatic disease

- Avoid repetitive stress-loading activities such as running.
- Extensor exercises for the back and abdominal muscle exercises may improve symptoms but will not correct kyphosis.
- Brace treatment usually prevents progression of kyphosis.
- Surgery is reserved for severe persistent pain, if there are severe or progressive deformities (>70°) or there is great concern about the appearance.

Fig. 20.1 Measurement of the degree of scoliosis by the Cobb method: 1, the lowest vertebra whose bottom tilts to the concavity of curve; 2, the erect perpendicular to line 1; 3, the highest vertebra whose top tilts to the concavity of curve; 4, the drop perpendicular to line 3; α, the intersecting angle. Curves less than 20° are considered to be mild, 20–40° are moderate, and above 40° are severe.

Spondylolysis and spondylolisthesis

- Spondylolysis is a defect in the pars interarticularis, most commonly seen at L5. It commonly appears as an isolated finding (4% preschool children and 6% at age 18 years).
- Spondylolysis is a risk factor for asymptomatic and symptomatic spondylolisthesis (slippage of one vertebra on another, see Figure 20.2).
- Progressive slippage is rare in children but can occur during the adolescent growth spurt.

Management

- On serial radiographs, if slippage is >25% (Grade II, III, or IV), then advise against contact sports or sports involving lumbar hyperextension.
- Advice should be given on regular abdominal muscle exercises, avoiding gaining abdominal obesity, and consider regular bracing.
- Surgery is considered for *progressive* vertebral slippage or Grade III/IV slip.

Fig. 20.2 Spondylolisthesis measured as a % slip of L4 on L5 (α/β). Grade I <25%, Grade II 25–50%, Grade III 50–75%, and Grade IV >75%.

Herniated disc

- This is infrequent in children. Most occur in children older than 11 years, and are often associated with scoliosis.
- Diagnose disc herniation by MR but be cautious in interpreting normal developmental changes in the growing spine.

Management

- Without nerve root impingement, management is conservative: short period of bed rest, adequate analgesics and NSAIDs, with early exercise-based rehabilitation regime.
- Over 50% improve with conservative treatment but reported results from surgery for significant nerve root lesion (i.e., persistent severe pain or neurological deficit) are very good.

Spinal tumors

- Although rare in children, spinal tumors frequently present with back pain (80% cases).
- It is important to recognize that painful scoliosis, radicular pain, night pain, stiffness, and effectiveness of NSAIDs are all features of spinal tumors (although none are specific).

Management
- Urgent radiographs (may be negative in early disease) and MRI are needed to delineate the nature of the problem and the clinician should consider bone scintigraphy or focal CT to identify posterior element tumors (e.g., osteoid osteoma).
- Adequate analgesia is required: NSAIDs—ibuprofen in recommended doses for weight may not be sufficient, consider naproxen 30 mg/kg/d for adolescents.
- Bed rest is not essential, but is wise if scans show there is risk of vertebral collapse or cord compression. If the latter is a worry, this should be discussed urgently with a pediatric spinal surgeon and radiation oncologist.
- Initiate a search for other tumors known to metastasize to spine (see Table 20.7).
- Investigation of adolescents on specific adolescent units is advisable, given the specific multidisciplinary input often needed.

Table 20.7 Primary spinal tumors in children and adolescents (see also Table 2.16)

Osteoid osteomas

Benign. Not uncommon. Mainly adolescents. Posterior vertebral bone usually. Pain can be severe. Discriminated from osteoblastomas by size (osteomas are <1.5 cm, osteoblastomas >1.5 cm) as histology is often identical. Lesions are associated with scoliosis (63% cases). Surgical excision is treatment of choice.

Aneurysmal bone cyst

Benign. Symptoms often triggered by vertebral collapse. Care when considering biopsy to discriminate from malignant lesions. Discuss in detail with musculoskeletal radiologist.

Eosinophilic granulomas

Benign—often occurs around age 10 years. Rare. Lytic lesion. May occasionally be multiple/disseminated—staging important. Symptoms often triggered by vertebral collapse. Cord and radicular compression can occur. Biopsy essential to discriminate from malignant lesions. Surgical excision or internal spine fixation not usually needed. Consider radiotherapy if cord compression threatened. Consider external brace fixation in all and monitor for spontaneous resolution. Disseminated lesions can be treated with chemotherapy.

Ewing sarcoma

Overall rarely affects spine (~10% cases). Can affect any part of spine including sacrum (latter cases often delayed diagnosis). Suspicion of it requires biopsy. Treat with combination chemotherapy and local radiotherapy. 5-years survival ~50%. Outcome better for tumor sizes <8 cm or localized disease.

Leukemia

Consider both ALL and AML in all cases of spinal osteopenia or single/multiple vertebral collapse. Notorious association with delayed diagnosis. Associated systemic symptoms may not necessarily be present but normal CBC at presentation unlikely (~10% cases only). Also look for eosinophilia and hypercalcemia and consider bone marrow aspirate.

Lymphomas

Rarely presents with back pain; however, known cause of persistent back pain. MR is imaging of choice. MR can show vertebral collapse and/or soft tissue paraspinal mass. Biopsy is diagnostic. Case reports of plasmacytomas presenting similarly.

Secondary malignant tumors

Neuroblastoma, rhabdomyosarcoma, Wilms tumor, retinoblastoma and teratoblastoma are known to present with back pain. Usually, biopsy triggers a search for the underlying primary neoplasm.

Complementary and alternative medicine in rheumatology

Introduction

The popularity of complementary and alternative medicine (CAM) among people with chronic diseases, including arthritis, is widely recognized. A 2002 study conducted by the National Center for Complementary and Alternative Medicine found that three out of every four adults in the United States have used CAM at some point. In some areas, up to one-third of arthritis sufferers have received CAM from CAM practitioners,[1] and the prevalence of CAM use has been reported at between 30–100% of patients with rheumatic disease.[2] Among the most popular are dietary approaches, herbalism, and acupuncture. Few interventions, however, have been studied in a robust way.

The prevalence of CAM use for chronic arthritis and pain chiefly mirrors that in other chronic diseases, and appears to be consistent across Western populations.

CAM is very popular despite a paucity of data. Using *homeopathy, complementary medicine* and *arthritis* to search for articles on CAM and arthritis in PubMed yields 1,080 articles (1950–2006); however, a Google search for "homeopathy" alone yields over 21 million hits (2012).

There may be no universal explanation for why patients use CAMs. Gender, age, income, education, degree of underlying psychological stress, and desire to regain greater self-control may all influence use. Published suggestions for CAM use also include dissatisfaction with conventional medicine or the belief that a philosophy associated with a particular CAM is desirable and aligns with the patient's own philosophy.

[1] Resch KL, Hill S, Ernst E. Use of complementary therapies by individuals with 'arthritis'. *Clin Rheumatol* 1997; 16: 391–5.

[2] Ernst E. Usage of complementary therapies in rheumatology: a systematic review. *Clin Rheumatol* 1998; 17: 301–5.

[3] Ernst E. Musculoskeletal conditions and complementary/alternative medicine. *Best Pract Res Clin Rheumatol* 2004; 18(4): 539–56.

[4] Weiner DK, Ernst E. Complementary and alternative approaches to the treatment of persistent Musculoskeletal pain. *Clin J Pain* 2004; 20(4): 244–55.

Herbal remedies (phytotherapy)[1]

- The likely mechanism of effect of most agents is on eicosanoid metabolism inhibiting either cyclooxygenase or lipoxygenase pathways.
- Most efficacy studies have methodological flaws—notably the failure to power studies sufficiently, given small differences in outcome versus placebo. Risk–benefit profiles are generally unknown.
- Adverse reactions similar to those from conventional medicines can occur, and include allergy and drug interactions.
- In most countries, few legal controls exist to ensure quality of herbal medicine constituents, and no legislative "medicine development" framework exists to reliably ensure safety and efficacy.

Phytodolor

This is a standardized extract of *Populus tremula* marketed for rheumatic pain. Reviews suggest studies overall show a reduction in pain in patients with OA (see Chapter 6) compared with placebo.

St. John's wort (Hypericum perforatum)

- St. John's wort has been shown in relatively robust trials to improve mild depression. This may relate to its effect on inhibiting synaptosomal uptake of 5-HT, dopamine, normetanephrine, glutamate, and GABA.
- Response in patients with arthritis or chronic pain may be due to improvements in mood, pain perception or coping strategies.
- St. John's wort increases the activity of cytochrome P450 3A4, which is responsible for the metabolism of many drugs. Concomitant administration results in decreased serum levels of cyclosporine and digoxin. St. John's Wort also decreases the anticoagulant effect of warfarin, and patients may require dose adjustment as a result.

Gamma linoleic acid (GLA)

- GLA is a plant-seed-oil derived, unsaturated fatty acid that suppresses production of Il-1β. It is contained in many different plant-seed oils (e.g., black currant-seed oil).
- Compared with placebo, 2.8 g/d GLA significantly improves symptoms and signs of active RA over 6 months.[2] However, virtually all plant-seed oil preparations that contain GLA are often taken at lower daily doses than those shown to be effective.

Devil's Claw (Harpagophytum procumbens)

- This may work by inhibiting cyclooxygenase or iNO synthase in joint tissues or by suppressing matrix metalloproteinase production.
- At 60–100 mg/day, *Harpagophytum* extract (harpagoside) has moderate but significant effects on back and joint pain associated with OA.[3]

---

[1] Soeken KL, Miller SA, Ernst E. Herbal medicines for the treatment of Rheumatoid arthritis: a systematic review. *Rheumatology* 2003; 42(5): 652–9.

[2] Zurier RB, Rossetti RG, Jacobson EW et al. Gamma-linolenic acid treatment of rheumatoid arthritis. A randomized placebo-controlled trial. *Arthritis Rheum* 1996; 39: 1808–17.

[3] Gagnier JJ, Chrubasik S, Manheimer E. Harpgophytum procumbens for osteo-carthritis and low back pain: a systematic review. *BMC complement Altern Med* 2004; 4: 13–23.

Physical and hands-on therapies

Acupuncture
- Acupuncture is commonly used to treat neck and back pain and is easily incorporated into primary care consultations.
- Meta-analyses suggest short-term efficacy for low back pain[1] but no overall effect for neck pain.[2]
- Controversy exists among acupuncturists as to the adequacy of acupuncture techniques used for back pain in published trials.
- No convincing evidence exists to suggest acupuncture should be used for long-term relief of symptoms in OA or RA.
- Serious complications of acupuncture exist (e.g., pneumothorax, hepatitis B, spinal cord injury, infection) but are rare. Complications may be underreported.[3,4]

Tai Chi
- In RA, tai chi has been shown to increase plantar flexion range and is associated with a higher level of participant enjoyment.
- Trials have shown few benefits in terms of outcome measures. It appears not to exacerbate RA,[5] and may help with fibromyalgia.

Reflexology
- This is one of the most frequently used CAMs.
- From the few controlled trials taken together, results do not suggest there is any specific therapeutic effect.

Spinal manipulation
- Of the most rigorous sham-controlled studies of manipulation (for any indication of back pain), none showed benefit compared with placebo.
- Studies suggest that about 50% of patients have side effects, although these are chiefly mild or transient.[6, 7]
- Reliable estimates of the incidence of serious adverse effects do not exist. Reported effects include vertebral arterial dissection, strokes, disc herniation, spinal fracture, cauda equina syndrome and worsening of undisclosed spinal inflammatory conditions (e.g., AS/SpA, discitis).
- Reports from neurologists suggest serious neurological lesions occurring after neck chiropractic are not infrequent.
- There is concern over excess radiation risk from overuse of radiographs ordered by practitioners.

[1] Ernst E, White AR. Acupuncture for backpain: a meta-analysis of randomized controlled trials. *Arch Intern Med* 1998; 158: 2235–41.

[2] White AR, Ernst E. A systematic review of randomized controlled trials of acupuncture for neck pain. *Rheumatology* 1999; 38: 143–7.

[3] Ernst E, White AR. Life-threatening adverse reactions after acupuncture? A systematic review. *Pain* 1998; 71: 123–6.

[4] Ernst E. Acupuncture—a critical appraisal. *J Intern Med* 2006; 259(2): 125–37.

[5] The Cochrane library. Issue 4. 2004.

[6] Ernst E. Prospective investigations into the safety of spinal manipulation. *J Pain Symptom Manage* 2001; 21: 238–42.

[7] Ernst E, Canter PH. A Systematic review of systematic reviews of spinal manipulation. *J R Soc Med* 2006; 99(4): 192–6.

Homeopathy

Homeopathy stems from the belief that tiny quantities of substances have a holistic therapeutic effect. There has been a great publicized debate about whether homeopathy is genuinely more effective than placebo, and whether conventional randomized studies are a relevant way of evaluating its effect. Reports in the medical and scientific literature invariably generate prolonged and sometimes fierce debate in the letters-to-the-editor pages for some time afterwards! Nevertheless, homeopaths are among the most frequently visited CAM practitioners by patients with arthritis.

- Meta-analyses of therapeutic trials suggest the clinical effects of homeopathic remedies cannot be fully explained by placebo effects alone.[1] However, the most robust methodological studies do not show any positive effects compared to placebo.[2,3]
- There is some evidence that short-term improvement in RA symptoms is superior to placebo.[4] A more robust methodological study, however, suggested no symptomatic improvement in RA over 3 months in patients stabilized on DMARDs and NSAIDs.[5]
- Summarizing four RCTs of homeopathy use in OA, there appears to be a positive effect, although firm conclusions cannot be reached.[6]
- One of the most frequently used homeopathic remedies is *Arnica montana*. A systematic review of its effects[7] suggests there is no proof of its effect.
- Preparations of *Echinacea* are believed by some to have significant immunomodulatory properties. Although this is a traditional treatment for a variety of ailments, some CAM practitioners advise that patients with autoimmune diseases avoid this supplement.

[1] Linde K, Melchart D. Randomized controlled trials of individualized homeopathy: a state-of-the-art review. *J Altern Complement Med* 1998; 4: 371–88.

[2] Ernst E, Pittler MH. Efficacy of homeopathic arnica: a systematic review of placebo-controlled clinical trials. *Arch Surg* 1998; 133: 1187–90.

[3] Ernst E. Are highly dilute homeopathic remedies placebos? *Perfusion* 1998; 1: 291–2.

[4] Jonas WB, Linde K, Ramirez G. Homeopathy and rheumatic disease. *Rheum Dis Clin* 2000; 26: 117–23.

[5] Fisher P, Scott DL. A randomized controlled trial of homeopathy in rheumatoid arthritis. *Rheumatology* 2001; 40: 1052–5.

[6] Long L, Ernst E. Homeopathic remedies for the treatment of osteoarthritis: a systematic review. *Br Homeopath J* 2001; 90: 37–43.

[7] Ernst E, Pittler MH. Efficacy of homeopathic arnica: a systematic review of placebo-controlled clinical trials. *Arch Surg* 1998; 133: 1187–90.

Other CAMs

Magnet therapy
- In one randomized study, patients wearing a magnet bracelet experienced reduction of hip and knee pain associated with osteoarthritis when compared to patients wearing dummy bracelets.[1]
- Other studies have indicated that magnets may relieve some forms of musculoskeletal pain, although this is controversial.

Dietary supplements
- Glucosamine and chondroitin sulfate supplements have long been used for the treatment of osteoarthritis, but the results of clinical trials have been mixed, and its use is falling out of favor.[2]
- Curcumin (turmeric) has anti-inflammatory properties, and may have some beneficial effects on arthritis.
- Other commonly used supplements by patients with arthritis and pain include cod liver oil, fish oil tablets, vitamins, and selenium.
- Although there is little available scientific evidence to support any recommendations regarding dietary modification, this form of intervention remains popular.

Hypnotherapy
- This is of long-standing interest in controlling pain.
- In studies, hypnotherapy has been shown to be effective at controlling anxiety.
- There is some evidence for efficacy in fibromyalgia patients.

Stress management/relaxation therapy
- Stress has been associated with an increased risk of sudden death, delay in wound healing, and higher rates of infection.
- Yoga, acupuncture, and meditation may improve quality of sleep, and decrease perceived stress, fatigue, and depression.
- Various studies suggest short-term benefit for patients with RA but proof of effects on measures of disease in the long term are absent.
- Methodological deficiencies in studies and absence of cost-effectiveness data suggest no firm conclusion can be drawn about the role of therapy in specific individuals or disease groups.

Spiritual healing
- A "therapeutic experience" transmitted by a therapist's touch, nontouch, prayer or "mental healing."
- Examples include therapeutic touch, reiki, distance healing, and intercessional prayer.

[1] Harlowe T et al. Randomised controlled trial of magnetic bracelets for relieving pain of osteoarthritis in the hip and knee. *BMJ* 2004; 18: 1450–4
[2] Clegg DO et al. Glucosamine, chondroitin sulfate, and the two in combination for painful knee osteoarthritis. *N Engl J Med* 2006; 354: 795–808.

- There is some evidence that "therapeutic touch" done by nurses can reduce anxiety in hospital patients. No data exist that compare this to talking to/informing patients about their condition.

Other

- Electrical stimulation increases grip strength in RA patients with hand muscle atrophy. Pulsed electrical stimulation can help knee OA symptoms. Data are weaker for an effect on pain from neck OA.
- Thermotherapy for RA—including wax and Faradic baths, hot and ice packs—have brief positive effects without any harmful effects.[1]
- Balneotherapy may be effective for the treatment of RA and low back pain.[2] Trial methodology has been poor, however—trials have generally not studied relevant outcomes.
- Rolfing, a form of deep tissue massage that attempts to stretch and open the fascia, may also benefit some patients with arthritis and chronic pain.

Further information

- National Center for Complementary and Alternative Medicine (NCCAM): http://nccam.nih.gov
- MD Anderson Complementary/Integrative Medicine: http://www.mdanderson.org/departments/CIMER
- Arthritis Foundation—*Arthritis Today* Supplement Guide: http://www.arthritis.org/at-supplement-guide.php
- Mayo Clinic: "Take a break to meditate": http://mayoclinic.com/health/meditation/MM00623

[1] Robinson VA, et al. Thermotherapy for treating rheumatoid arthritis. *Cochrane Database of Systematic Reviews* 2001, Issue 4. Art. No.: CD002826
[2] Pittler MH, Karagulle MZ, Karagulle M, Ernst E. Spa therapy and balneotherapy for treating low back pain: meta-analysis of randomized trials. *Rheumatology* 2006; 45: 880–4.

Chapter 22

Rheumatologic emergencies

For vertebral fracture, see Chapter 20.

Septic arthritis

Infection in a joint can progress rapidly and cause destruction of tissues and permanent deformity and disability. When septic arthritis is suspected, investigations should be prompt, appropriate antibiotics should be started without delay, and, where feasible, infected tissue should be removed. The epidemiology of infections is discussed in Chapter 17.

Suspecting infection

- Septic arthritis is uncommon but is more likely to occur in patients with established joint disease, with prosthetic joints, or with co-morbidities such as diabetes, chronic renal disease, or immunosuppression. Patients—especially the elderly—may not appear systemically unwell.
- The main differential diagnosis in adults is crystalline arthritis (see Chapter 15).
- Staphylococcal and streptococcal infections are the most common; septic arthritis from *H. influenzae* type b is no longer seen due to vaccinations. Gonococci cause almost 30% of cases in children >11 years.

Immediate management of adult joint sepsis (see Table 22.1)

- Immobilize the joint and provide adequate analgesia.
- Take blood for CBC, CMP, ESR, CRP, and cultures.
- Manage sepsis as appropriate and rule out infective endocarditis (especially in IV drug user (IVDU) or in those with known cardiac valve disease).
- Drain the joint completely (use at least an 18-gauge needle, since the fluid is viscous) and send the sample of joint fluid for Gram stain, culture, and for polarized light microscopy (LM). If the polarized LM demonstrates evidence of crystals and cultures are negative after 48 hours, then consider a diagnosis of a crystaline arthropathy.
- If minimal fluid is obtained, it should be sent for culture, since identification of an organism is most likely to change management.
- Joint fluid with a white blood cell count >50,000/mm^3 (mainly neutrophils) and a glucose <400 mg/L is highly suggestive of infection.
- Gonococcus is the most common cause of monoarthritis in a young, sexually active adult; women during menstruation may be at particular risk. Disseminated gonococcal infection (DGI) may present as a clinical triad of pustular skin lesions, tenosynovitis, or migratory arthralgias. The cutaneous manifestations are fleeting, and are not required to make this diagnosis.
- For a nongonococcal septic arthritis, consult orthopedics early to consider arthroscopic washout of knee, hip, or shoulder, and contact microbiology to arrange a Gram stain of joint fluid and set up cultures/special tests for atypical organisms (especially for a septic arthritis resistant to empiric antibiotics).

Table 22.1 Initial choice of antibiotics for septic arthritis based on Gram stain in adults. All antibiotics are given IV initially

Gram's stain result	Probable pathogen	Antibiotic choice
Gram-positive cocci Clusters	Staph. aureus (methicillin resistance suspected)	Nafcillin or Oxacillin (2 g q 4 h) Vancomycin (1 g q 12 h) Vancomycin (1 g q 12 h) Penicillin G (2.5 million U q 4 h)
Pairs and chains (urinary, biliary, bowel)	Staph. epidermidis Streptococci Enterococci	Penicillin G (2.5 million U q 4 h) [or Ampicillin (2g IV q 4 h)]+ gentamicin (1 mg/kg q 8 h)
Gram-negative cocci (hemorrhagic rash, meningitis)	N. gonorrhoeae N. meningtides	Ceftriaxone (2 g IV q 24 h) Cefotaxime (2 g IV q 8 h)
Gram-negative bacilli	Enterobacteriaceae Pseudomonas spp.	Ciprofloxacin (400 mg IV q 12 h) Cefotaxime (2 g IV q 8 h) Ceftazidime (2 g IV q 8 h) + Gentamicin 5mg/kg IV q 24 h
Polymicrobial		Clindamycin (600 mg IV q 6 –8 h)+ + ciprofloxacin (400 mg IV q 12 h)
No organisms seen (healthy young adult) (older adult, under- lying disease) (intravenous drug abuser)	N. gonorrhoeae Staphylococci Streptococci Enterobacteriaceae Staphylococci Pseudomonas spp. Enterobacteriaceae	Ceftriaxone (2 g IV q 24 h) Vancomycin and cefotaxime Vancomycin and ceftazidime

Source: Reprinted with modification from Parker, R. H. (1998). Acute bacterial arthritis. In Orthopedic Infections (ed. D. Schlossberg), p. 74. New York: Springer-Verlag.

- Empiric antibiotic treatment in the absence of a positive Gram stain in adults in a straightforward clinical scenario should be IV vancomycin 1 g q 12 h due to the risk of methicillin-resistant *S. aureus* (MRSA). For the elderly or immunocompromised patients, a third-generation cephalosporin (e.g., ceftriaxone 1 g IV q 12 h or q 24 h) should be added, given the possibility of gram-negative infection. Ceftriaxone alone may be reasonable empiric therapy for septic arthritis in areas where MRSA is not a concern. See Table 21.1.
- IVDU are at particular risk for MRSA. *Pseudomonas* should be suspected as well, particularly if the patient does not respond to empiric therapy.

Specific management in children (see Figure 22.1)

Prompt IV antibiotic therapy is essential. Initially treat according to the most likely organism for the patient's age: <3 months cover *S. aureus*, group B strep, and gram negative bacteria; for those 3 months to 2 years cover *S. aureus* and *S. pneumoniae*. Older children should be treated for staphylococcal and streptococcal infections, as in adults.

Postimmediate management of septic arthritis

- Review analgesia regularly.
- Rule out multiple foci of infection.
- Discontinue any immunosuppressants and consider stress-dose steroids if the patient is systemically unwell and has received chronic steroids.
- Adjust antibiotics according to culture sensitivities and in discussion with an infectious disease specialist.
- For affected weight-bearing joints, keep nonweight bearing until there is obvious improvement in pain and swelling, and you are confident the patient is on appropriate antimicrobials.
- Physical therapists should be involved early to help passive mobilization of joint before patient bears weight.
- There are little data regarding the optimum duration of antimicrobial therapy; therefore, the regimen should be individualized. Common protocols include IV antibiotics for 1–2 weeks followed by an oral antibiotic for an additional 2–4 weeks.

Reasons for no/poor improvement

- Consider that you may have the wrong diagnosis: think about crystalline arthritis, RA (see Chapter 5), and SpA monoarthritis (see Chapter 8).
- Consider that the infection has been successfully treated but that the slow progress is due to a superimposed crystal-induced or reactive autoimmune arthritis, foreign body, or background disease (e.g., RA).
- The antimicrobials may not be covering the infection. Consider multiple infecting organisms (reculture), atypical organisms (e.g., *M. marinum*, Lyme, fungal).

Gonococcal (GC) septic arthritis

- Cultures can be initially negative. If suspected, reculture blood but also urethra, cervix (80–90% positive), rectum, pharynx, pustules, and joint fluid. Send urine for GC nucleic acid detection.

- Use IV ceftriaxone 1 g q 24 h until clinical improvement is observed (as >5% organisms are penicillin resistant) then cefixime 400 mg q 12 h for 1–2 weeks (or a fluoroquinolone, depending on sensitivity testing).
- Because of increasing resistance, treatment with ciprofloxacin is no longer advisable.
- Consider empiric therapy for Chlamydia with doxycycline 100 mg daily for 7 days or one dose of azithromycin 1 g, and concurrent testing for HIV and syphilis.
- All sexual partners should receive one dose of ceftriaxone 250 mg IM and empiric treatment for Chlamydia (preferably azithromycin 1g).

Fig. 22.1 Management of suspected septic arthritis in the child.
Reproduced with the permission of Oxford University Press from the *Oxford Textbook of Rheumatology 3e*, edited by Isenberg, David et al.

Infections in patients taking anti-TNF-α drugs

Background

- Over the last decade, immunosuppressants that specifically inhibit the actions of TNF-α have become widely used to treat multiple rheumatic diseases.
- This class of drugs includes infliximab (Remicade®), etanercept (Enbrel®), adalimumab (Humira®), golimumab (Simponi®), and certolizumab (Cimzia®).
- The risk of infections is increased with anti-TNF-α use; the severity and type of infections associated with anti-TNF-α therapy also needs special consideration. Patients with a history of serious infections should not be treated with this class of drug.
- Patients treated with anti-TNF-α therapy are at particular risk for tuberculosis (TB), histoplasmosis, listeriosis, and other opportunistic infections.

Characteristics of infections

- Patients receiving treatment with anti-TNF-α therapy should be monitored closely for signs of infection, which should be evaluated aggressively.
- Disseminated fungal and viral infections can occur (see Table 22.2).
- Re-activation of latent infections may be a particular problem.
- Numerous reports of TB occurring with anti-TNF-α treatment make the following precautions prudent:
  - Patients with latent TB should be screened prior to initiation of therapy
  - Patients who travel to endemic areas and health care workers should be considered high risk
  - Screening should include intradermal injection of PPD, and consideration of chest radiograph given the possibility of anergy.
  - Induration of ≥5 mm should be considered a positive response for most patients with rheumatic disease
  - An interferon-γ release assay is also appropriate for screening for latent tuberculosis infection, and is not affected by prior BCG vaccination.
  - Patients with a positive PPD should receive oral isoniazid 300 mg daily with pyridoxine for 9 months (or alternate appropriate regimen)
- Reactivation of TB should be considered in febrile patients and those not screened for TB before anti-TNF-α treatment.
- Latent histoplasmosis should be considered in patients from endemic regions or history of potential exposure (e.g., spelunking, construction)
- The risk and severity of infections may be increased in those also taking other immunosuppressants, especially steroids.
- Patients may need a longer-than-normal course of antibiotics and need careful re-assessment before restarting anti-TNF-α drugs.

Table 22.2 The range of organisms and type of infections reported in the literature or witnessed by authors in association with anti-TNF-α treatment. Fatalities have occurred

Organisms		Nature of infection
Bacteria	M. tuberculosis	Disseminated
		Pulmonary
	Atypical mycobacteria	
	Listeriosis	Septicemia
		Septic arthritis
		Meningitis
	Staphylococcus	Septicemia
		Cavitating pneumonia
	Salmonella	Septicemia
		Septic arthritis
	Moraxella	Septic arthritis
	Actinobacillus	Septic arthritis
	Nocardia	
Viruses	Varicella	Disseminated
	H. simplex	Severe
	Hepatitis B	Reactivation
	CMV	Disseminated
Fungi/ yeasts	Candida	Septicemia
	Cryptococcus	Pneumonia
	Aspergillosis	Disseminated
	Sporotrichosis	Skin
	Pneumocystis	Disseminated
	Histoplasmosis	Pneumonia
		Disseminated
		Pneumonia
		Disseminated
Parasites	Leishmaniasis	Visceral

Acute SLE

Acute SLE will manifest either as a flare in patients with an established diagnosis or as the first presentation of the disease. Declining C3 and increasing dsDNA titers may predict acute disease flares in some (but not all!) patients. The reader is referred to Chapter 10 for SLE and Chapter 11 for antiphospholipid syndrome and catastrophic APS.

Diagnosing SLE in an acute medical context

- Consider SLE as a diagnosis in all young and middle-aged women who present with a history of joint pain, photosensitive rash, or pleuritic chest pain.
- Raynaud's phenomenon and recurrent mouth ulcers are non-specific, but may also appear in association with SLE.
- As labs usually do not test for ANA, C3/C4, or other serologies urgently, these tests may not be available when making an initial diagnosis of SLE.
- Inflammatory markers such as the ESR or CRP may not be a reliable indicator of SLE activity.

Acute SLE nephritis (adults)

- Check the BP accurately, creatinine, blood urea nitrogen, electrolytes, send urine for culture, a spot urine protein/creatinine ratio (as an estimate of proteinuria) and ultrasound the renal tract to rule out post-renal obstruction.
- Quantification of urinary protein and creatinine grades the severity of the renal lesion and guides the management approach (see Figure 22.2).
- Control BP. Often a diuretic, ACE inhibitor, or beta blocker are required.
- Biopsy can inform treatment decisions. Treatment will generally include steroids and oral mycophenolate mofetil (1.0–1.5 g bid) or IV cyclophosphamide (0.75 g/m² IV monthly).
- Steroid-induced osteoporosis and cardiovascular risk should be managed from the outset. Consider getting the following done early: DEXA scan, ECG, and fasting lipid panel.
- Daily calcium (1000–1500 mg) and vitamin D (800 IU) should be administered to all patients receiving steroids.
- Patients treated with cyclophosphamide must be counseled about infertility, malignancy, and hemorrhagic cystitis risks, the dose schedules (e.g., MESNA), monitoring (CBC at day 10 after and prior to IV pulse to check WBC nadir) and Pneumocystis prophylaxis (e.g., dapsone 100 mg po qd-qod) (see Figure 22.2).

Fig. 22.2 The management of adult renal SLE: treatment algorithm
Reproduced with the permission of Oxford University Press from the *Oxford Textbook of Rheumatology 3e*, edited by Isenberg, David et al.

Acute SLE involving heart and lung (adults)

- Cardiac and isolated pulmonary manifestations of SLE are rare, and in many patients with SLE, acute cardiac and pulmonary features may be due to other common conditions (see Table 22.3).
- CRP elevation may reflect infection or significant pleuropericardial SLE. Lupus pericarditis alone without evidence of cardiac compromise can be treated with NSAIDs and prednisone 20–40 mg daily for 2–4 weeks with subsequent steroid taper.
- If not due to cardiac failure, acute dyspnea in SLE may be due to intercurrent infection, pneumonitis, pulmonary vasculitis, pulmonary embolism, pulmonary hypertension, or dyspnea from pleuritic chest pain.
- Cyclophosphamide should be considered for severe or life-threatening manifestations of SLE.

Table 22.3 Important aspects in management of acute cardiopulmonary manifestations of SLE in adults

For initial clinical cardiac assessment, consider:	ECG, blood for CK, troponin, echocardiogram
For initial lung assessment, consider:	ABGs, CXR, spirometry, HRCT chest, V/Q scan
Pulmonary embolism	Especially important to consider in patients who are at high risk (e.g., immobility, recent surgery, nephrotic syndrome). Consider empiric anticoagulation early and check for lupus anticoagulant, APL antibodies, and complete thrombophilia screen.
Pulmonary vasculitis (very rare)	Features: severe dyspnea, CT with dependent infiltrates consistent with hemorrhage. Requires ICU and pulmonary physician support and consideration of plasma exchange.
Lupus pneumonitis	Requires high-dose steroids (methylprednisolone 1 g IV qd x 3 days followed by prednisone 1 mg/kg/day) and cyclophosphamide (750 mg/m² IV q month, followed by a remission maintenance regimen). AZA (up to 2.5 mg per kg/d) may be effective in some cases, although most would use cyclophosphamide in these cases.
Antiphospholipid syndrome	PE associated with APL syndrome in SLE requires lifelong anticoagulation.
Specific therapies	
Steroids	Assuming non-viral infections excluded or treated, most cardiopulmonary SLE manifestations respond to oral prednisone 0.5–1 mg/d (max 80 mg/d). Consider treatment with methylprednisolone 1g IV qd x 3 days if the clinical situation is extreme and IV steroids will not compromise clinical situation.
Mycophenolate	Mycophenolate mofetil (0.5 mg bid initially increasing after 1–2 weeks to 1–1.5 g bid) is the drug of choice for lupus nephritis, except for patients with rapidly progressive glomerulonephritis, for whom intravenous cyclophosphamide is still indicated.
Belimumab	Belimumab 10 mg/kg administered intravenously on days 0, 14, 28 and every 28 days afterwards decreases disease activity when added to standard-of-care therapies. Patients with anti-dsDNA antibodies and low serum complements are the most likely to respond. Belimumab should not be used for the treatment of lupus nephritis.
Bone protection	All patients treated with steroids require daily calcium (1 g) and vitamin D (800 IU). Most should also get bisphosphonate initially, which may be withdrawn if DEXA scan shows good BMD with all T scores >–1.5

Acute hematologic manifestations of SLE (adults)

- Many patients with SLE are Coomb's positive without having significant hemolysis, and do not need to be treated specifically for this.
- Features of hemolysis include fever, chills, anemia, elevated bilirubin in serum and urine, low serum haptoglobin and reticulocytosis.
- Acute thrombocytopenia is a relatively frequent presentation.
- If severe, both hemolytic anemia (Hb < 7 mg/dL) and thrombocytopenia (platelets < 25,000) require high dose prednisone 60–80 mg/day and intravenous immunoglobulin therapy.

Pediatric SLE—acute nephritis

- The most common lesion is diffuse proliferative GN (30–45% cases).
- One-third have hypertension, which may need aggressive management.
- All have microscopic hematuria and proteinuria > 500 mg/24 hours. However, up to one-third may have a normal serum albumin, and about 50% maintain a normal GFR.
- Prognosis and therapy of nephritis is guided by the active ISN-grade pathological lesion and chronicity index; thus biopsy is important.
- Management includes high dose steroids and cyclophosphamide 750 mg/m^2 IV monthly for 6–12 months, then quarterly IV cyclophosphamide or mycophenolate mofetil, especially in older children (see Figure 22.3).
- In acute fulminant renal disease consider plasmapheresis, although this is not routinely done.

Pediatric SLE—acute hematological manifestations

- Overt hemolysis occurs in <10%, thrombocytopenia in 15–45%.
- Bleeding is uncommon.
- Most with thrombocytopenia respond to steroids. IVIG can be used; rituximab may be beneficial in refractory cases, although this has not been well studied.
- A high index of suspicion is needed to diagnose catastrophic APLS. It is characterized by multiple organ thromboses and microangiopathic changes.
- All cases require working closely with hematologists as highly informed interpretation of detailed serial coagulation studies is required.
- The treatment of hematologic manifestations of SLE is shown in Figure 22.4.

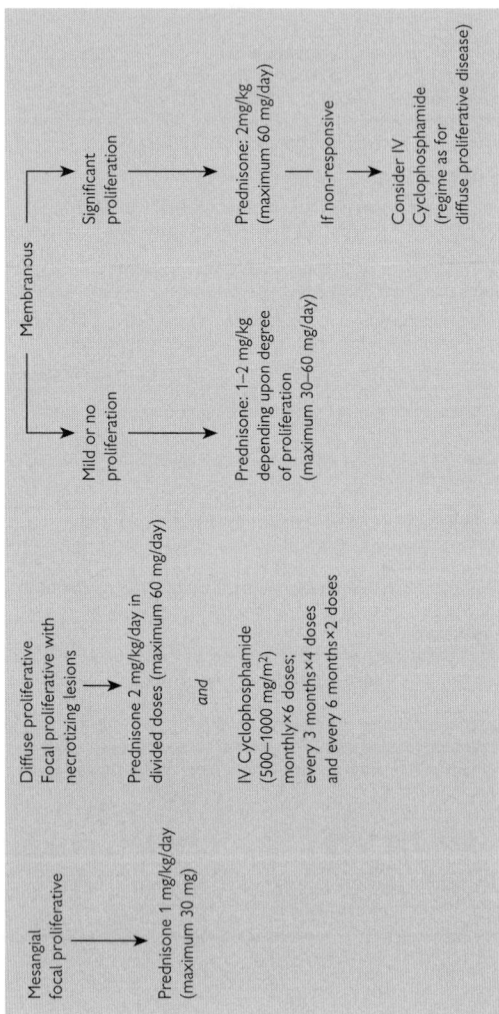

Fig. 22.3 Therapy flowchart for treating pediatric SLE nephritis.

Reproduced with the permission of Oxford University Press from the *Oxford Textbook of Rheumatology* 3e, edited by Isenberg, David et al.

Thrombocytopenia

↓

If unresponsive to
treatment of
systemic disease

↓

Prednisone:
  1 mg/kg/day
  (maximum 30 mg)
IV gammaglobulin

↓

Consider pulse
  cyclophosphamide
Splenectomy is
  very controversial

Anemia

↓

If unresponsive to
treatment of
systemic disease

↓

Prednisone:
  1–2mg/kg/day
  (maximum 60 mg)
Consider pulse
  methylprednislone

Leucopenia

↓

Usually marker of
  disease activity
If persistent consider
  other causes including
  drug-induced

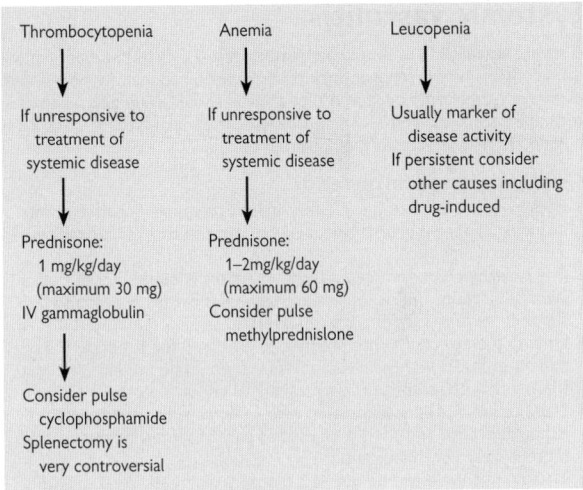

Fig. 22.4 Flowchart for treating pediatric hematologic manifestations of SLE.

Reproduced with the permission of Oxford University Press from the *Oxford Textbook of Rheumatology 3e*, edited by Isenberg, David *et al.*

Systemic vasculitis

A severe vasculitis flare should be treated aggressively because permanent damage from tissue ischemia may occur rapidly. Patients diagnosed with pulmonary capillaritis or glomerulonephritis should generally be treated with pulse steroids. The specific management of each type of vasculitis is outlined in relevant sections of Chapter 14.

Giant cell (temporal) arteritis

- Because giant cell arteritis (GCA) can lead to cranial ischemic events including blindness and stroke, it is important to treat empirically when suspicion is high.
- The prevalence of giant cell arteritis increases with age. Visual changes, jaw claudication, and diplopia in the setting of B-type symptoms all support the diagnosis of giant cell arteritis.
- Empiric therapy starts with prednisone 1mg/kg/d for 1 month; if the patient presents with visual complaints, it would be prudent to initiate treatment with methylprednisolone 1 g IV qd for 3 days.
- Daily aspirin has been associated with a decreased risk of cranial ischemic events, and should be used as part of standard therapy unless there is clear contraindication.
- Treatment should not be delayed; biopsy is diagnostically useful up to 2 weeks after steroid therapy is initiated.
- To optimize yield, temporal artery biopsy should be bilateral, with samples of at least 1.5 cm in length.

"Severe" vasculitis

- Patients with active vasculitis can quickly develop manifestations that threaten life or the function of a vital organ. These patients are sometimes referred to as having "severe" vasculitis.
- Severe manifestations of the small vessel vasculitides include pulmonary hemorrhage (or capillaritis) and glomerulonephritis. Severe manifestations of medium vessel vasculitis include mononeuritis multiplex (i.e., foot drop/wrist drop) or mesenteric angina/ischemia.
- When glomerulonephritis is suspected, renal biopsy can be very useful to confirm the diagnosis.
- Severe vasculitis is generally treated with pulse solumedrol 1g IV qd for 3 days, followed by prednisone 1mg/kg/d.
- Most patients with severe vasculitis will also be treated with oral cyclophosphamide 1.5–2.0 mg/kg/d. Lower doses should be used in the elderly or in patients with renal insufficiency.
- Cyclophosphamide places patients at risk for *Pneumocystis* infection, and appropriate chemoprophylaxis should be instituted.
- Oral cyclophosphamide should be administered in the morning in a single dose to minimize risk of hemorrhagic cystitis.
- In patients who are at high risk for infection, treatment with intravenous immunoglobulin or plasmapheresis may be appropriate.
- In patients who continue to decline despite immunosuppression, serious consideration should be given to the possibility that the patient has an infection mimicking a vasculitis flare.

Scleroderma (Scl) crises

Renal crisis

- This may manifest as an acute or subacute hypertensive crisis, usually within the first four years after diagnosis of diffuse scleroderma (dcSSc). It can be the presenting feature of SSc (Chapter 12).
- Glucocorticoids may place a patient with scleroderma at elevated risk of developing scleroderma renal crisis.
- An abrupt increase in BP >150/85 and new renal insufficiency are consistent with this diagnosis.
- Other manifestations include what would be expected with hypertensive emergency, such as microangiopathic hemolytic anemia, encephalopathy, and hypertensive retinopathy.

Acute Scl renal crisis management

- ACE inhibitors are the cornerstone of management of renal crisis. The patient should be treated with escalating doses of captopril until blood pressure is brought under control. ARB and calcium channel blockers can be added sequentially if captopril is inadequate.
- Fast drops in blood pressure should be avoided, as low perfusion pressures in abnormal renal vessels may worsen renal failure.
- Consult nephrology about hemodialysis if necessary.
- Prompt initial treatment often leads to re-establishment of good renal function.

Pulmonary hypertension

- Primary pulmonary arterial hypertension (PAH) occurs as a complication of lcSSc, although it can also occur in dcSSc (both as a primary feature and secondary to pulmonary fibrosis)
- Echocardiography can be used to screen for PAH; an RVSP > 40 mm Hg is suggestive, but the diagnosis must be confirmed by right heart catheterization.
- Decompensated PAH presents with subacute onset of signs and symptoms consistent with right heart failure, including peripheral edema and dyspnea.

Management of acute SSc-related primary PAH

- Patients with rapidly decompensating heart failure secondary to pulmonary arterial hypertension should be treated with supplemental oxygen, diuresis, and continuous IV prostacyclin.
- Diuretics decrease right ventricular preload, and can lead to significant symptomatic relief.
- A large pulmonary embolism can also result in rapidly worsening of pulmonary arterial hypertension, and should be considered in the appropriate setting.
- Management of subacute pulmonary arterial hypertension associated with SSc is discussed elsewhere.

Methotrexate-induced pneumonitis

This is rare but it can occur in any patient given methotrexate (MTX). Reports suggest the incidence ranges from <0.5% to 7% of patients (variation due to definition of condition). It is probably much rarer in children and adolescents compared to adults. Life-threatening pneumonitis requiring hospital admission probably occurs in <1% patients taking MTX. It is thought that mild pneumonitis resolves on drug withdrawal alone.

Patients at risk

- Most patients suffering from pneumonitis do so within the first few months of starting MTX or after a significant dose change.
- In patients on stable-dose MTX, blood levels may change in the setting of progressive renal insufficiency or low levels of folate.
- Consider the diagnosis in all patients on MTX with acute onset of dry cough, dyspnea, headache, and fever. The differential diagnosis lies between chest infection, acute pulmonary edema, or acute interstitial lung disease associated with the underlying condition.

Immediate management of severe toxicity.

- Stop MTX.
- Optimal therapy for methotrexate-induced pneumonitis has not been well defined. Folinic acid (15–25 mg po q6 h) may reverse methotrexate toxicity.
- Anecdotally, steroids accelerate recovery; in cases of severe decompensation, it is reasonable to treat with methylprednisolone 1g IV qd for 3 days, followed by prednisone 1mg/kg/d. Prednisone can be tapered over the subsequent 1–6 months, depending on disease severity.
- The remainder of management should be focused on identifying alternate causes for respiratory compromise (e.g., BAL and high resolution CT to exclude infection) and supportive care (e.g., supplemental oxygen, consideration of transfusion if anemia is present) Most patients with methotrexate-induced lung injury will recover, but may have chronic lung damage as a result.

Index